Studies in Computational Intelligence

Volume 1011

Series Editor

Janusz Kacprzyk, Polish Academy of Sciences, Warsaw, Poland

The series "Studies in Computational Intelligence" (SCI) publishes new developments and advances in the various areas of computational intelligence—quickly and with a high quality. The intent is to cover the theory, applications, and design methods of computational intelligence, as embedded in the fields of engineering, computer science, physics and life sciences, as well as the methodologies behind them. The series contains monographs, lecture notes and edited volumes in computational intelligence spanning the areas of neural networks, connectionist systems, genetic algorithms, evolutionary computation, artificial intelligence, cellular automata, self-organizing systems, soft computing, fuzzy systems, and hybrid intelligent systems. Of particular value to both the contributors and the readership are the short publication timeframe and the world-wide distribution, which enable both wide and rapid dissemination of research output.

Indexed by SCOPUS, DBLP, WTI Frankfurt eG, zbMATH, SCImago.

All books published in the series are submitted for consideration in Web of Science.

More information about this series at https://link.springer.com/bookseries/7092

Sofia Scataglini · Silvia Imbesi · Gonçalo Marques
Editors

Internet of Things for Human-Centered Design

Application to Elderly Healthcare

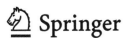

Editors
Sofia Scataglini
University of Antwerp
Antwerp, Belgium

Silvia Imbesi
Università degli Studi di Ferrara
Ferrara, Italy

Gonçalo Marques
Polytechnic of Coimbra, ESTGOH
Rua General Santos Costa
Oliveira do Hospital, Portugal

ISSN 1860-949X   ISSN 1860-9503 (electronic)
Studies in Computational Intelligence
ISBN 978-981-16-8490-6   ISBN 978-981-16-8488-3 (eBook)
https://doi.org/10.1007/978-981-16-8488-3

© The Editor(s) (if applicable) and The Author(s), under exclusive license to Springer Nature Singapore Pte Ltd. 2022
This work is subject to copyright. All rights are solely and exclusively licensed by the Publisher, whether the whole or part of the material is concerned, specifically the rights of translation, reprinting, reuse of illustrations, recitation, broadcasting, reproduction on microfilms or in any other physical way, and transmission or information storage and retrieval, electronic adaptation, computer software, or by similar or dissimilar methodology now known or hereafter developed.
The use of general descriptive names, registered names, trademarks, service marks, etc. in this publication does not imply, even in the absence of a specific statement, that such names are exempt from the relevant protective laws and regulations and therefore free for general use.
The publisher, the authors and the editors are safe to assume that the advice and information in this book are believed to be true and accurate at the date of publication. Neither the publisher nor the authors or the editors give a warranty, expressed or implied, with respect to the material contained herein or for any errors or omissions that may have been made. The publisher remains neutral with regard to jurisdictional claims in published maps and institutional affiliations.

This Springer imprint is published by the registered company Springer Nature Singapore Pte Ltd.
The registered company address is: 152 Beach Road, #21-01/04 Gateway East, Singapore 189721, Singapore

Preface

"To know how to grow old is the master-work of wisdom, and one of the most difficult chapters in the great art of living" wrote Henri-Frédéric Amiel. *Therefore*, it is necessary to know how to do it by helping us with a multidisciplinary approach that embraces the principles of human-centred design (HCD), technology and Internet of Things (IoT). These aspects that are seen sometimes as separate aspects are intertwined in this book creating new possibilities for the development of niche solutions for older users who are beginning to experience physical and cognitive decline but are still autonomous and need to preserve their autonomy for as long as possible.

IoT encompasses the use of novel systems that include new generation sensors and microcontrollers connected to the Internet. These systems can be used for several applications of ambient-assisted living (AAL), which is a critical topic concerning the world's population ageing. The combination between the needs expressed by older users and the opportunities offered by recent innovative technologies allows research institutions, stakeholders and academia to target and design new solutions for older users, safeguarding their well-being, health, and care and improving their quality of life. AAL architectures are created to meet the needs of older adults, with the aim of maintaining them autonomous for as long as possible. The work conducted by numerous researchers worldwide makes it possible to create novel architectures, algorithms and systems to improve older adults' life quality and well-being.

The book presents the state of the art of the IoT, applied to human-centred design (HCD) projects addressed to ageing users, from the perspective of health, care, and well-being. The current focus on the ageing population is creating new possibilities for the development of niche solutions for older users who are beginning to experience physical and cognitive decline but are still autonomous and need to preserve their autonomy for as long as possible. Moreover, it discusses and analyses the most recent services, products, systems and environments specifically conceived for older users, to enhance health, care, well-being and improve their quality of life. This approach is coherent with the percept of AAL or enhanced living environment, looking to the users' comfort, autonomy, engagement and health care.

This volume consists of eighteen chapters, divided into four sessions analysing aspects of HCD with older users looking at emerging technologies, products, services and environments in their actual application in different areas, always concerning the design for the elderly related to the IoT, such as the development of biomonitoring devices, tools for activity recognition and simulation, creation of smart living environments, solutions for their autonomy, assistance and engagement enhancing health, care and well-being.

The project touches the five continents involving different countries as Australia, Belgium, India, Italy, Malaysia, Mexico, Nigeria, Pakistan, Portugal, Sri Lanka, Sweden, UK, and USA.

To these authors, reviewers and book's managers, we would like to express our gratitude for their enthusiasm and professionalism to participate in a timely and favourable manner in this challenge.

We truly hope that the chapters in this book will contribute to fostering education, research and innovation among academics, stakeholders and research organisations.

Antwerp, Belgium Sofia Scataglini
Ferrara, Italy Silvia Imbesi
Coimbra, Portugal Gonçalo Marques

About This Book

The book presents the state of the art of the Internet of Things (IoT), applied to human-centred design (HCD) projects addressed to ageing users, from the perspective of health, care and well-being. The current focus on the ageing population is opening up new opportunities for the development of niche solutions aimed at the niche category of older users who are beginning to experience physical and cognitive decline but are still independent and need to maintain their autonomy for as long as possible. The combination between the needs expressed by older users and the opportunities offered by the recent innovative technologies related to the Internet of Things allows research institutions, stakeholders and academia to target and design new solutions for older users, safeguarding their well-being, health and care, improving their quality of life. This book discusses and analyses the most recent services, products, systems and environments specifically conceived for older users, in order to enhance health, care, well-being and improve their quality of life. This approach is coherent with the percept of AAL or enhanced living environment, looking to the users' comfort, autonomy, engagement and health care. The book describes and analyses aspects of HCD with older users looking to the emerging technologies, products, services and environments analysed in their actual application in different areas, always concerning the design for the elderly related to the IoT, just as the development of biomonitoring devices, tools for activity recognition and simulation, creation of smart living environments, solutions for their autonomy, assistance and engagement enhancing health, care and well-being. The book is intended for researchers, designers, engineers and practitioners in health care to connect academia, stakeholders and research institutions to foster education, research and innovation.

List of Reviewers

Alessandro Pollini, BSD Design, Via Lazzaretto 19, 20124 Milano, Italy
Awotunde Joseph Bamidele, Department of Computer Science, University of Ilorin, Ilorin, Nigeria
Daniele Busciantella Ricci, Design Research Lab, Department of Humanities, University of Trento, Italy
Elvira Maranesi, Scientific Direction, IRCCS INRCA, Ancona, Italy
Filippo Petrocchi, Department of Architecture, University of Ferrara, Italy
Francesco Pasquale, Department of Architecture, University of Ferrara, Italy
Giacinto Barresi, Rehab Technologies, Istituto Italiano di Tecnologia, Genoa, Italy
Jagriti Saini, National Institute of Technical Teacher's Training and Research, Chandigarh (160019), India
Laura Screpanti, Dipartimento di Ingegneria dell'Informazione (DII), Università Politecnica delle Marche, Ancona, Italy
Marco Gonçalves, Departamento de Desporto e Saúde, Escola de Saúde e Desenvolvimento Humano, Universidade de Évora, Largo dos Colegiais, 7000-727 Évora, Portugal
Comprehensive Health Research Centre (CHRC), Universidade de Évora, Largo dos Colegiais, 7000-727 Évora, Portugal
Mattia Corzani, Department of Electrical, Electronic, and Information Engineering, University of Bologna
Riccardo Berta, University of Genova, Italy
Roberta Bevilacqua, National Institute of Health and Science on Aging, IRCCS INRCA, Via S. Margherita 5, 60124 Ancona, Italy
Roberto Pasini, International Telematic University Uninettuno, Via Vittorio Emanuele II, 39, 00186 Rome, Italy
Silvia Gasparotto, University of the Republic of San Marino, Department of Economics, Sciences and Law, SM
Umer Asgher, Department of Robotics and Artificial Intelligence, School of Mechanical and Manufacturing Engineering, National University of Sciences and Technology (NUST), Islamabad, Pakistan

Contents

Aspects of Human-Centered Design in Older Adults

Inclusive Innovation Through Design for Services: A Service Ergonomics Perspective 3
Daniele Busciantella-Ricci, Carlos Aceves-Gonzalez, and Sofia Scataglini

Human-Centered Design for Older Users: A Design Methodology for the Development of Smart Devices and Systems Related to Health Care 25
Silvia Imbesi

Aging and Interaction: Designing for Active Living Experiences 39
Alessandro Pollini, Gian Andrea Giacobone, and Michele Zannoni

How to Enhance Elderly Care Products, Services, and Systems by Means of IoT Technology and Human-Centered Design Approach 63
Filippo Petrocchi

Digital Human Modelling: Inclusive Design and the Ageing Population 73
Russell Marshall, Erik Brolin, Steve Summerskill, and Dan Högberg

IoT-Enabled Biomonitoring Solutions for Elderly Health, Care and Well-Being

IoT-Powered Monitoring Systems for Geriatric Healthcare: Overview 99
Alexey Petrushin, Marco Freddolini, Giacinto Barresi, Matteo Bustreo, Matteo Laffranchi, Alessio Del Bue, and Lorenzo De Michieli

Neuro-Gerontechnologies: Applications and Opportunities 123
Giacinto Barresi, Jacopo Zenzeri, Jacopo Tessadori,
Matteo Laffranchi, Marianna Semprini, and Lorenzo De Michieli

Attention-Aware Recognition of Activities of Daily Living Based on Eye Gaze Tracking 155
B. G. D. A. Madhusanka, Sureswaran Ramadass,
Premkumar Rajagopal, and H. M. K. K. M. B. Herath

Internet of Things and Cloud Activity Monitoring Systems for Elderly Healthcare 181
Joseph Bamidele Awotunde, Oluwafisayo Babatope Ayoade,
Gbemisola Janet Ajamu, Muyideen AbdulRaheem,
and Idowu Dauda Oladipo

IoT Based Fall Detection System for Elderly Healthcare 209
Ahsen Tahir, William Taylor, Ahmad Taha, Muhammad Usman,
Syed Aziz Shah, Muhammad Ali Imran, and Qammer H. Abbasi

mHealth Apps for Older Adults and Persons with Parkinson's Disease 233
Mattia Corzani

IoT-Enabled Smart Elderly Living Environment and Their Autonomy for Ageing Well

An Experience of Co-Design with Elderly People in the HABITAT Project: Improving Older Users' Lifestyle with Assistive Home Systems 263
Giuseppe Mincolelli, Gian Andrea Giacobone, Michele Marchi,
Filippo Petrocchi, and Silvia Imbesi

From Driver to Passenger: Exploring New Driving Experiences for Older Drivers in Highly Automated Vehicles 277
Gian Andrea Giacobone

Remote Caring for Older People: Future Trends and Speculative Design 293
Oya Demirbilek

Innovative Street Furniture Supporting Electric Micro-mobility for Active Aging 313
Theo Zaffagnini, Gabriele Lelli, Ilaria Fabbri, and Marco Negri

IoT-Enabled Assistance and Engagement

Understanding the Acceptance of IoT and Social Assistive Robotics for the Healthcare Sector: A Review of the Current User-Centred Applications for the Older Users 331
Elvira Maranesi, Giulio Amabili, Giacomo Cucchieri, Silvia Bolognini, Arianna Margaritini, and Roberta Bevilacqua

Exoskeletons in Elderly Healthcare 353
Matteo Sposito, Tommaso Poliero, Christian Di Natali, Marianna Semprini, Giacinto Barresi, Matteo Laffranchi, Darwin Gordon Caldwell, Lorenzo De Michieli, and Jesús Ortiz

Video Games for Positive Aging: Playfully Engaging Older Adults 375
Sasha Blue Godfrey and Giacinto Barresi

About the Editors

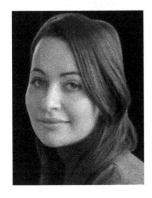

Sofia Scataglini is a Biomedical Engineer and Visiting Professor at the Department of Product Development at the Faculty of Design Sciences of Antwerp University. She holds a Joint Ph.D. in Applied Science between Politecnico di Milano and Belgian Royal Military Academy. Since 2014, she has been working as a Researcher at the Belgian Royal Academy and since 2018 at the Belgian Military Hospital Queen Astrid. She is a member of the Center for Health and Technology (CHAT), which is a multidisciplinary interfaculty Institute of the University of Antwerp.

Sofia Scataglini is a member of the Scientific Committee of the International Ergonomics Association (IEA) and co-chair of the IEA Technical Committee (TC) on Human Simulation and Virtual Environments. She is also the founder of the Digital Human Modeling by Women group (DHMW), which is dedicated to promoting women researchers around the world. In doing so, she organizes congresses related to Applied Human Factor and Ergonomics, IEA and Digital Human Modelling. She is also an active editor and reviewer of books, journals and scientific grants focusing on sensors, medicine, health and care, modelling and simulation, standardization, ergonomics, biomechanics and design. Sofia Scataglini is involved in different TC groups for standardization such as National, European (CENELEC) and International levels (ISO and IEC) for Ergonomics, Wearable, Smart textiles, PPE and clothing. Her research activities focus on research and design of products, systems, environments, and services for the health, care, and well-being of people using Co-Design and User-Centred Design methods combined with Ergonomics.

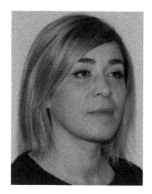

Silvia Imbesi has a master degree in Architecture and a bachelor degree in Industrial Design; she is now completing a Ph.D. program in Inclusive Design within the International Doctorate in Architecture and Urban Planning program (IDAUP) at the Department of Architecture of the University of Ferrara, in Italy, presenting a research on Inclusive Design for smart devices addressed to older users.

She is an expert of User Centered methodologies for the design of products, services and systems. She uses to develop design projects for niche users belonging to fragile categories, particularly in the field of healthcare devices related to the Internet of things.

Since 2009 Silvia Imbesi has worked as a freelance architect and designer, collaborating with other professionals, companies, industries and institutions for the development of projects and design research.

Starting from 2012 she collaborated with the University of Ferrara as Contract Professor and participated at several researches, as research fellow, regarding User Centered methodologies, inclusive devices related to the Internet of Things, innovative teaching methods, etc.

From 2016 to 2019 she participated in the Challenge Based Innovation program (CBI) of Cern (Geneve, Switzerland), since 2012 she develops human centered projects of applied research with Studio Lineaguida (Florence, Italy).

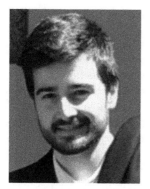

Gonçalo Marques holds a Ph.D. in Computer Science Engineering and is member of the Portuguese Engineering Association (Ordem dos Engenheiros). He is currently working as Assistant Professor lecturing courses on programming, multimedia and database systems. Furthermore, he worked as a Software Engineer in the Innovation and Development unit of Groupe PSA automotive industry from 2016 to 2017 and in the IBM group from 2018 to 2019. His current research interests include Internet of Things, Enhanced Living Environments, machine learning, e-health, telemedicine, medical and healthcare systems, indoor air quality monitoring and assessment, and wireless sensor networks. He has more than 80 publications in international journals and conferences, is a frequent reviewer of journals and international conferences and is also involved in several edited books projects.

Aspects of Human-Centered Design in Older Adults

Inclusive Innovation Through Design for Services: A Service Ergonomics Perspective

Daniele Busciantella-Ricci, Carlos Aceves-Gonzalez, and Sofia Scataglini

Abstract This chapter focuses on the relationships between Ergonomics and innovation through design from a service perspective. The aim is to underline how design for elderly users can be a resource for finding inclusive innovations that can be exploited for all the service users. This work underlines how Design for Inclusion represents a design resource for designing inclusive services for all—elderly users included. We outline the value of the Design for Inclusion approach in Service Design as a catalyst for finding inclusive innovations. From this perspective, knowledge fields such as Ergonomics, fields of design knowledge such as Inclusive Design, Design for All, Universal Design and design disciplines such as design for services play a crucial role. Therefore, the first part will offer theoretical discussions on the relationships between Service Design and Design for Inclusion. The second part will discuss the Inclusive Service Design approach by reporting studies and research experiences for designing services that mainly consider the elderly user's perspective. The third part frames the Service Ergonomics concept. Finally, we discuss how Design for Inclusion, the Inclusive Service Design approaches and the Service Ergonomics concept can contribute to the aim of this book from a holistic, inclusive and disruptive perspective.

Keywords Inclusive Service Design · Design for Inclusion · Inclusive innovation · Ergonomics · Service Design · Inclusive Design · Design for All

---

D. Busciantella-Ricci (✉)
Design Research Lab, Department of Humanities, University of Trento, Trento, Italy
e-mail: d.busciantellaricci@unitn.it

C. Aceves-Gonzalez
Ergonomics Research Center, Universidad de Guadalajara, Guadalajara, México
e-mail: c.aceves@academicos.udg.mx

S. Scataglini
Department of Product Development, Faculty of Design Sciences, University of Antwerp, Antwerp, Belgium
e-mail: sofia.scataglini@uantwerpen.be

© The Author(s), under exclusive license to Springer Nature Singapore Pte Ltd. 2022
S. Scataglini et al. (eds.), *Internet of Things for Human-Centered Design*,
Studies in Computational Intelligence 1011,
https://doi.org/10.1007/978-981-16-8488-3_1

1 Introduction

Design for innovation is a mantra and a buzzword of the last decades in the design thinking culture (e.g. [1–7]). Less attention has been given on the 'design for inclusive innovations' that should be one of the focus to reach social issues and facing systemic changes. Therefore, before entering the core of this work, it would be necessary to provide the assumptions that guided the development of this chapter. Indeed, the main contents and what we argue is described through in the following assumptions related to the Internet of Things (IoT) for human-centred design (HCD) and their applications to elderly healthcare. We argue:

(i) IoTs are essentially services [8–11] applied through products and systems according to flows and experiences that require design processes where users should be involved in every phase and where creativity and the design thinking should find applications and solutions; Service Design (SD) may help in understanding this perspective;

(ii) creating human-centred applications for elderly is more fruitful if inclusive approaches for designing are applied [12]; Inclusive Design (ID), Design for All (DfA), Universal Design (UD)—or in general terms 'Design for Inclusion'—may help on understanding this perspective;

(iii) designing for elderly in complex systems such as healthcare requires design disciplines that can consider levels of design related to services and systems [13–15] with design principles that emphasise at least contextual observations, collaborative design practices among the stakeholders (elderly included), and inclusive approaches in terms of emphasising the diversities; new approaches such as the Inclusive Service Design (ISD) approach [16, 17] may help on understanding this perspective.

Finally, this chapter proposes to take advantage of all these fields of studies both from the design culture and the Ergonomics culture by considering some kind of changes of the traditional perspectives such as:

- from an approach that focuses on elderly users to an approach that considers innovations for all;
- from an 'Ergonomics and/in/for design' approach to an 'innovation through Ergonomics design' approach;
- from a product-oriented approach to a service-system-oriented approach;
- from a human-centred approach to a truly inclusive and participative approach.

In general terms, the main goal of this chapter is to focus on how Ergonomics and design can create favourable conditions to foster inclusive innovations. SD is here underlined as a design discipline [18–21] to reach the goal of using Ergonomics for innovations through design. We argue that this can be useful for practitioners, researchers, designers and ergonomists that want to use these perspectives in applying human factors and Ergonomics with the aim to design products, services, systems and policies for all with a real HCD approach, comprised applications in the field of IoTs for elderly.

This chapter focuses on approaches and design disciplines that we suggest for designing IoT—in terms of products, services and systems—for elderly users through inclusive perspectives. We argue taking into consideration 'IoT for HCD' by focusing on 'application to elderly healthcare' calls into question fields of studies and practices of the design thinking culture (cf. [22–24]) as well as the Ergonomics field of knowledge. Designing for elderly users can be a resource for finding inclusive innovations that can be exploited for all the service users. Therefore, this chapter underlines how Design for Inclusion represents a design resource for designing inclusive services for all [12, 25]—elderly users included. The first part of the chapter will introduce basics of SD and create a link with the inclusive perspective in designing for inclusive services. A second part of the chapter will introduce the ISD approach and some practical implications in designing services for elderly through the Inclusive Service Blueprint tool. The last part of the chapter frames the 'Service Ergonomics' concept and underlines some implications of the perspective that we propose for the aim of this book.

2 Design for Inclusion and Service Design

According to the premises above, in this paragraph, we discuss the reasons we are introducing SD, Design for Inclusion and some perspectives that may help in merging these two domains of the design culture for the purpose of this book. It is well known that SD can frame its implications in services, policies and systems (cf. [26]). In addition, Design for Inclusion may create inclusive contexts for innovations [25, 27]. However, a better understanding on the relationships between SD and the Design for Inclusion is needed [12]. This is because the call of institutions and international organisations such as the European Commission (EC) through the Horizon Europe programme [28], the United Nations (UN) through the 2030 Agenda for Sustainable Development [29], or the Organisation for Economic Co-operation and Development (OECD) through specific initiatives (e.g. [30]), just to name a few, widely underlined the interest in supporting social cohesion, inclusive growths, inclusive societies and facing big challenges such as the climate change that requires inclusive and sustainable approaches for ideating, designing and developing projects (see [31–33]). We argue that a holistic perspective and a participatory and inclusive approach is required to address big global challenges for aiming inclusive innovations—also through IoT for human-centred applications that focus on elderly users in the healthcare system. Design for Inclusion and SD may simplify these needs and create fruitful connections for using multiple knowledge domains such as Ergonomics.

2.1 SD in Design for Inclusion and Design for Inclusion in SD

From a certain perspective, Design for Inclusion can work as an umbrella term to comprise approaches in designing for inclusive purposes (cf. [25, 34–38]). In the last decades, well-known approaches such as ID, UD and DfA are going to replace terms such as barrier free design, design for accessibility, or approaches that tend to stigmatise or focus on specific target groups of people; e.g. design for elderly, design for disability (cf. [39–45]). Also, this reinforced the main common principles of these three approaches (ID, UD and DfA) in using design strategies for contrasting stigmatisations, social exclusions, promoting social inclusion and adequately exploiting people diversity as a design resource (cf. [46]). These principles combine the three approaches under the common concept of 'Design for Inclusion'. In addition, about the ID, DfA and UD approaches, wider attention has been given to the design of physical and digital products, interfaces, spaces and build environment (cf. [40, 41, 44, 47, 48]), while, from an inclusive perspective, less attention has been given in those aspects characterise intangible things such as services, policies and systems.[1]

The application of Design for Inclusion approaches in designing services can be partially tracked down in making interfaces, Web applications or ICT systems more usable, comfortable, pleasurable and accessible for the wider range of people's needs (cf. [12, 49–53]). On one hand, the design of this kind of digital and physical products or integrated system is not always recognised as a part of the SD process. On the other hand, the design at this level of design contents is not fully representative of the whole complexity of the SD process. According to an inclusive approach, designing these types of design contents is not enough for facing an adequate design complexity and considering the whole inclusion aspects in front of the experiences, activities, infrastructures, products and policies of the entire service system. We argue designing inclusive services—also in IoT for elderly—requires basic knowledge on what a service and SD is and at least what kind of principles this design discipline should follow.

Therefore, before entering the core aspects of this chapter, an overview on the service term, SD definitions and principles are needed.

About the service term, multiple definitions are offered from several authors with different backgrounds. Indeed, Edvardsson, et al. [54] suggested that 'on a general level the service definition is a perspective'. For instance, a general perspective is offered by resources such as the Cambridge Dictionary [55] that associates the service meaning with the 'public need' domain and this noun is described as 'the fact that a system is working'; in alternative, it is described as a noun that indicates 'the act of dealing with customers in a shop, restaurant or hotel by taking their orders, showing or selling them goods, etc.' Also, according to the synthesis offered by Downe [56], a

---

[1] For instance, if one compares the results in searching "inclusive design", "design for all", "universal design" combined with "product design" on academic search engines, a greater amount of results can be actually found with respect to the same set of keywords combined with "service design".

service 'is simply something that helps someone to do something' and the challenge in designing a service resides in these relationships among the 'something', among the 'someone', and between the 'someone' and the 'something'. This is not so far from the definition that describes the service as 'an interaction between entities that co-create value, where the entities involved may be persons or nonpersons, such as government offices, educational institutions and possibly some form of automation' [57]. From a service system perspective, 'service is the application of resources (including competences, skills and knowledge) to make changes that have value for another (system)' [58].

Basically, it is also possible to see a service as a process [59]. According to Katzan [57], a service 'is a socially constructed temporal event that possesses a life cycle comprised of design, development, analysis and implementation, as with most technological innovations'.

According to Morelli et al. [26], the different definitions of the term 'service' refer to different interpretations of this term, i.e. (i) 'service as interaction between two or more people, characterised by unbalanced roles between server(s) and served' […]; (ii) 'service as an infrastructure that supports a certain kind of (service) activities' […]; (iii) 'service as a systemic institution […] that organises the activities and processes'.

One can also retrace a service definition on the assumption proposed by Kim [60] that assumed service as 'a system of collective action of parts connected to the whole for the purpose of achieving a shared goal'; therefore, service can be also interpreted as a system of participation [61]. In fact, with a broad perspective, 'services are systems that involve many different influential factors' [62]; and 'service design takes a holistic approach in order to get an understanding of the system and the different actors within the system' [62].

Therefore, after this brief introduction on the service term, what is SD?

By referring to the framework proposed by Kimbell [63], Morelli et al. [26] argue that the SD definition 'derived from such tensions define design, either from an engineering perspective—keeping the distinction between products and services, and interpreting design as a problem-solving activity—or from a design for services perspective, which looks at services as a value creation activity in an open-ended problem exploration involving different actors'. However, after several years from the first origin of the term from the marketing literature (see Shostack [59]), it is actually possible to identify several definitions of SD such as (here a non-exhaustive overview of the SD definitions):

- 'It aims to ensure that service interfaces are useful, usable and desirable from the client's point of view and effective, efficient and distinctive from the supplier's point of view' [64];
- 'Service design aims at designing services that are useful, usable and desirable from the user perspective, and efficient, effective and different from the provider perspective. It is a strategic approach that helps providers to develop a clear strategic positioning for their service offerings' [62];

- It is 'design for experiences that happen over time and across different touchpoints' (see servicedesign.org in [65]);
- 'Service design is the activity of organising and planning people, infrastructure, communication and material components of a service in order to improve its quality and the interaction between service providers and customers. It is a creative, viable and user-centred design process that is used by organisations to create value for their customers or users and serves as a competitive advantage for the service provider' [3];
- 'The systematic application of design methods and principles to the creation of service concepts for new or improved services' ([66] by also following [18]);
- 'Service design is a transdisciplinary design practice: it deals with complex systems that require different skills and capabilities across various forms of media and spheres of human interaction. Service design also requires a capability for critically analysing situated problems and formulating strategies for change. Several disciplines converge in the designing of services, including the arts, economics, the humanities and technology' [67];
- According to Stickdorn et al. [68], SD can be explained in many ways such as a mindset—therefore, as 'a collection of attitudes that determine our responses to various situations'—or, as a process that is driven by the design mindset, or as a toolset that lose much of their impact and may even make no sense without a process, mindset, and even common languages; or SD can be explained as a cross-disciplinary language—therefore as a common language among different disciplines—or as a management approach to both the incremental and radical innovations;
- 'Service design is the activity of working out which of these pieces need to fit together, asking how well they meet user needs, and rebuilding them from the ground up so that they do' [69];
- SD can be also described as 'a multidisciplinary field with a wide range of tools and methods for creating and improving service systems' [70].

About the principles of SD, we briefly provide an overview about some perspective from the literature generally service designers refer to. Among the authors that explicitly have taken positions on SD principles, we mention the followings:

- Mager [64] described SD as a work with a holistic approach; an interdisciplinary, co-creative practice that has a radical approach, and it is based on visual thinking;
- Stickdorn et al. [71] proposed the Service Design Thinking with five principles that describe SD as a user-centred, co-creative, sequencing, evidencing and holistic practice;
- Stickdorn et al. [68] by proposing a revision presented six principles highlighting that SD is a human-centred, collaborative, iterative, sequential, real and holistic practice;
- Downe [56] described fifteen principles of good services by emphasising what are those principles that make a service 'good'; so (i) a good service is easy to find; (ii) it explains its purpose; (iii) it sets the expectations a user has of it; (iv) it enables a user to complete the outcome they set out to; (v) it works in a familiar way; (vi) it

requires no prior knowledge; (vii) it is agnostic to organisational structures; (viii) it requires few steps; (ix) it is consistent throughout; (x) it should have no dead ends; (xi) it is usable by everyone, equally; (xii) it encourages the right behaviours from users and staff; (xiii) it should respond to change quickly; (xiv) it explains why a decision has been made; (xv) it makes easy to get human assistance.

Even if both Mager [64] and Stickdorn et al. [68, 71] introduce, respectively, the collaborative aspects and Stickdorn et al. [68] the HCD principles, none of them explicitly mention principles related to inclusive approaches in designing services. 'Human-centred' does not necessarily mean 'inclusive'. In contrast, Downe [56] explicitly mentions inclusive principles in designing services. Indeed, according to the eleventh principle, as Downe wrote, good services are usable by everyone regardless of their circumstances or abilities and in this case inclusion is a necessity, not an enhancement.

The need for inclusion in services is also declared by Fisk et al. [70] that introduced the 'service inclusion' paradigm and proposed the 'design for service inclusion' to move to socially inclusive service systems that require tools and methods for fostering service inclusion. Formally, 'service inclusion' is 'defined as an egalitarian system that provides customers with fair access to a service, fair treatment during a service and fair opportunity to exit a service' [70]. Also, according to Fisk et al. [70], service inclusion 'should be a moral imperative for service organisations, systems and nation-states'. We argue that design for service inclusion means creating the condition to design a service in an inclusive way about the whole complexity and in all the dimensions of a service system. It means considering that inclusion in good services 'is about more than just accessibility' [56]. Therefore, to design an inclusive service, we need to 'start to think in terms of "inclusion" of a full spectrum of needs instead' by considering 'how all these needs will affect each user across each channel, rather than just looking at the experience of a digital service' [56]. Addressing inclusion in SD for creating inclusive service systems also means innovating through diversity, personalisation, collaboration and ethics. Therefore, it also means to address SD with an Inclusive Design 3.0^2 level that focuses on service experience and user diversity, and moving forward to the Inclusive Design 4.0 that focuses on system and personalisation features.

However, taking a truly inclusive approach in designing services is not easy and should not be confused with approaches that address specific target users only. Eventually, like in the spirit of the Inclusive Design 4.0, finding inclusive solutions with specific target users should be useful for finding creative solutions for everybody.

---

[2] Hua Dong and Sharon Cook proposed the Evolving Inclusive Design model [72] to summarize the Inclusive Design research over the years. In this model, Inclusive Design 1.0 (1994) focuses on user capabilities; Inclusive Design 2.0 (2004) focuses on interfaces, interactions and processes; Inclusive Design 3.0 (2014) focuses on services and user diversity; Inclusive Design 4.0 (2024) focuses on systems and personalization features.

For the aim of this book, we argue this model may help to understand the level of complexity in designing inclusive services and we suggest using it to map your own approach in designing services through inclusive approaches.

2.2 Understanding Design for Inclusion and SD Relationships: A Proposal

According to the perspectives described in the previous paragraph, for understanding the relationship between SD and Design for Inclusion, we propose to consider four categories that can describe how these two fields can be interrelated. Therefore, the following categories are based on research works [12, 25] that proposed a framework based on the assumptions that consider a reasonable relationship between ID and SD.

The first of the four categories is named 'Inclusive Service Design'. This category is based on the ISD approach [16, 17] where principles and methods of ID, Ergonomics and SD are used for designing services.

The second category is named 'Design for Inclusive Services'. It is the design for an inclusive design result that in this case is an inclusive service rather than focusing on the methods and the theoretical framework of the design process.

The third category is named 'Service Design for Inclusion'—or we also named this category 'Service Design for All'. This means that SD is used for democratising design or at least democratising SD as a strategic tool for inclusion.

The fourth and last category is named 'Inclusive Design for Service Design'. In this category, an inclusive process is used to design services through the ID field of knowledge. In other words, about the fourth category, the ID attitude, praxis, approaches and methods are used to design services.

These categories can describe a theoretical framework for understanding how to design services by taking advantage of possible relationships between SD and the Design for Inclusion approaches. They can also frame some basic knowledge for SD approaches with a holistic and widely inclusive perspective. According to the results of the previous work, the first category can be fully described with the ISD approach as defined by Aceves-Gonzalez [16, 17] or with design approaches that address the need for SD to provide a more inclusive approach for including potentially excluded users and taking into consideration the diversity as a value in the design process. About the second category, not sufficient literature has been found for supporting the hypothesis behind this category. About the third category, 'Service Design for Inclusion' finds tangibility in those works that consider the contemporary SD discipline as a collaborative and inclusive practice; and from those perspectives that consider services and SD as a tool to alleviate social issues. About the 'Inclusive Design for Service Design'—the fourth category—it is represented by those works where a Design for Inclusion attitude is adopted to contemplate more inclusive services. It is the case where known approaches such as ID, DfA, UD are applied for designing services with inclusive features and values.

Although these four categories are still the subject of several discussions in our work, they offer a perspective to understand possibilities for framing strategies and approaches in designing for consciously orienting the design of services toward inclusive paradigms. If we also consider what we introduced in the previous paragraph through the four categories, it is possible to identify approaches for designing services with a Design for Inclusion perspective. And they can also support or integrate the design for 'service inclusion' paradigm from a design perspective. However, we argue the categories presented in this chapter offer an overview on the different possibilities a practitioner may use to find its own approach for designing inclusive services. And this is particularly useful for those practitioners, researchers and designers that are engaged in designing products-services based on the IoT systems for elderly.

Therefore, to also offer a tangible perspective in what designing for inclusive services means–especially with experimentation on the ageing population contexts—a focus on the ISD approach is offered by the following paragraphs.

3 Inclusive Service Design

ISD emerged from a research project [16] in the aging population context, where it had been recognised by the World Health Organization (WHO) [73] that in both developed and developing countries, people claimed that their city was not designed for older people and the provision of commercial and public services showed problems in meeting older people's needs. Data from the WHO report suggested that along with the need for an accessible built environment, there is a compelling need for inclusive services that can be used by a broader range of users. Services in which providers are able to understand how they can better respond to users irrespective of their age or capabilities. Inclusive services, as defined at the British Standard BS 18477 [74], are those which are available, usable and accessible to all customers equally, regardless of their personal circumstances.

As the population ages the need for inclusive services increases, representing a challenge for the design disciplines in terms of providing knowledge and tools for the evaluation, design and improvement of such types of services. With this in mind, the integration of ISD was the main contribution from Aceves-González's research project [16]. ISD is an approach that integrates theory, principles and methods from Ergonomics, ID and SD for evaluating and designing better (more inclusive and effective) services. Providing knowledge and tools for the evaluation, design and improvement of inclusive services is the primary goal of the ISD approach. ID and SD are intimately connected to the idea of developing better services. It has been highlighted the potential that these two approaches have to individually transform services into more functional, usable, desirable and viable ones [62, 75], but explicitly considering their integration as a facilitator of designing better services is a novel way to see that potential. In addition, ISD suggests Ergonomics (or human factors), the scientific discipline concerned with the understanding of interactions among humans and other elements of a system [76] as the underpinning discipline of the approach.

Initially, the ISD framework was used to evaluate bus service use by younger and older people in a city in Mexico [77, 78], which allowed identifying the gaps between what older passengers want and expect and what service operators do. It was possible to contrast how using the service imposes greater difficulties to older people given their capabilities reduction. The research then focussed on visualising and communicating the findings to stakeholders. An Inclusive Service Blueprint was developed to graphically represent the level of difficulty in using the service by younger and older people across the door-to-door journey and to highlight areas for service improvements [16].

Although the research was undertaken in the context of the bus service in Mexico, the approach and outcomes from ISD may be applicable for designing inclusive services in other contexts around the world.

3.1 An Inclusive Service Blueprint

Within SD there is a broad range of visualisation tools, one of the most valuable for representing service research is service blueprinting. Service blueprinting is a method introduced by Shostack [59, 79] and developed by Kingman-Brundage to visualise service processes [80]. As defined by the Design Council [81] 'a Service Blueprint is a detailed visual representation of the total service over time—showing the user's journey, all the different touchpoints and channels, as well as the behind the scenes parts of a service that make it work.

A Service Blueprint is an extremely useful tool for SD [82] because it is more precise than verbal definitions and less subject to misinterpretation [79]. Furthermore, this tool is relatively simple. Its graphical representations are easy to understand by all stakeholders involved—customers, managers and frontline employees—to assimilate, utilise and even adapt to meet different necessities according to each service.

However, an important point of note is that one of the core issues for Service Blueprints is to put users in the centre of design activities [82, 83].

A typical blueprint seems to under-emphasise that users are diverse and possess various capabilities, needs and desires, which present specific challenges to the design of services. This potential gap in service blueprinting encouraged the development of an Inclusive Service Blueprint [16] that considered the needs of a broader range of users and provided a sense of inclusiveness to this tool.

According to [16] developing, an Inclusive Service Blueprint aims to accomplish the following objectives:

- To visualise and communicate the differences in using a service for different group of users, for instance, younger and older people,
- To help in demonstrating visually how the gap between personal abilities and environmental demands become wider for older people.
- To provide a means for contrasting the ideal service and the younger and older user experience within the existing service.
- To detect and visualise the points of interaction associated with higher level of difficulty, particularly for older users; and therefore to provide a set of priorities for designing a more inclusive bus service,

- To visually represent that by addressing older people's needs in improving the service, the needs of younger people might be considered as well.

The Inclusive Service Blueprint was devised considering the typical format of a blueprint, including the onstage and backstage divided by the visibility line. It can be seen from Fig. 1 that backstage retained exactly the same components of a typical blueprint: invisible contact, employee actions, line of internal interaction and support processes (Fig. 2).

However, two adaptations were applied to the onstage. First, the section of physical evidence was removed from the top and integrated in the same section of touchpoints and staff activities. Second and more significant, the line of interaction was used to represent the level of difficulty in using the service by younger and older people, and the gap between what users need and what service organisations do (Fig. 3).

It is essential to mention that while this Inclusive Service Blueprint represents a bus service in Mexico, it can be applied to analyse and design inclusive services in many other contexts such as healthcare, tourism, finance, and of course, digital services.

4 The Service Ergonomics Concept

In this chapter, we argue about how SD applied to health and addressed to a population—or to a specific population such as the elderly users—bring an innovative paradigm in design creating a societal inclusive change.

In this context, the Inclusive Service Blueprint can be used to analyse the implications that older users may have in different contexts and environments such as taking a bus. These relations are not always taking into considerations as people are working as researchers in a mechanism to look in a specific detail such as a design output, a chair (e.g. of the bus), or the IoT connection to pay the ticket in the bus (e.g. contactless service), without thinking the entire system behind and the critical constraints that can interact with this system. As a consequence, people are not working in a multidisciplinary context with a multidisciplinary team. But they are looking to a specific micro-area without wondering if this is a subsystem of a system such as, for instance, the entire actions flow for the elderly users in taking the bus. They are not even wondering if the entire mechanism of the system is working. And this creates consequences for the users that are part of this system.

The Service Design Blueprint can solve this issue creating a better understanding of the criticalities that older users can have during a task such as taking a bus. However, sometimes, it is considered just as a SD tool, and it is not seen as a 'service system' tool addressed by SD researchers. In this chapter, we aim to describe how SD can be used by a multidisciplinary team with different backgrounds to foster innovation in research that, even if applied to older users, can be extended to the entire population of a service system.

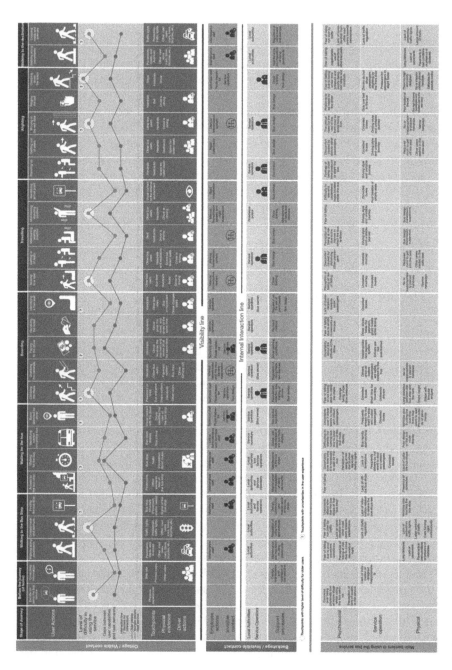

Fig. 1 Inclusive service blueprint

Inclusive Innovation Through Design ...

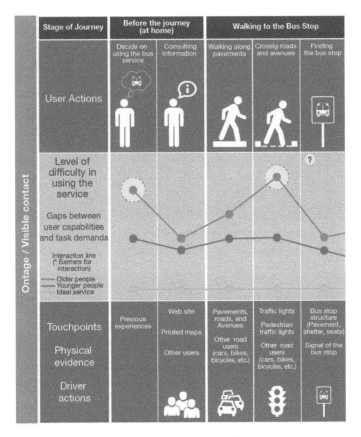

Fig. 2 Inclusive service blueprint: a portion above the visibility line

We argue that SD can be seen as an 'ergonomic system' that is already part of a research project, which, however, is not always being considered or is latent. This system can sustain the entire system of the research work that can involve different actors. Therefore, we can say that this system is a sustainable system that creates sustainability in every design process also addressed to a technology, an action or a task using a service.

As we asserted at the beginning of this chapter, IoTs are services that for instance can be used to connect smart devices with users such as the elderly (e.g. smart clothing) [84]. But, this can be considered a limited way to see SD in older users' context. SD as an 'ergonomic system' is able to create sustainable systems that can study the relationship between the human needs and other systems or subsystems. In some way, it is considered as an ergonomic system that can understand, visualise and interpret the human needs and their relationship with system and subsystem. This can be translated in a new way to foster innovation in design for/in Ergonomics where we frame the concept of 'Service Ergonomics' as an Ergonomics domain engaged in studying the relationship between the service system and the human needs. This

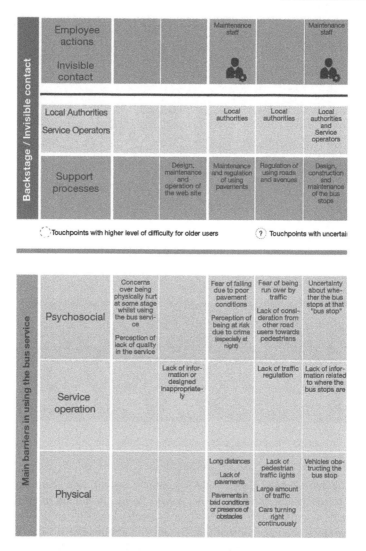

Fig. 3 Inclusive service blueprint: a portion below the visibility line

should be a field of study where design is considered as a strategic driver for inclusive innovations.

In other words, Service Ergonomics:

- uses HCD as a strategy (cf. [85–88]);
- concerns a service system perspective [89–91];
- refers to Ergonomics 4.0 [92, 93];
- adopts the ISD approach.

5 Discussion

Through this chapter, we proposed to use SD as a strategy to reach inclusive innovations. SD was presented as a discipline to be also applied with inclusive approaches such as the four categories that describe the relationships between Design for Inclusion and SD. Also, the ISD approach has been presented as particularly useful to find inclusive solutions by taking advantages from Ergonomics, ID and SD through a holistic approach. In this context, the Inclusive Service Blueprint tool has been presented through applications in the bus transportation systems with a study that focused on elderly users. Finally, we presented the Service Ergonomics concept with the aim to frame all those reflections under a common domain driven by a holistic, systemic and inclusive approach.

Firstly, the design of IoT services and systems for HCD applied to elderly healthcare can take advantage of the SD discipline and the Design for Inclusion approach by considering at least one of the categories that we presented in paragraph 2. According to this perspective, designing services for elderly users mean considering the users' diversities and needs as creative instruments to find solutions for as many users as possible like in the Design for Inclusion philosophy. In this perspective, the ISD approach is an innovative and consolidated approach that can be useful to apply this philosophy for designing services for all. The ISD approach highlights how inclusive innovations can be reached through the design of services. ISD may help designers, researchers and ergonomists in addressing challenges in the healthcare system through both a SD and an inclusive perspective. Therefore, it is useful for applications with elderly users in the healthcare system by considering IoT as services to be designed with a truly inclusive human-centred approach. At the same time, within the ISD domain, the Inclusive Service Blueprint is a tool that can be used in every stage of the design process to understand, define, improve and deliver a service where the elderly journey is the focus of the service experience. The Inclusive Service Blueprint may also help to find inclusive solutions from the analysis of these experiences. IoTs designed with the help of the Inclusive Service Blueprint can facilitate the identification of inclusive solutions that are exploitable for as many users as possible—elderly included. About the application of this tool in the healthcare system, even if service blueprinting shares some similarities with tools that generally consider the user journey—such as the patient journey map [94–100]—the Inclusive Service Blueprint allows creating a detailed visual representation of the service over time from a holistic/systemic perspective. Furthermore, the Inclusive Service Blueprint focuses on the diversity of characteristics and abilities of all those who participate in the service—patients and staff—and therefore on their inclusion. From a design perspective, it also complements well with other SD tools such as the stakeholder map [68, 101] to ensure the participation of all stakeholders, and it might be more comprehensive than a care pathway to get stakeholders' feedback.

In this perspective, the needs of the elderly, the patients, and the staff, as users that participate in the whole service may be used as creative drivers to identify inclusive service experiences and support the creation of inclusive service systems. Also, this is how the healthcare service system can take advantage of a design for service inclusion paradigm.

Finally, the Service Ergonomics concept has been introduced for the first time as a domain where HCD as a strategy, the service system perspective, the Ergonomics 4.0 and the ISD approach converge under a unique domain. Service Ergonomics fosters inclusive innovations by studying the relationship between the service system and the human needs and by adopting Ergonomics and design in the field of the services as systems to be designed. Service Ergonomics describes the complexity of the service system through the service experience of the users. This new Ergonomics domain encourages inclusive innovations through design. If applied to the healthcare systems, it can potentially transform the practices of designing for specific users—such as the elderly—to the design of a healthcare system where elderly is an active part of the whole population of the service system. At the same time, Service Ergonomics is the field of study that allows to consider the design of IoT products in terms of services and systems where elderly, patients (such as in the case of the healthcare system), staff and families of the patients may interact in the whole service system and participate to the design (or redesign) of the service by giving inputs and feedback and by co-creating opportunities like in a real human-centred and open system.

Regarding the Service Ergonomics concept and the ISD approach, the increase of the applications and further research and development experiences represent both the limits and future works in this field of study. The ISD approach is a promising approach that will be also useful to consider the renewed global interests on big challenges such as social inequalities, climate changes and healthcare conditions. Even if this approach is finding quite new experimentations, further occasions to research and develop related tools such as the Inclusive Service Blueprint are needed.

The Service Ergonomics concept has been coined here for the first time as a new Ergonomics domain. Therefore, the search for theoretical frameworks, cases, and empirical research activities is required.

6 Conclusion

In conclusion, Service Ergonomics serves as an orientation perspective to find ways to exploit the design thinking culture in order to design inclusive innovations. This is even more crucial where complexities come from elderly needs and the design context is the healthcare system. If IoTs are recognised as services, Service Ergonomics can be adopted as a perspective to understand what are those new services to address elderly needs in the healthcare system by IoT solutions. Also, adopting a Service Ergonomics perspective increases the chances to find inclusive innovations from the elderly to the whole population needs. It means exploiting the focus on the elderly needs as a creative stimulus to find service solutions for all. Practically, in designing IoTs for elderly in the healthcare system, the Service Ergonomics perspective can favour the use of approaches such as the ISD and tools such as the Inclusive Service Blueprint. Therefore, through this chapter, we emphasised:

- the relationship between SD and Design for Inclusion;
- the relevance on using the ISD approach;
- the Service Ergonomics perspective.

These three macro-contents should be considered by designers and researchers engaged in designing IoTs for elderly in the healthcare system. If not, IoTs will remain products that only will focus on specific users (such as a sample of elderly users with very specific needs) by creating stigmatisation, losing the chance to address system complexity and decreasing the possibility to create solutions that work for several needs and markets. By coining the term 'Service Ergonomics', we also followed the idea that an IoT solution studied around the elderly people's needs can ethically and sustainably work in complex systems such as the healthcare system. And this is why we considered the need to describe the Service Ergonomics concept in the fourth paragraph. However, we also consider that the limits of this work should be also addressed for comprehensively understanding and describing the Service Ergonomics perspective as a way that ensures inclusive innovations through design for services.

References

1. Cantamessa, M., Cascini, G., Montagna, F.: Design for innovation. In: Marjanovic, D., Štorga, M., Pavkovic, N., Bojcetic, N. (eds.) Proceedings of the 12th International Design Conference DESIGN 2012, May 21–24, 2012, Dubrovnik, Croatia, pp. 747–756. Faculty of Mechanical Engineering and Naval Architecture, University of Zagreb, Croatia (2012)
2. Design Council: Design for innovation: Facts, figures and practical plans for growth. Design Council. https://www.designcouncil.org.uk/sites/default/files/asset/document/Design ForInnovation_Dec2011.pdf (2011). Accessed 03 Sept 2021
3. Dervojeda, K., Verzijl, D., Nagtegaal, F., Lengton, M., Rouwmaat, E., Monfardini, E., Frideres, L.: Design for Innovation: Service design as a means to advance business models. Business Innovation Observatory. European Commission (2014)
4. Hernández, R.J., Cooper, R., Tether, B., Murphy, E.: Design, the language of innovation: a review of the design studies literature. She Ji: J. Des. Econ. Innov. **4**(3), 249–274 (2018)
5. Plambeck, E.L., Taylor, T.A.: Implications of breach remedy and renegotiation design for innovation and capacity. Manage. Sci. **53**(12), 1859–1871 (2007)
6. Whicher, A., Walters, A.: Mapping design for innovation in Wales & Scotland. Cardiff Metropolitan University (2014)
7. European Union. Interreg Europe: Design for Innovation. https://www.interregeurope.eu/design4innovation/. Accessed 02 Sept 2021
8. Brincat, A.A., Pacifici, F., Mazzola, F.: Iot as a service for smart cities and nations. IEEE Internet Things Mag. **2**(1), 28–31 (2019)
9. Deng, D.J., Pang, A.C., Hanzo, L.: Recent advances in IoT as a service (IoTaas 2017). Mobile Netw. Appl. **24**(3), 721–723 (2019)
10. Giacobbe, M., Di Pietro, R., Minnolo, A.L., Puliafito, A.: Evaluating information quality in delivering IoT-as-a-service. In: 2018 IEEE international Conference on Smart Computing (SMARTCOMP), pp. 405–410. IEEE (2018)
11. Świątek, P., Rucinski, A.: IoT as a service system for eHealth. In: 2013 IEEE 15th International Conference on e-Health Networking, Applications and Services (Healthcom 2013), pp. 81–84. IEEE (2013)

12. Busciantella-Ricci, D., Rizo-Corona, L., Aceves-Gonzalez, C.: Exploring boundaries and synergies between inclusive design and service design. In: Di Bucchianico, G., Shin, C., Shim, S., Fukuda, S., Montagna, G., Carvalho, C. (eds.), Advances in Industrial Design. AHFE 2020. Advances in Intelligent Systems and Computing, vol. 1202, pp. 55–61. Springer, Heidelberg (2020)
13. Jones, P.H.: Systemic design principles for complex social systems. In Metcalf, G.S. (ed.), Social Systems and Design, pp. 91–128. Springer, Heidelberg (2014)
14. Jones, P.H., Van Patter, G.K.: Design 1.0, 2.0, 3.0, 4.0: The Rise of Visual Sensemaking. NextDesign Leadership Institute, New York (2009)
15. Young, R.A.: An integrated model of designing to aid understanding of the complexity paradigm in design practice. Futures **40**(6), 562–576 (2008)
16. Aceves-Gonzalez, C.: The application and development of inclusive service design in the context of a bus service. Doctoral dissertation (©Carlos Aceves Gonzalez) (2014)
17. Aceves-Gonzalez, C., Cook, S., May, A.: Improving bus travel through inclusive service design. In: Soares, M.M., Rebelo, F. (eds.) Ergonomics in Design: Methods and Techniques, pp. 431–444. CRC Press, Boca Raton (2016)
18. Holmlid, S., Evenson, S.: Bringing service design to service sciences, management and engineering. In: Service Science, Management and Engineering Education for the 21st Century, pp. 341–345. Springer, Heidelberg (2008)
19. Mager, B.: Service Design: A Review. Köln International School of Design (2004)
20. Manzini, E.: Design, When Everybody Designs: An Introduction to Design for Social Innovation. MIT press (2015)
21. Moritz, S.: Service Design: Practical Access to an Evolving Field. MSc thesis, Köln International School of Design (2005)
22. Altman, M., Huang, T.T., Breland, J.Y.: Design thinking in health care. Preventing Chronic Dis. **15** (2018)
23. Lorusso, L., Lee, J.H., Worden, E.A.: Design thinking for healthcare: transliterating the creative problem-solving method into architectural practice. HERD: Health Environ. Res. Design J. **14**(2), 16–29 (2021)
24. Thies, A.: On the value of design thinking for innovation in complex contexts: a case from healthcare. IxD&A (Interaction Design and Architecture(s)) J. **27**, 59–171 (2015)
25. Busciantella-Ricci, D., Aceves-Gonzalez, C.: Framing design for inclusion strategies for service design. In: Shin, C.S., Di Bucchianico, G., Fukuda, S., Ghim, Y.G., Montagna, G., Carvalho, C. (eds.), Advances in Industrial Design. AHFE 2021. Lecture Notes in Networks and Systems, vol. 260, pp. 371–379. Springer, Cham (2021)
26. Morelli, N., De Götzen, A., Simeone, L.: Service Design Capabilities. Springer Nature, Heidelberg (2021)
27. Foster, C., Heeks, R.: Policies to support inclusive innovation. In: Development Informatics Working Paper (61) (2015)
28. European Commission: Horizon Europe Strategic Plan (2021–2024). European Commission, Directorate-General for Research and Innovation. https://op.europa.eu/en/web/eu-law-and-publications/publication-detail/-/publication/3c6ffd74-8ac3-11eb-b85c-01aa75ed71a1 (2021)
29. United Nations: Transforming our World: The 2030 Agenda for Sustainable Development. United Nations https://sdgs.un.org/publications/transforming-our-world-2030-agenda-sustainable-development-17981 (2015)
30. Organisation for Economic Co-operation and Development (OECD): Putting people's well-being at the top of the agenda. OECD Centre on Well-being, Inclusion, Sustainability and Equal Opportunity (WISE). https://www.oecd.org/wise/Peoples-well-being-at-the-top-of-the-agenda-WISE-mission.pdf (2020)
31. C40 Cities Climate Leadership Group: Inclusive Climate Action in Practice—How to Jointly Tackle Climate Change and Inequality: Case Studies from Leading Global Cities. C40 Cities https://c40.my.salesforce.com/sfc/p/#36000001Enhz/a/1Q000000MdxP/6_TozntO.AKisUzkWS0FsogewLcfYu89XOCICwJoL5g (2019)

32. European Commission: The New European Bauhaus: Shaping more beautiful, sustainable and inclusive forms of living together. https://europa.eu/new-european-bauhaus/index_en. Accessed 02 Sept 2021
33. Luna-Galván, M., Vargas-Chaves, I., Franco-Gantiva, A.: Towards an inclusive approach for climate change adaptation strategies: the case of the plan 4C in the City of Cartagena de Indias. Eur. J. Sustain. Dev. **6**(3), 457–457 (2017)
34. Di Bucchianico, G.: Design for inclusion. Different approaches for a shared goal. In: Shin, C.S., Di Bucchianico, G., Fukuda, S., Ghim, Y.G., Montagna, G., Carvalho, C. (eds.), Advances in Industrial Design. AHFE 2021. Lecture Notes in Networks and Systems, vol. 260. Springer, Heidelberg (2021)
35. Garay-Rondero, C.L., Salinas-Navarro, D.E., Calvo, E.Z.R.: Design for inclusion and diversity: developing social competencies in engineering education. In: Di Bucchianico, G., Shin, C., Shim, S., Fukuda, S., Montagna, G., Carvalho, C. (eds.), Advances in Industrial Design. AHFE 2020. Advances in Intelligent Systems and Computing, vol. 1202, pp. 85–92. Springer, Heidelberg (2020)
36. Langdon, P., Lazar, J., Heylighen, A., Dong, H. (eds.): Designing for Inclusion: Inclusive Design: Looking Towards the Future. CWUAAT 2020. Springer, Heidelberg (2020)
37. Reed, D.J., Monk, A.: Design for inclusion. In: Clarkson, P.J., Langdon, P., Robinson, P. (eds.), Designing Accessible Technology, pp. 53–63. Springer, Heidelberg (2006)
38. Reinert, A., Ebert, D.S.: Humane design for inclusion. In: Black, N.L., Neumann, W.P., Noy, I. (eds.), Proceedings of the 21st Congress of the International Ergonomics Association (IEA 2021), Volume II: Inclusive Design, pp. 307–316. Springer, Heidelberg (2021)
39. Cassim, J., Coleman, R., Clarkson, J., Dong, H.: Why inclusive design? In: Coleman, R., Clarkson, J., Dong, H., Cassim, J. (eds.), Design for Inclusivity. A Practical Guide to Accessible, Innovative and User-Centred Design, pp. 11–21. Gower (2007)
40. Clarkson, J., Coleman, R.: Inclusive design. J. Eng. Des. **21**(2–3), 127–129 (2010)
41. Clarkson, P.J., Coleman, R.: History of inclusive design in the UK. Appl. Ergon. **46**, 235–247 (2015)
42. Coleman, R., Lebbon, C., Clarkson, P.J., Keates, S.: From margins to mainstream. In: Clarkson, J., Coleman, R., Keates, S. (eds.), Inclusive Design: Design for the Whole Population. Springer, Heidelberg (2003)
43. Ostroff, E.: Universal design: an evolving paradigm. In: Preiser, W.F.E. Smith, K.H. (eds.), Universal Design Handbook, 2nd edn., pp. 34–42. McGraw-Hill (2011)
44. Persson, H., Åhman, H., Yngling, A.A., Gulliksen, J.: Universal design, inclusive design, accessible design, design for all: different concepts—one goal? On the concept of accessibility—historical, methodological and philosophical aspects. Univ. Access Inf. Soc. **14**(4), 505–526 (2015)
45. Zhu, H., Gruber, T., Dong, H.: Value and values in inclusive design. In: Gao, Q., Zhou, J. (eds.), Human Aspects of IT for the Aged Population. Technologies, Design and User Experience. HCII 2020. Lecture Notes in Computer Science, vol. 12207. Springer, Heidelberg (2020)
46. European Institute for Design and Disability (EIDD): The EIDD Stockholm Declaration. European Institute for Design and Disability (EIDD). https://dfaeurope.eu/wordpress/wp-content/uploads/2014/05/stockholm-declaration_english.pdf (2004)
47. Harding, J.: Moving inclusively through transport buildings: a cross-disciplinary design case study. In: Langdon, P., Lazar, J., Heylighen, A., Dong. H. (eds.), Designing for Inclusion: Inclusive Design: Looking Towards the Future. CWUAAT 2020. Springer, Heidelberg (2020)
48. O'Neill, J.L.: Accessibility for all abilities: how universal design, universal design for learning, and inclusive design combat inaccessibility and ableism. J. Open Access Law **9**(1), 1–15 (2021)
49. Bue Lintho, O., Begnum, M.: Towards inclusive service design in the digital society: current practices and future recommendations. In: DS 91: Proceedings of NordDesign 2018, Design in the Era of Digitalization, Linköping, Sweden, 14–17 August (2018)
50. Darzentas, J.S., Darzentas, J.: Accessible self-service: a driver for innovation in service design. In: ServDes, 2014 Service Future, Proceedings of the fourth Service Design and Service

Innovation Conference, Lancaster University, United Kingdom, 9–11 April 2014, pp. 143–153. Linköping University Electronic Press (2014)
51. Lazar, J., Wentz, B., Akeley, C., Almuhim, M., Barmoy, S., Beavan, P., Beck, C., Blair, A.,Bortz, A., Bradley, B., Carter, M., Crouch, D., Dehmer, G., Gorman, M., Gregory, C., Lanier, E., McIntee, A., Nelson, Jr. R., Ritgert, D., Rogers, Jr. R., Rosenwald, S., Sullivan, S., Wells, J., Willis, C., Wingo-Jones, K., Yatto, T.: Equal access to information? Evaluating the accessibility of public library web sites in the State of Maryland. In: Langdon, P., Clarkson, J., Robinson, P., Lazar, J., Heylighen, A. (eds.), Designing Inclusive Systems, pp. 185–194. Springer, Heidelberg (2012)
52. Scandurra, I., Sjölinder, M.: Participatory design with seniors: design of future services and iterative refinements of interactive eHealth services for old citizens. Medicine 2.0 **2**(2), e12 (2013)
53. Spinelli, G., Jain, S.: Designing and evaluating web interaction for older users. In: Evaluating Websites and Web Services: Interdisciplinary Perspectives on User Satisfaction, pp. 176–202. IGI Global (2014)
54. Edvardsson, B., Gustafsson, A., Roos, I.: Service portraits in service research: a critical review. Int. J. Serv. Ind. Manag. **16**(1), 107–121 (2005)
55. Cambridge Dictionary: Service. https://dictionary.cambridge.org/dictionary/english/service. Accessed 09 Jul 2021
56. Downe, L.: Good Services: How to Design Services that Work. BIS Publishers (2020)
57. Katzan, H., Jr.: Essentials of service design. J. Service Sci. (JSS) **4**(2), 43–60 (2011)
58. Maglio, P.P., Vargo, S.L., Caswell, N., Spohrer, J.: The service system is the basic abstraction of service science. IseB **7**(4), 395–406 (2009)
59. Shostack, G.L.: How to design a service. Eur. J. Mark. **16**(1), 49–63 (1982)
60. Kim, M.: An inquiry into the nature of service: a historical overview (part 1). Des. Issues **34**(2), 31–47 (2018)
61. Kim, M.: Service is not perishable: nurturing ongoing participation with conceptual models. Des. Issues **36**(4), 56–71 (2020)
62. Mager, B., Sung, T.J.D.: Special issue editorial: designing for services. Int. J. Des. **5**(2), 1–3 (2011)
63. Kimbell, L.: Designing for service as one way of designing services. Int. J. Des. **5**(2), 41–52 (2011)
64. Mager, B.: Service design as an emerging field. In: Miettinen, S., Koivisto, M. (eds.) Designing Services with Innovative Methods, pp. 28–43. University of Art and Design, Helsinki (2009)
65. Clatworthy, S.: Service innovation through touch-points: development of an innovation toolkit for the first stages of new service development. Int. J. Des. **5**(2), 15–28 (2011)
66. Feldmann, N., Cardoso, J.: Service design. In: Cardoso, J., Fromm, H., Nickel, S. Satzger, G., Studer, R., Weinhardt, C. (eds.), Fundamentals of Service Systems, pp. 105–135. Springer, Heidelberg (2015)
67. Penin, L.: An Introduction to Service Design: Designing the Invisible. Bloomsbury Publishing (2018)
68. Stickdorn, M., Hormess, M.E., Lawrence, A., Schneider, J.: This is Service Design Doing. O'Reilly Media (2018)
69. Downe, L.: What we mean by service design. Blog Government Digital Service (2016). https://gds.blog.gov.uk/2016/04/18/what-we-mean-by-service-design/. Accessed 09 Jul 2021
70. Fisk, R.P., Dean, A.M., Alkire, L., Joubert, A., Previte, J., Robertson, N., Rosenbaum, M.S.: Design for service inclusion: creating inclusive service systems by 2050. J. Serv. Manag. **29**, 834–858 (2018)
71. Stickdorn, M., Schneider, J.: This is Service Design Thinking: Basics-Tools-Cases. BISPublishers (2011)
72. Loughborough University. Evolving Inclusive Design. https://www.youtube.com/watch?v=pzl1dKCMGLw. Accessed 09 Jul 2021
73. WHO: Global Age-friendly Cities: A Guide. WHO. http://www.who.int/ageing/age_friendly_cities_guide/en/. (2007)

74. BS 18477:2010. Inclusive Service Provision—Requirements for Identifying and Responding to Consumer Vulnerability. BSI (2010)
75. Clarkson, J., Coleman, R., Hosking, I., Waller, S.: Inclusive Design Toolkit (1st edn.). University of Cambridge, Cambridge (2007)
76. International Ergonomics Association (IEA): Definition of Ergonomics. https://iea.cc/ (2000)
77. Aceves-González, C., Cook, S., May, A.: Bus use in a developing world city: implications for the health and well-being of older passengers. J. Transp. Health **2**(2), 308–316 (2015)
78. Aceves-González, C., May, A., Cook, S.: An observational comparison of the older and younger bus passenger experience in a developing world city. Ergonomics **59**(6), 840–850 (2016)
79. Shostack, G.: Designing services that deliver. Harv. Bus. Rev. **62**, 133–139 (1984)
80. Fließ, S., Kleinaltenkamp, M.: Blueprinting the service company. J. Bus. Res. **57**(4), 392–404 (2004)
81. Design Council: Design methods for developing services. An introduction to service design and a selection of service design tools. Design Council (2015)
82. Polaine, A., Løvlie, L., Reason, B.: Service Design: From Insight to Implementation. Rosenfeld Media (2013)
83. Bitner, M.J., Ostrom, A.L., Morgan, F.N.: Service blueprinting: a practical technique for service innovation. Calif. Manage. Rev. **50**(3), 66–95 (2008)
84. Imbesi, S., Scataglini, S.: A user centered methodology for the design of smart apparel for older users. Sensors **21**(8), 2804 (2021)
85. Design Council: Design for public good. Design Council (2013)
86. Nusem, E., Wrigley, C., Matthews, J.: Developing design capability in nonprofit organizations. Des. Issues **33**(1), 61–75 (2017)
87. Ramlau, U.H.: In Denmark, design tops the agenda. Des. Manage. Rev. **15**(4), 48–54 (2004)
88. Wrigley, C., Straker, K.: Design thinking pedagogy: the educational design ladder. Innov. Educ. Teach. Int. **54**(4), 374–385 (2017)
89. Katzan, H.: Principles of service systems: an ontological approach. J. Service Sci. (JSS) **2**(2), 35–52 (2009)
90. Maglio, P.P., Spohrer, J.: Fundamentals of service science. J. Acad. Mark. Sci. **36**(1), 18–20 (2008)
91. Vargo, S.L., Maglio, P.P., Akaka, M.A.: On value and value co-creation: a service systems and service logic perspective. Eur. Manag. J. **26**(3), 145–152 (2008)
92. Aiello, G.: Ergonomics 4.0: the role of human operator in the future smart production environment. Acta Ergonomica **1**(1), 1–4 (2020)
93. Paul, G., Briceno, L.: A conceptual framework of DHM enablers for ergonomics 4.0. In: Congress of the International Ergonomics Association, pp. 403–406. Springer, Heidelberg (2021)
94. Gregory, M.: A possible patient journey: a tool to facilitate patient-centered care. Semin. Hear. **33**(1), 9–15 (2012)
95. Joseph, A.L., Kushniruk, A.W., Borycki, E.M.: Patient journey mapping: current practices, challenges and future opportunities in healthcare. Knowl. Manage. E-Learning: Int. J. **12**(4), 387–404 (2020)
96. McCarthy, S., O'Raghallaigh, P., Woodworth, S., Lim, Y.L., Kenny, L.C., Adam, F.: An integrated patient journey mapping tool for embedding quality in healthcare service reform. J. Decis. Syst. **25**(sup1), 354–368 (2016)
97. Meyer, M.A.: Mapping the patient journey across the continuum: lessons learned from one patient's experience. J. Patient Experience **6**(2), 103–107 (2019)
98. Sijm-Eeken, M., Zheng, J., Peute, L.: Towards a lean process for patient journey mapping—a case study in a large academic setting. In: Pape-Haugaard, L.B., Lovis, C., Cort Madsen, I., Weber, P., Hostrup Nielsen, P., Scott, P. (eds.), Digital Personalized Health and Medicine. Studies in Health Technology and Informatics Series, pp. 1071–1075. IOS Press (2020)
99. Simonse, L., Albayrak, A., Starre, S.: Patient journey method for integrated service design. Des. Health **3**(1), 82–97 (2019)

100. Trebble, T.M., Hansi, N., Hydes, T., Smith, M.A., Baker, M.: Process mapping the patient journey: an introduction. Bmj **341** (2010)
101. Morelli, N., Tollestrup, C.: New representation techniques for designing in aSystemic perspective. In: Design Inquiries, Nordes 07 Conference (2007)

Human-Centered Design for Older Users: A Design Methodology for the Development of Smart Devices and Systems Related to Health Care

Silvia Imbesi

Abstract Considering the current aging society and innovation brought by the Internet of Things, it is important to design and develop new innovative smart solutions using available technologies and design research knowledge, in order to allow older people to be as autonomous as possible, improving their quality of life. The design of smart devices and systems, following a human-centered approach and addressed to older users with particular needs, can be developed following an innovative re-designed methodological process aiming to reduce the project's complexity and maximize its level of usability. The suggested methodological strategy divides the iterative design process in several design cycles, where every cycle is composed of the stages of planning, analyzing, creating, and verifying. The PASSO project is reported as practical example of the experimented methodological strategy.

Keywords Human-Centered Design · Design methodologies · Older users · Smart Systems · Smart Devices · Internet of Things · PASSO project

1 Introduction

The aging trend affecting populations of most of developed countries all over the world has consolidated in recent years, creating a growing attention to the consequences and implications of this demographic trend. Although the problems afflicting an aging population have been studied for a long time [1], it is in the last few years that international entities or institutions such as the World Health Organization (WHO) have asked for attention to this change taking place. Particularly, WHO published in 2015 the "World Report on Aging and Health" introducing the concept of "active aging" and emphasizing the importance of health promotion and diseases prevention throughout life, especially in old age, as effective strategies to face the aging trend [2].

S. Imbesi (✉)
Department of Architecture, University of Ferrara, Ferrara, Italy
e-mail: silvia.imbesi@unife.it

© The Author(s), under exclusive license to Springer Nature Singapore Pte Ltd. 2022
S. Scataglini et al. (eds.), *Internet of Things for Human-Centered Design*,
Studies in Computational Intelligence 1011,
https://doi.org/10.1007/978-981-16-8488-3_2

One of the obvious negative consequences pending on public systems is the foreseeable increase in public spending in the fields of welfare and health care, due to the increase of older people no longer self-sufficient and in need of medical assistance.

To mitigate these effects, health promotion and primary prevention measures are needed to maintain and increase abilities of the elderly in daily activities. Constancy in physical exercise and the presence of stimuli that provide emotional and motivation are the prerequisites for healthy aging, as well as a social involvement of the person [3].

2 Older Users and the Internet of Things

Typically, aging is associated with a physical and cognitive decline, bringing changes that would require some adaptations to the person's daily habits and environment in order to facilitate everyday life. Critical events that could incur or the slow loss of personal abilities may lead to a significant loss of autonomy and to the necessity of satisfying new growing needs regarding both the emotional and functional fields.

In light of previous considerations, it is important to design and develop new innovative solutions using available technologies and design research knowledge, in order to ensure elderly people an adequate health care allowing them to be as autonomous as possible and involved in social life [4].

The Internet of Things (IoT) is a novel paradigm consisting in the pervasive presence around us of a variety of "things" as objects and devices, able to interact and cooperate with each other and with the user, to improve her/his daily life's quality [5].

In the context of aging populations, domotics, assisted living, e-health, and telemedicine are just some possible applications of the pervasive role that IoT is actually gaining in our lives.

The connection between common objects linked to a system and the ability to read and interpret the user's behaviors allows the intelligent system to collect data and to exchange information with the person. These elements can improve the level of comfort, security, care, and usability of objects and environments related to the elderly [6].

In detail, some possible applications of the Iot in the healthcare sector that could bring advantage to older people are related to technologies for tracking, for identification and authentication, for data collection, and for sensing [7]. Tracking technologies aim to identify the person in motion; this can be done in real-time positioning tracking or in correspondence of important locations in the environment. Identification and authentication is usually related to the satisfaction of requirements of security procedures and safety issues. Automatic data collection and transfer is often used to reduce processing time and increase data accuracy, integrating data from different sources and creating network possibilities. Sensing enables the possibility of collection of real-time information on the user's health parameters, with the consequent possibility of monitoring at distance for medical purposes [6].

IoT seems to be crucial in healthcare applications addressed to aging users, with great potentialities to have an impact even on other categories of people directly or indirectly related to them.

Currently, computing is related to computer-based systems which are usually embedded in the person's daily environment and can be accessed everywhere (ubiquitous); information and communication technology is a great part of ubiquitous computing [8]. These instruments seem to be very effective in developing services for older people, because of their ability of providing accessibility to healthcare providers, e.g., to check some aspects of the person's health status.

Developing smart systems addressed to older people facilitates them in daily activities maintaining autonomy and avoiding risks. Ubiquitous computing allows the automation of performed daily activities due to the removal of motor and cognitive barriers and the addition of facilities provided by innovative technologies related to the IoT [9].

One of the main issues in the design of IoT to products, services, and processes is the development of communication instruments able to facilitate the interaction by using a natural language and natural shapes. An easy interaction is strictly related to the usability and accessibility of every project: Specifically, in the design of smart systems, a good interaction design allows users to take advantage from new technologies related to the IoT, even if they are affected from limitations related to disabilities, social status, or ignorance [10].

3 Human-Centered Design and Usability

In light of the previous considerations, one of the key aspects in designing for aging people is the attention to project aspects related to usability where the user's point of view plays a determinant role [11].

For a large amount of older users, technology is perceived as difficult and challenging when not specifically conceived for them as final users of the developed devices or systems. Usually, problems are related to a project's lack of usability that implies difficulties for the elderly in learning and operating, making the person frustrated in using the developed design solutions [12].

Hence, in addition to functional aspects, it is fundamental to conceive systems able to adapt themselves to people's needs, requirements, and expectations. Thus, designing smart devices and systems considering primarily technological aspects and functional requirements, as the traditional machine-centered approach suggests, is no longer effective when the design is addressed to the elderly [13].

In the described perspective, it becomes necessary to shift from a machine-centered to a human-centered approach, giving a special focus to issues concerning the user's abilities and capabilities and preferences related to the specific context. Generally, devices and environments are conceived for users without disabilities and impairments, but there are some niche categories of people who have to face physical or cognitive limitations and to ask for personal assistance to support their daily routines. Older people are a growing group of users belonging to this category, presenting special requirements related to the decline of some physical functions and mental abilities.

Limitations coming through aging can be partially offset by the use of human-centered technologies able to improve people's quality of life by establishing a correspondence between users' needs and project's requirements [14].

According to international standards [15], human-centered design (HCD) suggests a design process that considers and involves users since the early stages of the research, investigating their psychophysical characteristics and behaviors during their daily routine in the primary environment, in order to define main needs and difficulties in achieving several goals [16]. In this perspective, multidisciplinary project teams are expected to plan processes including older users' voices in order to improve projects usability through the application of inclusive design methodologies.

4 PASSO Project's Methodology

This paper describes a human-centered process applied by the author to the ongoing design research project called Parkinson's Smart Sensory-cues for Older-users (PASSO). This project develops a system providing sensory cues to train the walk of older people affected by Parkinson's disease (PD) [17], a disease causing impairments that often impact on functional independence, well-being, and health-related quality of life [18].

The aim of this design research project is to create a wearable gait rehabilitation solution by integrating smart glasses and earphones into a smartphone-based gait monitoring system. That should allow health professionals to elaborate personally tailored rehabilitation programs adaptable on individual patients' sensory preferences, cognitive aspects, and medical knowledge. Specifically, the system provides visual and vibratory cues by smart glasses and auditory cues by earphones [19].

The PASSO project, as said before, followed a HCD approach. The author, starting from existing models [20], elaborated an improved HCD design methodology which shown to be very effective in complex design processes keeping in consideration both qualitative factors related to people and quantitative factors related to technologies.

The process has been divided in several iterative design cycles, each one composed of four stages [21]. In the PASSO project, the traditional stages have been renamed as plan, analyze, verify, and create (Fig. 1).

In the following part of the chapter, the author will explain the applied methodology without being too specific on the current project, but keeping it as general guidelines, adaptable to other design research projects.

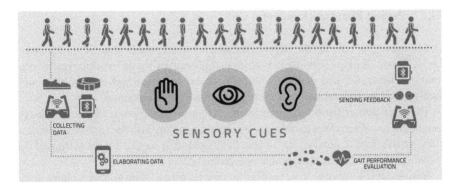

Fig. 1 Schematization of the PASSO project. Smart devices submit smart cues for gait rehabilitation to older users affected by Parkinson's disease

4.1 Stage 1: Planning

The first stage of each cycle was the planning one: in this first part of the project are taken important decisions about strategies to be used in the whole design process.

4.1.1 Multidisciplinary Team Composition

It is fundamental to define which abilities should be included in the team in order to gain the project success. The right mix of competences allows the research project to be effective and usable, giving a valid answer to specific needs addressed to aging people, usually related to the improvement of autonomy in daily activities.

In this project, as in most ones regarding the design of smart devices and systems, three main groups of professionals were recognized as fundamental in relation to set objectives and process development.

- Designers (user research, usability, HCD methodology, interaction design, product design, visual design, etc.);
- Technical operators (biomedical engineering, computer science and technology, informatics, etc.);
- Medical operators (neurology, physiatry, physiotherapy, geriatrics, etc.).

Depending on the project resources, it is possible to enlarge the team including specialists on specific fields. These professionals can work with the multidisciplinary team for the whole process or be consulted for specific technical parts of the project.

4.1.2 Project Plan Development

The project plan reflects the approach chosen for the whole project, in this case the HCD one. It helps defining strategies and objectives for the work development, setting deliverables and communication between the team and stakeholders and, finally, helps in the evaluation of human and non-human resources.

The main aim of the project plan is the definition of the project to be developed and the choice of activities to be included in the design process due to their usefulness in the satisfaction of older users' needs. In this phase, it starts even the setting of the project goals, defined as measurable objectives [22].

Besides, it is important to set project invariants related to available technologies, budget, professionals' skills, etc.

Every time an aim has been set, it is important to specify how the team will unambiguously verify the achievement of this objective.

4.1.3 Choice of Users

The users that need to be chosen belong to three categories: primary users, secondary users, and stakeholders [23].

Primary users are a niche category of elderly (usually affected by a specific problem in carrying out a specific activity) that are going to personally use the smart devices and/or the system app. They must be considered as final users, and their lack of satisfaction can invalidate the project's results.

Secondary users are people who will take advantage from the project even if it is not addressed to them. Some typical examples are the person's relatives and caregivers helped by a system improving the final user's independence or doctors and healthcare professionals taking care of him/her that can obtain much more feedback on daily routine and health status.

Stakeholders are not strictly related to the use of the device but have interest in its success for other reasons. Some examples are decision makers of the public healthcare system that could obtain a decrease of public expenses improving autonomy and quality of life of aging people; companies realizing the developed smart devices that need to have feasible products accepted by costumers; research institutions using this research project's results for other aims, etc. [24].

4.2 Stage 2: Analyzing

In this second phase, the multidisciplinary team analyzes users and technologies in order to set objectives and constraints regarding qualitative and quantitative project aspects.

4.2.1 Users Analysis

The multidisciplinary team needs to know more about primary users, secondary users, and stakeholders.

Primary users could have difficulties in being concentrated on this kind of activities for a long amount of time, so it would be desirable not to bother them with boring texts and difficult tasks, but to elaborate flexible activities that can be modify and adapted to the specific older person basing on his/her reactions.

Some of the HCD tools can be suitable for the applications in the field of aging people. Individual general interviews and contextual interviews demonstrated to be one of the most efficient tools for the users' analysis of a project for aging people [25]. General interviews allow to build the project scenario, describing the person's habits, environment, predisposition to use innovative technologies, etc., while contextual interviews are related to the smart device, or service, or system, that is going to be designed in the research project, and aim to get feedback on existing technologies, or to evaluate the development of new ones [26]. Focus groups are recommended only if involving few people and for a short time. Activities like card sorting, heuristic evaluation, and usability tests should be submitted only to users able to face these activities in a serene way.

The final output of the users' analysis is the elaboration of the list of needs expressed by the different users considered within the project process [11].

4.2.2 Technologies Analysis

Considering the design of a device belonging to an existing typology of products, it is useful to make a benchmarking analysis to evaluate positive and negative aspects of similar devices developed with available technologies, possibly matching them with the list of users' needs, in order to evaluate which requirements is able to satisfy each design aspect [27]. At this stage, it is important to evaluate also which are innovative technologies that can be used in the project, considering the amount of human, economical, and technological effort they request.

The analysis of technologies aims to set the project's invariants that will considerably influence the process development.

4.3 Stage 3: Creating

Starting from information collected from the previous stages, in this phase are developed design and technological solutions to be tested in the next step of the process.

4.3.1 Design Solutions

Developed design solutions aim to satisfy most significant users' needs, which have been selected and hierarchized by the whole multidisciplinary team and some users, in order to include different points of view and interests in the choice of the project requirements.

Co-design is successfully used in HCD design processes, because it allows designers to work with users, having a contribution in making prototypes of possible simple solutions that will be the starting point of a more complex project [28].

Every designer and each design process need to have a specific creating strategy correlated to the ongoing research project. Available HCD design tools are a huge number, but they must be selected considering the team abilities, the project's resources, the potential involvement of older users, the research project's output (device, service, system, etc.).

4.3.2 Technological Solutions

The development of feasible technological solutions is fundamental for the project's success. Technological innovation is strongly related to design opportunities and can determinate design choices' value. Technology determines design boundaries giving project invariants and available resources, but at the same time, choices related to design can suggest new ways of developing innovation, creating, e.g., new typologies of products [10].

At this step of the process, it can also be useful to set a list of measurable parameters connected to possible technological solutions, in order to evaluate in a second moment how effective and functional are the elaborated ideas, making a scientific comparison possible by evaluating significant measurable parameters.

4.3.3 Prototyping

The prototyping phase finalized the creating phase, matching design and technical solutions for the development of a device, a service or a system. Prototypes are not only a tool to make the project accessible for the multidisciplinary team and users, but are a real tool to work on possible different solutions and to compare their effectiveness [29].

It is also possible to prototype only some parts of the projects, just to deepen a specific aspect or to find solution to a critical issue.

Co-design workshops can be very useful at this stage to make prototypes a tool of work for users and team.

4.4 Stage 4: Verifying

In the last part of the HCD process, developed solutions are evaluated both from a qualitative and from a quantitative point of view. This final step will be the starting point for the following design cycle.

4.4.1 Testing with Users

The multidisciplinary team needs to set protocols in order to verify if the project satisfies selected human and technological requirements. This phase aims to collect data on older users' performance and personal feedback.

The testing protocols need to set a path, context conditions, parameters that need to be collected and how to collect them, how to prepare the user and what to communicate him/her on the incoming tests, what to ask him/her in order to get his/her feedback, etc. [30].

Particular attention should be given to the choice of participants to the set experimentation: In order not to bother people with physical and cognitive impairments, it should be evaluated a short and flexible protocol that can be modified at the moment maintaining coherence with other patients' trials.

4.4.2 Quantitative and Qualitative Evaluations

Quantitative and qualitative collected data are analyzed in order to evaluate if the submitted tests gave a satisfactory functional and human feedback.

There are actually many HCD tools that can be useful to represent and compare the previous stage's outputs, and for a correct choice of them, it is fundamental to evaluate previously which are the performing areas the team wants to focus on.

An instrument that was considered very useful in the hierarchization of different aspects is quality function deployment (QFD), a tool that collects in a matrix users' needs and device/system's measurable characteristics, in order to express a degree of correlation between them [31]. The QFD results help the multidisciplinary team to understand which are needs whose satisfaction will particularly boost the whole project and which characteristics implementations can lead to needs satisfaction [32]

4.4.3 Plan Implementation

Quantitative and qualitative evaluations are compared and discussed by the multidisciplinary team to decide which considerations will be the starting point of next HCD cycle. In this phase, it is important to remember the general project's objectives and chose a low number of statements and considerations as results of the current cycle.

This choice will make it easier, in a second moment, to merge outputs deriving from the different HCD cycles.

4.5 Iterative Process

The cited four HCD stages can be iteratively repeated several times, due to complexity of the project and to the design elements of the whole design project.

The HCD cycles can be in linear relationship, that is when every cycle is consequent to a previous one, using its only output as input; otherwise, cycle can have multiple correlations, that is, when a cycle is consequent to several previous ones, needing the output of several cycles as input.

In the PASSO project were identified four HCD design cycles: it was decided to start with the design of sensory cues, than the results of this cycle were used as starting point for two of the following the cycles that are the one for the design of smart devices for the submission of sensory cues and the one defining rehabilitation elements and protocols. Finally, the last cycle, dedicated to the development of the whole rehabilitation system, used as inputs both the results of the two previous ones (Fig. 2).

Making this kind of methodological abstraction is useful in order to have a large vision of the process, to understand which are the most important information we

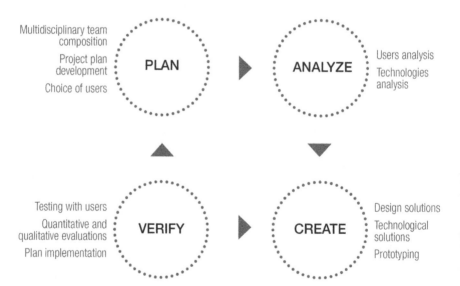

Fig. 2 Schematization of the four stages identified as HCD iterative process components. The stages that will be analyzed in the following paragraphs are plan, analyze, verify, and create. These steps can be repeated in the design process multiple times, as the project development suggests

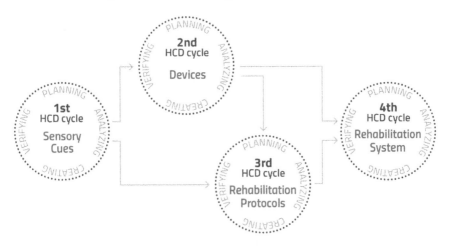

Fig. 3 Schematization of the four cycles used for the development of the PASSO project: design of sensory cues, devices, rehabilitation protocols, and rehabilitation system

need to have to continue the project, and to be consistent and coherent with the established project goals (Fig. 3).

5 Conclusions

The PASSO project has been used as an example to show the methodological strategy of a design research project developing a smart system for the implementation of older users' autonomy by rehabilitating their gait. Its design process was divided into four HCD cycles, each one developing an element of the project: sensory cues, smart devices, rehabilitation protocols, and rehabilitation system. Every cycle was organized into four stages: plan, analyze, create, and verify.

The experimented HCD methodology has proven to be effective in reducing the complexity of this multidisciplinary design process involving both human aspects related to quality and technological aspects related to quantity that are usually difficult to compare. It also optimized the interrelation between constraints deriving from technological characteristics and requirements resulting from the users' analysis.

The contribution given by the design discipline in this kind of applied research projects aims to increase the accessibility to technology, but also the level of autonomy that every older user can achieve.

This approach seems to be applicable in other different kinds of design research projects addressed to elderly with particular needs, giving an innovative contribution to HCD methodologies as a managing tool to collect and combine data to evaluate and choose design solutions.

References

1. Roth, M.: Problems of an ageing population. Br. Med. J. **1**, 1226–1230 (1960)
2. WHO World Health Organization: World Report on Aging and Health. WHO Press, Geneva, Switzerland (2015)
3. Kulik, C.T., Ryan, S., Harper, S., George, G.: From the editors Aging populations and management. Acad. Manag. J. **57**, 929–935 (2014)
4. Majumder, S., Aghayi, E., Noferesti, M., Memarzadeh-Tehran, H., Mondal, T., Pang, Z., Deen, M.J.: Smart Homes for elderly healthcare-recent advances and research challenges. Sensors **17**, 249 (2017)
5. Giusto, D., Iera, A., Morabito, G., Atzori L., (eds.): The Internet of Things. Springer, Heidelberg (2010). ISBN: 978-1-4419-1673-0
6. Atzori, L., Iera, A., Morabito, G.: Internet of Things: A survey. Comput. Netw. (2010)
7. Vilamovska, A.M., Hattziandreu, E., Schindler, R., Van Oranje, C., De Vries, H., Krapelse, J.: RFID Application in Healthcare—Scoping and Identifying Areas for RFID Deployment in Healthcare Delivery, RAND Europe, February 2009
8. Tatsuya, Y.: The ubiquitous home. Int. J. Smart Home**1**(I) (2007)
9. Aghajan, H., Augusto, J.C., López-Cózar, R.: Human-Centric Interfaces for Ambient Intelligence. Elsevier (2009)
10. López-Cózar, R., Callejas, Z.: Multimodal dialogue for ambient intelligence and Smart environments. In: Handbook of Ambient Intelligence and Smart Environments. Springer, Heidelberg (2010)
11. Mincolelli, G., Marchi, M., Imbesi, S.: Inclusive design for ageing people and the Internet of Things: understanding needs. In: Di Bucchianico, G., Kercher, P. (eds.), Advances in Design for Inclusion. AHFE 2017. Advances in Intelligent Systems and Computing, vol 587. Springer, Cham (2018)
12. Kurnianingsih, L.E. Nugroho, W.L., Lazuardi, R.: Ferdiana and Selo: perspectives of human centered design and interoperability in ubiquitous home care for elderly people. In: Makassar International Conference on Electrical Engineering and Informatics (MICEEI), pp. 118–123 (2014)
13. Callejas, Z., López-Cózar, R.: Designing smart home interfaces for the elderly. In: SIGACCESS Access. Comput., 95, September 2009, pp. 10–16 (2009)
14. Imbesi, S., Mincolelli, G.: Design of Smart Devices for older people: a user centered approach for the collection of users' needs. In: Ahram, T., Karwowski, W., Vergnano, A., Leali, F., Taiar, R. (eds.), Intelligent Human Systems Integration 2020. IHSI 2020. Advances in Intelligent Systems and Computing, vol. 1131. Springer, Cham (2020)
15. ISO 9241–210: 2010 Ergonomics ofHuman-SystemInteraction—Part 210: Human-Centred Design for Interactive Systems. Available online: https://www.iso.org/standard/52075.html. Accessed on 1 Mar 2019
16. Jokela, T., Iivari, N., Matero, J., Karukka, M.: The standard of user-centered design and the standard definition of usability: analyzing ISO 13407 against ISO 9241–11. In: Proceedings of the Latin American Conference on Human-Computer Interaction (CLIHC '03). Association for Computing Machinery, New York, NY, USA, pp. 53–60 (2003)
17. https://passocues.wordpress.com/. Accessed on 28/05/2021
18. Peterson, D.S., Horak, F.B.: Neural control of walking in people with Parkinsonism. Physiology **31**(2), 95–107 (2015)
19. Imbesi, S., Corzani, M., Lopane, G., Chiari, L., Mincolelli, G.: User-centered design of cues with smart glasses for gait rehabilitation in people with Parkinson's disease: a methodology for the analysis of human requirements and cues effectiveness. In: Cassenti, D., Scataglini, S., Rajulu, S., Wright, J. (eds.), Advances in Simulation and Digital Human Modeling. AHFE 2021. Advances in Intelligent Systems and Computing. Springer, Cham (2021)
20. https://www.usability.gov/how-to-and-tools/resources/ucd-map.html. Visited on 28/05/2021

21. Harte, R., Glynn, L., Rodríguez-Molinero, A., Baker, P., Scharf, T., Quinlan, L., ÓLaighin, G.: A human-centered design methodology to enhance the usability, human factors, and user experience of connected health systems: a three-phase methodology, JMIR Hum Factors (2017)
22. Imbesi, S., Mincolelli, G., Petrocchi, F.: How to enhance aging people's wellness by means of human centered and co-design methodology. In: Cassenti, D., Scataglini, S., Rajulu, S., Wright, J. (eds.), Advances in Simulation and Digital Human Modeling. AHFE 2020. Advances in Intelligent Systems and Computing, vol. 1206. Springer, Cham (2021)
23. Mincolelli, G.: Customer/User centered design. Analisi di un caso applicativo, Maggioli, Rimini (2008)
24. Mincolelli, G., Imbesi, S., Marchi, M., Giacobone, G.A.: New domestic healthcare. Co-designing assistive technologies for autonomous ageing at home. Design J. **22**(sup1), 503–516 (2019)
25. Goodman, E., Kuniavsky, M., Moed, A.: Observing the User Experience: A Practitioner's Guide to User Research (2nd edn). Morgan Kaufmann Series in Interactive Technologies (2003)
26. https://medium.com/user-research/never-ask-what-they-want-3-better-questions-to-ask-in-user-interviews-aeddd2a2101e#.izil93jqf. Visited on 28/05/2021
27. Mincolelli, G., Imbesi, S., Giacobone, G.A., Marchi, M.: Internet of Things and elderly: quantitative and qualitative benchmarking of smart objects. In: Di Bucchianico, G. (eds.), Advances in Design for Inclusion. AHFE 2018. Advances in Intelligent Systems and Computing, vol. 776. Springer, Cham (2019)
28. Mincolelli, G., Imbesi, S., Marchi, M., Healthcare, G.A.G.N.D.: Co-designing assistive technologies for autonomous ageing at home. Design J. **22**(sup1), 503–516 (2019)
29. Mincolelli, G., et al.: UCD, ergonomics and inclusive design: the HABITAT Project. In: Bagnara, S., Tartaglia, R., Albolino, S., Alexander, T., Fujita, Y. (eds.), Proceedings of the 20th Congress of the International Ergonomics Association (IEA 2018). IEA 2018. Advances in Intelligent Systems and Computing, vol. 824. Springer, Cham (2019)
30. König, H., Ulrich, A., Heiner, M.: Design for testability: a step-wise approach to protocol testing. In: Kim, M., Kang, S., Hong, K. (eds.), Testing of Communicating Systems. IFIP—The International Federation for Information Processing. Springer, Boston, MA (1997)
31. Mincolelli, G., Giacobone, G.A., Marchi, M., Imbesi, S.: New collaborative version of the quality function deployment: practical application to the HABITAT Project. In: Ahram, T., Karwowski, W., Vergnano, A., Leali, F., Taiar, R. (eds.), Intelligent Human Systems Integration 2020. IHSI 2020. Advances in Intelligent Systems and Computing, vol. 1131. Springer, Cham (2020)
32. Mincolelli, G., Imbesi, S., Zallio, M.: Collaborative quality function deployment. A methodology for enabling co-design research practice. In: Di Bucchianico, G. (eds.), Advances in Design for Inclusion. AHFE 2019. Advances in Intelligent Systems and Computing, vol. 954. Springer, Cham (2020)

Aging and Interaction: Designing for Active Living Experiences

Alessandro Pollini, Gian Andrea Giacobone, and Michele Zannoni

Abstract Over the last century, the life expectancy of the worldwide population has been increasing due to significant improvements in housing and healthcare. As a result, the number of older people in the worldwide population will continue to grow rapidly. Considering this, the concept of active living is an important strategy that can enhance healthy lifestyles by staying mentally, socially and physically active during aging. In this concept, digital technology can be a great tool that can help people to pursue those benefits. However, it seems that older people are particularly susceptible to the negative effects of technology directly caused by poorly designed products and user interfaces. For these reasons, this paper wants to discuss age-related changes and characteristics that usually impact the user experience, in order to delineate background information of those problems and then propose design methods and practices that can help designers to develop accessible and age-friendly products and interfaces. We use the concept of active living to verify if and how the existing products on the market are fostering the values of an active lifestyle, promoting independence, empowerment, self-esteem and self-efficacy. We conclude by exploring new conceptual and methodological design guidelines through scenario-based design for inspiring future research in this field.

Keywords Active living · User-centered design · Human–computer interaction · User experience · User interface

---

A. Pollini (✉)
BSD Design, Via Lazzaretto 19, 20124 Milano, Italy
e-mail: alessandro.pollini@bsdesign.eu

G. A. Giacobone
Department of Architecture, University of Ferrara, Via Quartieri 8, 44121 Ferrara, Italy
e-mail: gianandrea.giacobone@unife.it

M. Zannoni
Department of Architecture, University of Bologna, Viale del Risorgimento 2, 40136 Bologna, Italy
e-mail: michele.zannoni@unibo.it

© The Author(s), under exclusive license to Springer Nature Singapore Pte Ltd. 2022
S. Scataglini et al. (eds.), *Internet of Things for Human-Centered Design*,
Studies in Computational Intelligence 1011,
https://doi.org/10.1007/978-981-16-8488-3_3

1 Introduction

Population is gradually aging with a global life expectancy that has increased by more than 6 years between 2000 and 2019, from 66.8 years in 2000 to 73.4 years in 2019 [1]. This phenomenon is coupled with a dramatic gap involving low-income countries, where life expectancy is 16 years lower than for people in high-income countries. Life expectancy, quality of life, and equitable access to information technologies do represent in our perspective intertwining assets of healthy aging and active living.

As the population ages, important questions are coming into view [2]: *How might we better support seniors to lead active and independent lives in their homes, communities, and neighborhoods? Can we make services and products for seniors easy to use and navigate?*

Ergonomics and interaction design for elderly people has been widely addressed at the theoretical and methodological level [3–5]; at the cognitive level, with an extensive production of reviews of the changes that aging makes to the human factors [6–9] and at the exploratory and research level dealing with projects on novel interaction paradigms and multiple devices [10]. The benefits of staying mentally, socially, and physically active as we age are well known [11]. Digital technology can help with that. But everything changes when products and services thought for the elderly are poorly designed, especially since interacting with a computer is no longer about sitting in front of a desktop. Computers have become deeply engrained in nearly every activity of everyday life: "We carry them, wear them, and may even have them implanted within us" [12]. And it seems paradoxical how older adults can be particularly susceptible to the ill effects of unusable digital devices and user interfaces. While older people have not grown up with technology in the way that today's children have, most have had significant experience with it in their working lives and, later, in their personal lives [13].

Much of the research on age and technology use has been conducted from the perspective of usability, user experience, accessibility, and adoption. Such research projects are concerned with measures like frequency of use, performance, efficiency, and accuracy [14–18]. In particular, several researches suggest that many older adults have difficulty using contemporary consumer products due to their complexity both in terms of functionality and interface design [19].

This chapter focuses on the experiential nature of the interaction with digital technology for aging population. As other interaction design and human factors' specialists [2], we would like to continue to explore what are the characteristics of product design for the elderly and to understand how to enhance user experience for older adults. In particular the authors will focus on a purposeful and well thought-through design approach, shaped by participatory, user-centered, and critical design traditions.

Even though the authors refer to designing interactions for elderly people, this should not be taken as implying a uniform "elderly people" group [20]. Because of the great heterogeneity of individual traits and diversity of life experiences according to the onset and progression of aging, the "older" group is the least uniform of the developmental stages. Age-related declines in cognitive and sensory-motor function occur slowly and at varying intensities from individual to individual. In other words, compared to the younger population, variability in older adults is significantly larger [21–23].

The definition of older people is now replaced by more articulated concepts, such as primary aging (the changes due to aging, without becoming ill), secondary aging (characterized by the onset of chronic diseases, which affect the individual's adaptation to the environment), and tertiary aging (the period immediately preceding the term of existence, characterized by a rapid decline of the skills of the individual) [11]. From the point of view of an interaction designer, it is not age itself that is the issue but some of the effects of aging such as reduced vision, reduced manipulative ability, decreased autonomy, and cognitive effects that lead to declines in memory, reasoning ability, and speed of learning as well as the psychological correlates, like loss of self-efficacy.

Thus, in order to design for older people, it became relevant that designers empathize and sensitize themselves to the realities of elderly people [24], especially regarding what does "active living" mean for them and how they could establish and maintain "active living." This involves studying the literature on aging and active living; developing a vision on what is the main design scope; and understanding the rationale behind successful products and their design for older users. The objective of the chapter is to define a critical work on the domain and to propose a possible theoretical and methodological framework to support design studies and practices for the benefit of older people.

We will at first investigate active living as a concept with its own peculiar psychological aspects. Those factors will be then adopted as evaluation criteria to review the design of current products for older people. Last section of the chapter will provide support for an holistic approach to active living that would encompass the purely functional approach to design. Active living will be in fact validated through scenario-based design [25, 26] and will allow us to identify conceptual and methodological design guidelines for inspiring future research in this field.

2 Active Living Concept

2.1 Active Living in the Literature

The World Health Organization defines active aging [27] as "the process of optimizing opportunities for health, participation, and security in order to enhance quality of life as people age including those who are frail, disabled, and in need of care." As a policy framework, active aging allows people to realize their potential for physical, social, and mental well-being throughout the life course and to participate in society.

The state of well-being is a multifaceted phenomenon that refers to an individual's subjective feelings, and exploring perspectives of older adults on aging well is developing to be an important area of research [28]. Even though "active aging," "successful aging," "healthy aging," "positive aging," "productive aging," and—in relation to technology—"silver surfing," are just a few of the terms in use for naming this field [29]. Aging well is conceptualized using different contemporary theoretical frameworks in the last decades, including healthy aging, positive aging, productive aging, active aging, and successful aging [30].

This chapter will focus on the multidimensional approach and subjective definition to active living. In the last 50 years, the importance of understanding the needs and wishes of older people has been extensively treated [31]. In considering planning for quality long-term care for older persons, Lawton defined the concept of quality of life (QoL) as "the multidimensional evaluation, by both intrapersonal and social-normative criteria, of the person-environment system of the individual" [32, 33] aiming at the improvement of older people in daily life activities and individual well-being [33–35]. Among QoL indicators, there are autonomy, comfort, relationship, and security.

The state of well-being is a multifaceted phenomenon in the older population which generally involves happiness, self-contentment, satisfying social relationships, and autonomy [36]. The sense of well-being refers to an individual's feelings, in this case, based on how older persons perceive the concept of well-being. The term "subjective well-being" is frequently used and strongly characterized by the interplay between individual characteristics and qualities of people's social environment [37].

We are proposing, in line with the "good aging" definition, a multidimensional concept, which is based on the meaningful integration of five main elements: (a) healthy nutrition, (b) daily physical exercise, (c) regular cognitive and mental activities, (d) maintaining social contacts inside and outside the family, and (e) keeping an active interest in society.

Such elements are tightly interwoven since maintaining good physical health and functioning plays an important role in facilitating mobility and enables older adults to perform more integrated functional tasks which include activities of daily living, fulfilment of social roles, and recreational activities. Furthermore good cognitive health is linked to social connectedness, independence, and life activities, and it might be preserved and enhanced by maintaining an intellectually engaged and physically active lifestyle [28, 38].

2.2 The Active Living Concept

The active living concept, which we propose, has been investigated from both a scientific literature and a user research perspective in the international research project *RESILIEN-T, Technology driven self-management for building resilience among people with early stage cognitive impairment*, funded under AAL2018 that is currently being carried out in Italy, The Netherlands, Switzerland, and Canada

(RESILIEN-T) on aging and resilience. We hypothesize that crucial psychological aspects need to be taken into account to shape a meaningfully rich active living definition that does integrate factors such as cognition, functioning, and physical action.

In particular, we want to highlight the need for older people to dynamically reframe their condition and capabilities over time: they need to be aware of, and also to accept, the personal conditions that they are making experience of, in terms of autonomy, use of tools, personal care, and self-management.

For people, active living may be defined as living an active and meaningful life, in order to be able to maintain independence and self-efficacy in daily activities. By optimizing opportunities for participation in paths of health, safety, and socialization, which improves the quality of life and implements the potentials for physical and mental well-being [11]. Functional and objective conditions of people need to be considered in combination with their intimate and subjective experience, since the ability to act into the world is equally important to trust and self-esteem, acceptance, and wish to share personal needs, limits, and abilities. Therefore, as designers, rather than aiming to develop "innovative technologies that serve well-defined purposes" such as "optimal health and independence" [39], the approach that we will take is in line with the "resourceful aging" framework [10, 40] which focuses on empowering older people to age resourcefully.

We identified the following factors as main dimensions of older people experience: (a) empowerment, (b) perceived self-efficacy, and (c) autonomy.

2.2.1 Empowerment

The notion of empowerment [41] is foundational in our approach since it does represent the overall scope of an intervention. The empowerment is a multidimensional concept constituted by several components including supporting older people to keep their current levels of mental functioning; by preventing possible decay in cognitive and social skills; by coping with adverse events and negative experiences; and by exploiting latent resources [11]. That is why, in order to empower older people to live independently, designers should make sure that older people can adapt and configure devices according to their personal circumstances in a way that their independence can be supported and be constantly renegotiated [10, 42]. Renegotiation of self-image may support the idea of iterative empowerment pathways as structured, organized, and goal-oriented paths for a healthy population integrating multiple levels of skill support.

2.2.2 Perceived Self-efficacy

Self-efficacy can be defined as a personal judgment of "how well one can execute courses of action required to deal with prospective situations" [43] and of own capabilities to produce designated level of performance. Perception of self-efficacy results from a reciprocal interaction between interpersonal factors, behavior, and the external environment. Self-efficacy is considered both as a predictor and as an outcome of social and physical interaction. Staying active is reportedly connected to self-efficacy since it implies good physical functioning and the ability to autonomously reach a goal. In general, individuals with high perceived self-efficacy are determined and show more effort across a broader range of tasks than people with a lower level of self-efficacy.

2.2.3 Autonomy

Staying independent was viewed as a major characteristic of aging well. Beyond the participants' living status (alone or with family), the importance of being independent was connected with the autonomous status of the older adults. A major concern that was frequently mentioned in the RESILIEN-T user research was not being or becoming a burden to others. In particular, along with the interactive discussions in all groups, target users involved in the user research reflected on the necessity of staying independent in performing their daily life activities including both personal and instrumental activities.

We have used the active living dimensions to verify if and how the existing products on the market are fostering the values of an active lifestyle, promoting independence, empowerment, self-esteem, and self-efficacy.

3 Products for Elderly People: The-State-of-the-Art

On the basis of the above considerations, the phenomenon of the aging population leads to many important social changes that are highlighting the necessity of finding new design solutions to support older people in living longer and healthier in their homes, communities, and neighborhoods. In this perspective, rapid advances in technology are contributing to enhance the concept of active living since the development of assistive environments have the opportunity to offer a series of benefits that can increase the older people's quality of life according to cognitive, physical, and relational factors.

The Internet of Things and the development of recent technologies, such as sensor networks, Artificial Intelligence, and Machine Learning algorithms, have great chances to improve the self-independence, autonomy, and participation in social life and skills of the elderly. In particular, these systems may be able to collect and integrate qualitative and quantitative data from multiple sources, and may extend the interaction modalities by utilizing tracking of daily routines and targeted suggestions, reminders, or activities.

Unfortunately, nowadays, many products and services that are already available on the market do not fully satisfy such requirements because they can only partially cover the active living, or even demonstrate one single function. Moreover, these products often put end-users in a condition where they have no option but to passively undergo the operation of technology [42]. On the contrary, as examined before, the concept of active living lays on the multidimensionality of different human necessities, which, if well supported, are able to increase the quality of the elderly's health and independence.

For this reason, this section focuses on seven specific case studies because they share common characteristics—for instance all of them are screen-based multifunctional systems for senior care—that are capable of empowering older people under the concept of active living, specifically investigating particular interactions that can match with their main necessities and capabilities. The analyzed products are **Pillo Health, ElliQ, Lumin, Compaan, GrandCare, Claris Continuum,** and **Cutii**.[1] The main products' characteristics are focused on health monitoring, telepresence, physical and cognitive training, and many other services that enable older people to keep themselves autonomous, active, healthy, and socially connected.

We might state that the projects that have been analysed in this research, even though not providing comprehensive and rich Active Living scenarios, do implement some of the concept components, by focusing on empowerment, perceived self-efficacy or autonomy. The four factors that help to understand each project are: how the product take care of their users beyond the mere functional aspect of health monitoring; how they help users to stay connected with their relatives or friends; how the system is proactive in stimulating the users to stay healthy and active during the day; how the system is able to friendly dialog with their user and create a social bond with them through its natural interactions (Table 1).

3.1 Characteristics of the Products

All products are characterized by a tablet-based digital application, but only **Lumin, Compaan, GrandCare,** and **Claris Continuum** specifically refer their morphological aspects to the size of that device, while **Pillo Health, ElliQ,** and **Cutii** are interactive objects that integrate the tablet in their physical products. Referring to the form of those products, **Pillo Health** has the peculiarity to incorporate in its morphological aspect a medical dispenser that can be activated with its digital service. The peculiarity of **ElliQ** is a physical element incorporated in the tabletop product that abstractly simulates a human bust, to which the system uses to dynamically interact with the elderly as an artificial companion. **Cutii**, instead, acts as a companion robot that has the ability to navigate autonomously around the older people's domestic environment.

---

[1] For more information see: Pillo Health https://pillohealth.com/; ElliQ https://elliq.com/; Lumin https://mylumin.org; Compaan https://www.uwcompaan.nl/; GrandCare https://www.grandcare.com/; Claris Continuum https://www.clarishealthcare.com/; Cutii https://www.cutii.io/en/ (accessed August 3th 2021).

Table 1 Schematic analysis of the selected products

Products	Pillo health	ElliQ	Lumin	Compaan	GrandCare	Claris Continuum	Cutii
Morphology	Smart object	Smart object	Tablet-based app	Tablet-based app	Tablet-based app	Tablet-based app	Companion robot
Purpose	Social companion Recreational device and medical device	Social companion Recreational device	Device for telepresence Recreational device	Homecare service Recreational device and medical device	Homecare service Recreational device and medical device	Homecare service Recreational device and medical device	Social companion Recreational device
Personal care	Self-management app Health monitoring Connection for external medical devices	Self-management app	Self-management app	Self-management app Health monitoring Connection for external medical devices	Self-management app Health monitoring Connection for external medical devices	Self-management app Health monitoring Connection for external medical devices	Self-management app
Social connection	Remote calls Text messaging Multimedia file sharing	Remote calls Text messaging Multimedia file sharing	Remote calls Text messaging Multimedia file sharing	Remote calls Text messaging Multimedia file sharing	Remote calls Text messaging Multimedia file sharing	Remote calls Text messaging Multimedia file sharing	Remote calls Text messaging Multimedia file sharing
Coaching	Health and medical reminders Encouraging activities through health plans	Health and medical reminders Encouraging activities proactively through daily routines or behaviors	Health and medical reminders	Health and medical reminders Encouraging activities through health plans	Health medical reminders Encouraging activities through assignments	Health and medical reminders Encouraging activities through health plans	Health and medical reminders Encouraging activities through real animators

(continued)

Table 1 (continued)

Products	Pillo health	ElliQ	Lumin	Compaan	GrandCare	Claris Continuum	Cutii
Identity and *role*	Visual interaction Natural dialog and voice interaction Facial expression and facial recognition	Visual interaction Natural dialog and voice Interaction Facial expression and facial recognition	Visual interaction	Visual interaction	Visual interaction	Visual interaction	Visual interaction Natural dialog and voice interaction Facial expression and facial recognition

While **Lumin**, **ElliQ**, and **Cutti** are intended for recreational and social uses, **Pillo Heath**, **Compaan**, **GrandCare**, and **Claris Continuum** are devices designed for medical purposes as well. In fact, those products are able to monitor some vital signs and biometric parameters, such as blood pressure, heart rate, glucose, weight, or breath, that can be useful for the older people, and also for formal or informal caregiving, to control chronic diseases or prevent future health issues. In particular, those products can increase their functionalities by allowing other external medical devices to be connected with their digital services in order to increase the elderly's monitoring of health conditions. All products enable visual interactions, but **ElliQ**, **Pillo Heath,** and **Cutti** are the only artifacts that make the dialog with their users more natural by using voice interaction. Again, to empathize with that interaction model and mimic human behaviors, these products utilize anthropomorphic aspects as well, which express nonverbal signals. In fact, to communicate with older people, **ElliQ** simulates human body language through the motion of its artificial human bust while **Pillo Health** and **Cutti** use facial expressions.

3.2 Analysis of the Products

The methodology used to analyze the products avoids to creating detailed benchmarking by only examining the mere functional features of the case studies. Rather, it focuses on many interaction aspects that, when harmonized in a consistent and goal-oriented design, may increase the active living's user experience and allow the older users empowerment, the perceived self-efficacy, and the autonomy. Recurring interaction patterns among the case studies allowed the analysis to identify four design themes that trace new reflections to enrich studies and practices in this field. The four design themes are: (1) personal care, (2) social interaction, (3) coaching, and (4) identity and role.

- **Personal Care**

Personal care helps the elderly to live healthier and longer because monitoring a series of health parameters or performing activities that maintain an active lifestyle permit them to prolong their physical, social, and mental well-being over time. Considering this, all examined products, especially **Compaan, GrandCare**, and **Claris Continuum**, have high monitoring accuracy. However, the technical and analytical data representation refers only to a passive and quantitative analysis of the elderly's health conditions without offering additional advice from a qualitative perspective. In that case, product perception decreases the feeling of autonomy because the service may run the risk of considering the elderly as patients rather than independent people giving full control of the system to technology. This is because the products force their users to follow their pre-setting options based on reminders or alert messages that omit any willingness of choice. For this reason, the result is a passive scenario in which the elderly are perceived as passive entities who are constantly at risk and, thus, continuously in need of help. Indeed, older people's independence becomes affected by the decisions of their informal or formal caregivers who are in charge of control of their health condition through a dedicated dashboard as available on **Compaan, GrandCare,** and **Claris Continuum**. That consequence may be stressed by **GrandCare** because it offers activity monitoring features that could make users feel constantly under surveillance.

The same issue on passive interaction appears on the elderly self-management. All artifacts provide a calendar for scheduling their own activities, though they focus mostly on managing health or medical reminders, which, in turn, transform the service into a medical experience where users are perceived as passive entities. Moreover, this condition is empathized by the absence of engaging recreational activities or social activities. In fact, all products provide only default applications already installed on the system, which offer information and service provision without a proper interactivity, i.e., reading a weather forecast, reading a journal newspaper, or listening to radio music.

Again, all the products encourage personal care by providing mnemonic games or physical exercises for supporting older people to keep their current levels of mental and physical functioning. However, the activities present poor engagement because they are delivered through basic video tutorials or virtual games embedded in the tablet application.

Although it does not provide any monitoring service, **Cutii** is the only system that offers human interaction by allowing older people to perform physical or cognitive exercises with some animators who propose to them ludic, cultural, or fitness activities in real time via video call. None of the products considers nutrition as a qualitative value for caregiving as reported in the definition of good aging.

Finally, although the products can manage monitoring of a single person—or multiple users such as **Pillo Health, Compaan, GrandCare,** and **Claris Continuum**—they provide a single caregiving experience. Therefore, none of these projects incentive a participatory and shared use of the service as could happen for an elderly couple, for example.

Social Connection

Social connection is an important value of active living because it permits older people to be socially included by enabling them to sustain relationships with their family or friends over time. The quality of social connection depends on the way an individual remains connected to the others [44]. For this reason, the analysis reports that all products give attention to social connection by giving people the ability to connect themselves with relatives or friends through their digital interfaces.

However, although maintaining people socially active is satisfied from a functional perspective, delivering qualitatively social interactions is always limited to video calls, text messages, emails, or sharing multimedia files. Moreover, **Pillo Health, GrandCare,** and **Claris Continuum** overshadow social connection because it is perceived as an additional functionality of the caregiving service. Considering this, none of the products suggest a level of interactivity able to stimulate meaningful rich social interactions, inside or outside of the domestic environment, or cultivate contextual, endure relationships with their family or friends. In addition, all products tend to provide remote communication rather than creating an experience that stimulates relationships in presence.

Coaching

Coaching is a powerful element to empower people in increasing their health and well-being by periodically stimulating them with new challenging goals to accomplish or particular suggestions that encourage interests toward new other recreational activities. This theme can be supported by giving the products a proactive approach that is able to engage the elderly in personalized activities, encourage good behaviors or interests in new hobbies, limiting, at the same time, sedentary lifestyle, or poor care of one's own health or well-being.

However, only **ElliQ** and **Cutii** provide such technology. Apart from those products, none of the other services takes advantage of that technology because they only collect data to set up notifications only for medical reminders or health issues based on a statistical prediction on the elderly's health conditions. In addition, those products encourage physical activity only by providing health exercise plans, without the intent proactively motivating users with personalized tips or suggestions. Moreover, **GrandCare** does not offer a proper quality of coaching as the motivations it sends to the users are perceived as assignments instead of recommended activities. In that way, the product may affect the elderly's self-independence because the motivational advice may be perceived as an obligation rather than an invitation.

The most advanced level of proactivity is provided by **ElliQ**, which is the only product that encourages physical and cognitive activities based not only on monitoring the elderly's vital signs but also on their daily behaviors or routines. In addition, compared to the others that focus only on health and fitness, **ElliQ** is the only system that promotes recreational and ludic activities. However, proactivity currently refers only to passive actions such as listening to music based on the elderly's perceived mood (it uses facial recognition). The same happens to **Cutii**, which uses its proactivity only to change facial expression according to the elderly facial recognition. Considering this, none of the products offers active support in cultivating interests in recreational activities, such as a personal hobby or passion. Again, all products do not provide proactive interactions that promote recreational activities outside the domestic environment.

Identity and Role

As reported in the literature [45], designing, not only usable and intuitive functions, but also morphological and interactive elements that stimulate human emotions, are key tenets to successful product development. Using human morphology can help products to increase the level of acceptance of new technologies or trust and reliability in particular interactive systems. Moreover, those elements confer to the artifact an identity and a precise role—for our case as a caregiver assistant or companion—within the elderly's everyday life.

However, **Lumin, Compaan, GrandCare,** and **Claris Continuum** do not offer any meaningful element of interaction that emotionally engages with users. On the contrary, they show an aseptic user experience since the interactions with the system are mediated by a visual interface on a tablet screen that acts as a mere communication bridge between the users and those who take care of them. Instead, **Pillo Health, ElliQ,** and **Cutii** are able to play on the elderly's emotional aspects because they try acting as a digital companion during the caregiving experience. In fact, the ability of the products transforms the products into actor agents [46] that actively respond to human behaviors. This consequently generates a sense of animism [47] that confers to the artifact a particular personality and identity. This type of agency is also supported by the introduction of anthropomorphic elements, such as verbal dialog and voice control to interact with the elderly. These elements, indeed, can provide additional benefits to the elderly because they can increase their perceived sense of self-efficacy since the natural feedback of language helps them to easily understand the accomplishment of their tasks.

3.3 Discussion of Results Toward Active Living

Most of the examined products support the concept of active living mostly from a gerontology perspective since the products have great capabilities in health monitoring, but they present operational lacks in the social, ludic, and emotional dimensions. In fact, the products offer good qualities of empowerment, but they are focused mostly on compensating the capabilities of older people rather than creating a system that really enhances their autonomy, self-independence and self-esteem. Considering this, coaching is a good opportunity to foster resourceful aging, but, apart from **ElliQ**, all the products focus mainly on taking care of the elderly's health parameters, missing the chance of stimulating qualitative aspects of their lives such as promoting new hobbies, social activities, or cultivating their own passions.

From the user experience perspective, the products delimitate the interaction with the elderly to a tablet touch screen. Only **Pillo Health, ElliQ,** and **Cutii** assume a physical identity that imitates human behaviors to elicit emotional interaction. Due to the use of voice control, they increase the elderly's sense of autonomy and self-efficacy as the natural interaction of verbal dialog makes communication more intuitive.

Finally, all the products relegate their functionalities only to the domestic environment, consequently limiting the chance to enrich the quality of the active living experience in a wider space of social interaction. However, all products offer good functionalities to support the elderly in aging well, which in turn can be considered a scaffold for developing future generations of interactive systems based on the concept of active living.

The state-of-the-art analysis allows us to focus on the development of a conceptual and methodological framework to design for older people. There might be several approaches to ideate services and interactions for elderly people. The majority of the existing products follow a proper functional approach, where the design defines features and functions, such as the calendar, the video call, and the cognitive exercises.

On the contrary, we would promote the centrality of the design of the human experience, by means of scenario-based design describing motivations, attitudes, sense making, and individual and social activities for supporting goal-directed action.

Furthermore, most products in the present analysis foster the capability of reading, understanding, and interpreting quantitative data as key to human activity. In fact a common strategy of the analyzed products is to enhance motivation through data, trends and statistics provision, as well as medical reminders, and assignments and exercises' plans. According to this perspective, motivation is thought to have arisen on the basis of stimuli coming from quantitative measures, such as frequency or data logging. Also we are interested in exploring how to support people in creating their own meaning from information, how motivation can be fostered even on the basis of subjective variability and how it can be possible to promote human contact and social exchange.

4 Rethinking Active Living: An Holistic Approach to the Elderly Experience

For a better understanding of the active living concept and a contribution at the methodological level, the envisioning scenarios and the user personas which stemmed out from the RESILIEN-T user research have been presented in the following paragraph.

During the early stages of the design process, the scenarios are used to understand how personas will take advantage of the designed solution to carry out their tasks. One of the most important conditions when we design is to start from real users, and personas and scenarios represent useful tools to build models of their experience. In particular, the personas consist in a detailed description of a potential user. It allows us to clarify needs, objectives, characteristics, context of use, and so on. Moreover personas are useful to describe subjective variables such as skills, typical activities, concrete motivations, and objective aspects including why an action is done.

"Scenarios use storytelling to explore design ideas by grounding them in a real context. Their focus is on the relationship between people and the designed product or service, their objectives, the context, and potential social implications." [48]. In other words, scenarios refer to interaction stories used as representative cases of real situations. The purpose of a scenario is to express in detail a situation and to document the actions performed by users point by point. We propose the envisioning scenarios to imagine the characteristics of the future experience of the users, as it will be transformed by the adoption of a novel interactive system.

In the envisioning scenarios, the only interactive and functional features of the system may be caught. We propose the user personas and the envisioning scenarios to describe the active living experience as might be supported by the interactive system that is currently under ideation in the RESILIEN-T.

4.1 Active Living Scenarios and Personas

Persona 1: Elizabeth—The autonomous patient
"What I enjoy the most is being with others, it's just wonderful!"

Themes: Memory, Mobility, Social Relations.

User Profile: Elizabeth is 74 years old and lives alone since her husband passed away a few years ago. Nevertheless Beth is a determined and dynamic woman. She is constantly on the move. Beth handles all her daily activities, such as grocery shopping and housework. She is also very active in the social field. She likes to do things for others, like getting groceries for her neighbors. When she gets out, she prefers to walk, but in case of necessity she uses a bus, which is another opportunity to socialize! She has no relevant age-related physical problem but she recently noticed that her memory is getting worse. She loves meeting up with her friends, especially to play bridge. Once a month, she goes to the theater. Elizabeth is quite capable with technology. She uses a tablet to search for online recipes and to consult the theater's program. She also uses a smartphone to communicate with her family.

Envisioning Scenario: Beth does not want to give up, she wants to maintain her independence, so she starts using the RESILIEN-T system. Beth has filled in her full profile into the system, including her interests, contacts, and recurring meetings.

Beth heard that tomorrow evening there will be a performance and sets the appointment on the calendar. The system checks the events organized in town and compares the collected data with those recorded by Elizabeth. The system detects a gap among data: a similar event will take place in two days. So it offers further information on the theater program and asks her: "Are you sure your event is correct? Do you want to check?". The RESILIEN-T also suggests to book the ticket and to invite her friends, so she calls Adele and Grace, and then, she buys tickets for everyone. On the day of the performance, the system asks questions related to mobility in order to stimulate Beth to plan the activity: "How will you reach the theater?" "Do you want to take pictures during the show to create a memento of this evening?".

When she gets home, the system asks how the soiree went and it proposes to Elizabeth to create a "memento" of the evening by adding photos, videos, and personal notes, in order to populate her own digital album of memories.

Persona 2: James and Margaret—The affectionate couple

"Travelling keeps us young and alive!"

Themes: Self-esteem, Support, Technology.

Users' Profile: James and Margaret Murphy are a very close couple. James is 68 years old and Margaret is 65. They love to travel and have visited many places, particularly South America. They are planning a trip to Vietnam next summer. James and Margaret have been married for 30 years and they have two grown-up children, Robert and Melanie, who do not live close to them. Despite the distance, they use Skype and other social networks to communicate with each other.

Margaret is starting to have some memory problems. For example, she started forgetting to bring the keys, when leaving home. James tries to support and to reassure his wife. James and Margaret are familiar with technology: they use smartphones and tablets to plan their trips and to keep updated. They say that they learn something new every day! They are very grateful for what life has given them and love their home, family, and friends. James and Margaret want to spend the rest of their lives together.

Envisioning Scenario: Margaret and James continue to divide the household tasks. Today, they have decided to split the responsibilities: Margaret will get groceries. The system helps Margaret to plan her activity and at the same time stimulating her cognitive activity. "Which of these foods do you have to buy?" "Where do you prefer to buy these foods?" showing the nearby shops on the map. Once the shopping list is completed and she has decided the itinerary, Margaret goes out. James continues to propose new activities to Margaret. In the afternoon they will go for a walk in the park. Since Margaret wears RESILIEN-T's smartwatch, the system monitors and collects data about her physical activity.

Persona 3: Giorgio—The proud patient

"I like to spend time on my own!"

Themes: Nutrition, Autonomy, Physical Activity.

User Profile: Giorgio is 78 years old and used to live alone after getting divorced in 2001. Until his retirement 5 years ago, he was an important lawyer. He has always been proud and charismatic man, and he rejects the idea of getting old. Giorgio appreciates loneliness, and he prefers to spend his days painting, reading, and listening to music. He has a few friends who visit him occasionally. Giorgio has one daughter, Sarah, who lives a few kilometers away from him. He usually goes out close to home or when his daughter Sarah picks him up by car to take a ride.

Giorgio is not interested in technology. His daughter gave him a mobile phone that he uses to communicate with his family. He has been living with diabetes since 2016. He is overweight, and he leads a sedentary life. Moreover, he does not follow a healthy diet, and this would also increase his risk of vascular problems. And as if that was not enough, he has had problems with his memory. Despite these challenges, Giorgio wants to maintain his independence and he is convinced he does not need help.

Envisioning Scenario: Giorgio starts to use the RESILIEN-T system to try to keep himself active and allow his daughter to get reassured when he is alone at home.

Sarah synchronized the blood glucose measuring system with the system. It shows in real time the data just measured relating to Giorgio's blood glucose, so that it can keep a report. In addition, the system supports Giorgio with food recommendations. The system also tries to encourage Giorgio toward social interactions and to keep on moving, proposing to him to join the local association of passionate for painting. "Next Friday there will be an art class, near your home. Are you interested in it?" "On

21st June will open the exhibition "Edgar Degas: A Strange New Beauty. I thought you might be interested!".

Giorgio becomes curious and decides to visit the exhibition. Since we believe that the active living concept is subjective, in the following paragraph, we will provide a comprehensive active living validation activity description that has been carried out in a dedicated research involving the Italian, Swiss, Canadian, and Dutch panels.

4.2 Active Living Scenarios Validation

The user experience validation has allowed us to enter into the details of how to design for older people and how people would interact with services in order to accomplish their personal objectives. Eight sessions have been carried out in the RESILIEN-T project: two sessions for each of the pilot countries of the project, Italy, Canada, Switzerland, and Netherlands. The research and design methodology proposed in the project integrates methods and techniques from a broad range of disciplines, from ethnography and psychology, to user-centered and participatory design.

4.2.1 Validation Methodology

The validation has been made through the validation sessions aiming at active living concept exploration and finalization by presenting the envisioning scenarios to the participants in order to start focusing on both older people and formal/ informal caregivers' daily life experience and situations. This activity was inspired by storytelling methodologies and allowed the participants to share personal opinions and perspectives.

The validation sessions were organized by a storytelling and UX statement method. The envisioning scenarios have been shown and the stories have been told to participants in order for them to reflect on their own personal experiences. Each story has been also disentangled in order to define a UX statement to be used in the discussion with participants.

The statement cards are an efficient tool to start discussions around experiential topics. By using scenario-inspired statements, the participants freely discuss the statement. It aims to trigger participants to react, whether they agree or disagree, without being the "owner" of the statement. The discussion is meant to lead to the placing of the statement card as "true" or "false," and to foster validation of statements as acceptable and feasible.

As example you have the Elizabeth envision scenario with the statements defined for Module 1 below:

1. Beth does not want to give up, she wants to maintain her independence, so she starts using the RESILIEN-T system. Beth has filled in her full profile into the system, including her interests, contacts, and recurring meetings.

Statement 1: I think I can also enter the description of my interests and preferences in the tool and manage a new appointment on the digital calendar.

2. Beth heard that tomorrow evening there will be a performance and sets the appointment on the calendar. The system checks the events organized in the town and compares the collected data with those recorded by Elizabeth. The system detects a gap among data: a similar event will take place in two days. So it offers further information on the theater program and asks her: "Are you sure your event is correct? Do you want to check?".

Statement 2: I believe that a tool for checking my calendar and confirming the scheduled event, could be useful.

3. The RESILIEN-T also suggests to book the ticket and to invite her friends, so she calls Adele and Grace and then she buys tickets for everyone. On the day of the performance, the system asks questions related to mobility in order to stimulate Beth to plan the activity: "How will you reach the theater?" "Do you want to take pictures during the show to create a memento of this evening?". When she gets home, the system asks how the soiree went and it proposes to Elizabeth to create a "memento" of the evening by adding photographs, videos, and personal notes, in order to populate her own digital album of memories.

Statement 3: I believe that a reminder tool for planning my appointments and sharing my photographs would be valuable and stimulating.

Statement 4: I would like to have a tool that encourages me to relate to others and cultivate my friendships.

4.2.2 Validation Results

This paragraph describes the validation session results as lived by participants. They have generally shown interest in RESILIEN-T scenarios and upcoming development from the project, and all the participants were extremely collaborative, engaged, and easy going.

Participants have been engaged and stimulated to take part with questions and proposals and for validating the interactions strategies. The users participated in a proactive way, proposing interesting ideas on how to improve the service. The workshops were useful to understand the real needs of users, their motivations, habits, but above all their concerns and frustrations. Users have positively participated at the validation of the scenarios, emphasizing the aspects of the project that are most relevant and useful to them.

The subjective nature of the exploration confirmed some of the assumptions the researchers had in mind:

- Older people's attitude toward technology needs to be investigated and verified through research: they are not necessarily interested in technology and personal attitude is based on prior experience with technology as well as anxiety or enthusiasm with digital services and tools;

- participants to the research largely appreciated to have useful, efficient, and efficacious aids, in particular for self-management, memory, and planning;

By elaborating the results obtained from the UX Statement, we may re-defined the active living concept as an experiential notion described as follows:

Active Living Re-defined As An Iterative, Continuous and Empirical Process

Active living is a healthy life to stay fit and cultivate personal hobbies and interests, like for example cooking, driving, painting, and reading. Active living is also connected with sharing personal interests and personal experiences. Action and interests go together with maintaining social relationships and social contacts: negotiating ideas and values, discussing personal opinions with other people on different topics is considered essential for a healthy life. Active living does also refer to living in a couple since older people living with husband or wife quite frequently tighten their lives together, by helping each other, sharing duties, and taking specific responsibilities over each other. Use of personal and social spaces, proximity and presence of the others, and overall lifestyle should be also taken into account as part of the concept.

5 Conclusion

There is an existing gap between the original vision behind the products that have been analyzed (see Par. 4) and the reality of how they have been designed or implemented at service level. And this gap is also reflected in the fact that even though older people are now surrounded by "beneficial, empowering, and magical new technologies" [49], many found little everyday advantage or pleasure in using them; they were ambivalent about ICT, citing it as irrelevant to their everyday.

Sackmann and Winkler make a further distinction between the 'first-level' and 'second-level' digital divide. The "first-level" divide is the difference in possession or access, and the "second-level" divide refers to different operational knowledge or modes of use [50]. The concern is that with such rapid advances in technology, this divide could result in disadvantage.

Due to the subjective nature of the experience, the diversity of the target, and the ambivalent approach to technology, an integrated, iterative, participatory, and user-centered approach is required to fill the gap among ideation and implementation of solutions. In fact, the design for intuitive use by older people involves understanding domain-specific prior experience and competence of the user; actual motivation, values, and scopes, and to design interfaces that project prior and current experience into a sustainable aging perspective, within the context of the active living.

The methodological proposal explained in Par. 4 follows a user-centered interaction design approach, aiming at properly addressing real target users' needs, ethical and cross-cultural dimensions, and at monitoring and validating the psycho-social impact of the proposed solution. All the involved target groups (elderly people and caregivers) are considered to be part of a continuous, iterative, consultative design process. A participatory design approach ought to be applied aiming at fostering:

- Diverse participation, perspective taking, and inclusive decision-making,
- Mutual learning, discussion of assumptions, and generation of new concepts,
- Iterative actions to achieve a final design of an artifact that answers to the participants' requirements and ideas.

For this reason, validation sessions are foundational: in fact "validation aids to create a common knowledge base among designers, users, and other stakeholders" about elderly people goals, needs, weaknesses, and expectations. Furthermore, the validation process could also nurture a positive impact on older people because it "fosters social interaction and enhances empathic connections between participants" [51]. In this regard, the suggested design process has a recursive nature and iteratively embraces these fundamental phases:

- User research and analysis, meaning identifying users' daily habits, their lifestyle (nutrition, physical activity, and social relationships),
- Generative and explorative phase, meaning collecting ideas and merge them into few scenarios and design concept,
- Experimental phase—prototyping and refining concrete mockups of product,
- Evaluation and assessment in validation session: the results are submitted, discussed, and improved together with the users.

References

1. World Health Organization: WHO Methods and Data Sources for Life Tables 1990–2019. WHO Press, Geneve (2020)
2. Johnson, J., Finn, K.: Designing User Interfaces for an Aging Population: Towards Universal Design. Morgan Kaufmann, Cambridge (2017)
3. Nielsen, J.: Usability Engineering. Morgan Kaufmann, Amsterdam (1994)
4. Nielsen, J.: 10 Usability Heuristics for User Interface Design, https://www.nngroup.com/articles/ten-usability-heuristics/. Last accessed 16 June 2021
5. Fisk, A.D., Rogers, W.A., Charness, N., Czaja, S.J., Sharit, J. (eds.): Designing for Older Adults: Principles and Creative Human Factors Approaches. CRC Press, Boca Raton (2009)
6. Kline, D.W.: Aging effects on Vision: Impairment, Variability, Self-Report and Compensatory Change. In: Schaie, K.W., Charness, N. (eds.) Impact of Technology on Successful Aging, pp. 85–99. Springer, New York (2003)
7. Morrell, R.W., Holt, B.J., Dailey, S.R., Feldman, C., Mayhorn, C.B., Echt, K.V., Podany, K.I.: Older Adults and Information Technology: A Compendium of Scientific Research and Web Site Accessibility Guidelines. National Institute on Aging, Washington (2001)
8. Hawthorn, D.: Possible implications of aging for interface designers. Interact. Comput. **12**, 507–528 (2000). https://doi.org/10.1016/S0953-5438(99)00021-1
9. Schieber, F.: Human factors and aging: Identifying and compensating for age-related deficits in sensory and cognitive function. In: Schaie, K.W., Charness, N. (eds.) Influences of Technological Change on Individual Aging, pp. 42–84. Springer (2003)

10. Giaccardia, E., Kuijerb, L., Nevenc, L.: Design for resourceful ageing: intervening in the ethics of gerontechnology. Presented at the Future Focused Thinking - DRS International Conference 2016, 27–30 June, Brighton, United Kingdom June 25 (2016). https://doi.org/10.21606/drs.2016.258
11. Antonietti, A., Balconi, M., Catellani, P., Marchetti, A.: Empowering skills for an active ageing and healthy living. Stud. Health Technol. Inform. **203**, 157–171 (2014)
12. Sellen, A., Rogers, Y., Harper, R., Rodden, T.: Reflecting human values in the digital age. Assoc. Comput. Mach. **52**, 58–66 (2009). https://doi.org/10.1145/1467247.1467265
13. Haddon, L.: Social exclusion and information and communication technologies: lessons from studies of single parents and the young elderly. New Media Soc. **2**, 387–406 (2000). https://doi.org/10.1177/1461444800002004001
14. Czaja, S.J., Charness, N., Fisk, A.D., Hertzog, C., Nair, S.N., Rogers, W.A., Sharit, J.: Factors predicting the use of technology: Findings from the center for research and education on aging and technology enhancement (create). Psychol. Aging **21**, 333–352 (2006). https://doi.org/10.1037/0882-7974.21.2.333
15. Hernández-Encuentra, E., Pousada, M., Gómez-Zúñiga, B.: ICT and older people: beyond usability. Educ. Gerontol. **35**, 226–245 (2009). https://doi.org/10.1080/03601270802466934
16. Mitzner, T.L., Boron, J.B., Fausset, C.B., Adams, A.E., Charness, N., Czaja, S.J., Dijkstra, K., Fisk, A.D., Rogers, W.A., Sharit, J.: Older adults talk technology: technology usage and attitudes. Comput. Hum. Behav. **26**, 1710–1721 (2010). https://doi.org/10.1016/j.chb.2010.06.020
17. O'Brien, M.A., Olson, K.E., Charness, N., Czaja, S.J., Fisk, A.D., Rogers, W.A., Sharit, J.: Understanding technology usage in older adults. In: Proceedings of the 6th International Society for Gerontechnology, pp. 1–5. Pisa (2008)
18. Olson, K.E., O'Brien, M.A., Rogers, W.A., Charness, N.: Diffusion of technology: frequency of use for younger and older adults. Ageing Int. **36**, 123–145 (2011). https://doi.org/10.1007/s12126-010-9077-9
19. Reddy, G.R., Blackler, A., Popovic, V.: Adaptable interface framework for intuitively learnable product interfaces for people with diverse capabilities. In: Blackler, A. (ed.) Intuitive Interaction, pp. 113–127. CRC Press (2018). https://doi.org/10.1201/b22191-6
20. Hawthorn, D.: Designing effective interfaces for older users. https://researchcommons.waikato.ac.nz/handle/10289/2538 (2006)
21. Zajicek, M.: Interface design for older adults. In: WUAUC'01: proceedings of the 2001 EC/NSF workshop on Universal accessibility of ubiquitous computing: providing for the elderly, pp. 60–65. Association for Computer Machinery, New York (2001). https://doi.org/10.1145/564526.564543
22. Gudur, R.: A framework to understanding factors that influence designing for older people. In: International Association of Societies of Design Research Conference 2019: Design Revolutions, pp. 1–15 (2019)
23. Czaja, S.J., Boot, W.R., Charness, N., Rogers, W.A.: Designing for Older Adults: Principles and Creative Human Factors Approaches. CRC Press, Boca Raton (2019)
24. Kolko, J.: Thoughts on Interaction Design: A Collection of Reflections. Morgan Kaufmann, Burlington (2010)
25. Carroll, J.M. (ed.): Scenario-Based Design: Envisioning Work and Technology in System Development. Wiley, New York (1995)
26. Carroll, J.M.: Making Use: Scenario-Based Design of Human-Computer Interactions. The MIT Press, Cambridge (2000)
27. World Health Organization: Active Ageing: A Policy Framework. WHO Press (2002)
28. Halaweh, H., Dahlin-Ivanoff, S., Svantesson, U., Willén, C.: Perspectives of Older Adults on Aging Well: A Focus Group Study. J. Aging Res. **2018**, 1–9 (2018). https://doi.org/10.1155/2018/9858252
29. Bowling, A.: Aspirations for Older Age in the 21st Century: What is Successful Aging? Int. J. Aging Human Dev. **64**, 263–297 (2007). https://doi.org/10.2190/L0K1-87W4-9R01-7127

30. Foster, L., Walker, A.: Active and successful aging: a European policy perspective. Gerontologist **55**, 83–90 (2015). https://doi.org/10.1093/geront/gnu028
31. Lawton, M.P., Brody, E.M.: Assessment of older people: self-maintaining and instrumental activities of daily living. Gerontologist **9**, 179–186 (1969). https://doi.org/10.1093/geront/9.3_Part_1.179
32. Lawton, M.P.: A multidimensional view of quality of life in frail elders. In: The concept and measurement of quality of life in the frail elderly, pp. 3–27. Elsevier, New York (1991). https://doi.org/10.1016/B978-0-12-101275-5.50005-3
33. Sloane, P.D., Zimmerman, S., Williams, C.S., Reed, P.S., Gill, K.S., Preisser, J.S.: Evaluating the quality of life of long-term care residents with dementia. Gerontologist **45**, 37–49 (2005). https://doi.org/10.1093/geront/45.suppl_1.37
34. Lawton, M.P., Weisman, G.D., Sloane, P., Calkins, M.: Assessing environments for older people with chronic illness. J. Ment Health Aging. **3**, 83–100 (1997)
35. Lawton, M.P.: Emotion in later life. Curr. Dir. Psychol. Sci. **10**, 120–123 (2001). https://doi.org/10.1111/1467-8721.00130
36. Kunzmann, U., Little, T.D., Smith, J.: Is age-related stability of subjective well-being a paradox? Cross-sectional and longitudinal evidence from the Berlin aging study. Psychol. Aging **15**, 511–526 (2000). https://doi.org/10.1037/0882-7974.15.3.511
37. McNulty, J.K., Fincham, F.D.: Beyond positive psychology? Toward a contextual view of psychological processes and well-being. Am. Psychol. **67**, 101–110 (2012). https://doi.org/10.1037/a0024572
38. Bourassa, K.J., Memel, M., Woolverton, C., Sbarra, D.A.: Social participation predicts cognitive functioning in aging adults over time: comparisons with physical health, depression, and physical activity. Aging Ment. Health **21**, 133–146 (2017). https://doi.org/10.1080/13607863.2015.1081152
39. Bouma, H., Fozard, J.L., Bronswijk, J.E.M.H.V.: Gerontechnology as a field of endeavour. Gerontechnology **8**, 68–75 (2009). https://doi.org/10.4017/gt.2009.08.02.004.00
40. Kitazaki, M., Nicenboim, I., Giaccardi, E., Kuijer, L., Neven, L., Lopez, B.: Connected resources: a research through design approach to designing for older people's resourcefulness. Presented at the Proceedings of the 4th Biennal Research Through Design Conference 2019 (2019). https://doi.org/10.6084/M9.FIGSHARE.7855868.V2
41. Perkins, D.D., Zimmerman, M.A.: Empowerment theory, research, and application. Am. J. Community Psychol. **23**, 569–579 (1995). https://doi.org/10.1007/BF02506982
42. Giaccardi, E., Nicenboim, I.: Resourceful ageing: Empowering older people to age resourcefully with the Internet of Things. Newnorth Print, Bedfordshire (2018)
43. Bandura, A.: Self-efficacy mechanism in human agency. Am. Psychol. **37**, 122–147 (1982). https://doi.org/10.1037/0003-066X.37.2.122
44. Eccola: Esteban Ortiz-Ospina and Max Roser (2020)—Loneliness and social connections. Published online at OurWorldInData.org. Retrieved from: https://ourworldindata.org/social-connections-and-loneliness
45. Norman, D.A.: Emotional Design: Why We Love (or Hate) Everyday Things. Basic Books, New York (2005)
46. Cila, N., Smit, I., Giaccardi, E., Kröse, B.: Products as agents: metaphors for designing the products of the IoT age. In: Proceedings of the 2017 CHI Conference on Human Factors in Computing Systems, pp. 448–459. ACM, Denver (2017). https://doi.org/10.1145/3025453.3025797
47. Marenko, B.: Neo-animism and design: a new paradigm in object theory. Des. Cult. **6**, 219–241 (2014). https://doi.org/10.2752/175470814X14031924627185
48. Rosson, M.B., Carroll, J.M.: Usability Engineering: Scenario-Based Development of Human-Computer Interaction. Academic Press, San Francisco (2002)
49. Selwyn, N., Gorard, S., Furlong, J., Madden, L.: Older adults' use of information and communications technology in everyday life. Ageing Soc. **23**, 561–582 (2003). https://doi.org/10.1017/S0144686X03001302

50. Sackmann, R., Winkler, O.: Technology generations revisited: The internet generation. Gerontechnology. **11**, 493–503 (2013). https://doi.org/10.4017/gt.2013.11.4.002.00
51. Wang, G., Marradi, C., Albayrak, A., van der Cammen, T.J.M.: Co-designing with people with dementia: a scoping review of involving people with dementia in design research. Maturitas **127**, 55–63 (2019). https://doi.org/10.1016/j.maturitas.2019.06.003

How to Enhance Elderly Care Products, Services, and Systems by Means of IoT Technology and Human-Centered Design Approach

Filippo Petrocchi

Abstract Nowadays world is characterized by two significant factors: a progressively ageing society and the digitalization process. While the first phenomenon is mainly due to the ageing of the Baby Boomer generation (those born between 1946 and 1964), as well as to increased longevity and the decrease of birth rate (Aguiar and Macário in Transp Res Proced 25:4355–4369, 2017 [1]; WHO, 2014 [2]), the digitalization process is spreading all over the world thanks to the enormous evolution of the Internet and Information Communication Technology (Gartner Information Technology Glossary: Definition of Digitalization, 2021 [3]). The related changes of these factors can be considered from two perspectives. On the one hand, they are a harbinger of possibilities and opportunities, but on the other hand, they also involve a high potential of exclusion, especially for fragile categories, such as elderly people. In this situation, the role of Human-centered design (HCD) is not only to design products and services that meet the needs of the elderly, but also to support an inclusive society where the elderly can actively age and continue their economic, social, and cultural routines. In particular, this contribution investigates the role of HCD in leveraging IoT technologies to enhance the elderly care scenario on three different levels: products, services, and systems. Finally, based on these three levels, the role of HCD methodology is discussed in relation to the context of elderly care and IoT technology.

Keywords Human-centered design · Design research · Design methodology · IoT · Elderly care

1 Introduction

Nowadays world is characterized by a progressively ageing society. For the first time in human history, most people can easily reach their sixties and beyond. By 2050, the world's population aged 60 years and older will nearly double, from 900 million

F. Petrocchi (✉)
Department of Architecture, University of Ferrara, Ferrara, Italy
e-mail: filippo.petrocchi@unife.it

© The Author(s), under exclusive license to Springer Nature Singapore Pte Ltd. 2022
S. Scataglini et al. (eds.), *Internet of Things for Human-Centered Design*,
Studies in Computational Intelligence 1011,
https://doi.org/10.1007/978-981-16-8488-3_4

in 2015 (12% of the world population) to an expected total of 2 billion (22% of the world population). This is also confirmed by the pace of ageing population, which is mainly due to the ageing of the Baby Boomer generation (those born between 1946 and 1964), as well as to increased longevity and the decline of birth rates [1]. The situation is worsened by the fact that ageing is not equally widespread. For example, the percentage of French elderly people has doubled from 7 to 14% in more than 100 years, while in Brazil and China the same growth is expected to be reached in less than 25 years [2].

In addition to this ageing population process, another factor to consider is the digitalization process, which, according to Gartner Information Technology Glossary, is the use of digital technologies to change a business model and provide new revenue and value-producing opportunities [3]. This disruptive phenomenon permeates at all levels of society, and elderly care is certainly not an exception. Thanks to the recent development of Information and Communication Technology (ICT) and the Internet of Things (IoT), there are new possibilities to face and solve elderly issues.

The combination of ageing society, digitalization, and IoT technology can be seen all over the world, and it comes with challenges and opportunities.

For instance, a challenge might be the fact that, in the future, the potential number of people needing hospital services will raise, resulting in overcrowded hospital facilities [4].

Furthermore, by 2030, more than 60% of the Baby Boomer generation will likely face at least one chronic condition. Consequently, managing these chronic conditions, along with a patient's level of disability, will increase the financial demands on health care systems [5].

Together with challenges, there are also new opportunities of business for those companies that can understand this large-scale demographic shift and embrace emerging opportunities in advance [6].

Possible strategies to address elderly care issues have already been proposed by several international authorities. The World Health Organization has promoted the *Global strategy and action plan on ageing and health* [7], aiming collecting evidence-based actions, maximizing functionality and, by 2020, establishing the evidence and partnerships required to support the Decade of Healthy ageing from 2020 to 2030. Specifically, the strategy focuses on five key objectives: commitment to action on healthy ageing in every country; developing age-friendly environments; aligning health systems to the needs of older populations; developing sustainable and equitable systems for providing long-term care and improving healthy ageing measurement, monitoring, and research.

On a similar direction, the European Commission has co-financed the Active and Assisted living programme [8], which has the purpose to create a better quality of life for older people in the digital world and to strengthen industrial opportunities in the field of healthy ageing technology and innovation.

In line with the WHO and the European Commission's actions, technology can be considered as a lever to enhance every health service guiding the transition from the current health care system to a digital health care, which is also referred to as e-health [9].

Nevertheless, while Information technology seems to be the ideal tool to guide the transition to e-health, there are still too many elderly people who can't use it, causing a significant underutilization. As a result, many seniors miss the opportunity to enhance their quality of life by means of Internet-based service delivery [10].

Furthermore, even though the IoT field is characterized by great innovation and development, the adoption of elderly care services is quite limited. This low adoption rate is mainly related to a design which is too much focused on technological development and lacks social and human comprehension. Hence, there is a mismatch between users' expectations and available services [11].

To recap, if we consider ageing society, digitalization, related challenges and opportunities, international policies and technology acceptance of elderly people in ICT, we can assume that HCD is a promising field to facilitate the users' comprehension and effectively foster the transition from current society to a more ageing and inclusive one. The aim of this contribution is to analyze several cases on different levels of design, highlighting and discussing the impact that HCD approach can have in the elderly care scenario.

2 Human-Centered Design

Created as an alternative to purely technology-driven innovation, Human-centered design is a multidisciplinary innovation process, based on user involvement at all stages of the process.

In contrast with the technological approach, the HCD considers the user not only as a passive consumer that buys products, but also as an active participant whose behaviours, goals, and needs are implemented at all phases of the process [12].

Focussing on elderly care, Design research has largely accepted the challenge of products and services for older people. In the last decade, the number of research and projects focussing on seniors and their assistance and monitoring has constantly increased [13].

Furthermore, according to Donald Norman, one of the most important experts of Human-centered design, design for elderly people is not only an interesting sector for research but also a promising sector for designers for three reasons: it is a growing market, due to demographic transition; it is populated by wealthy people; these users are willing to invest money in products and services that can enhance their quality of life [14].

3 Case Studies

Given the constant growth of HCD applications in the field of elderly care, this article underlines the validity of HCD methodology and its scalability. Therefore, the author has conducted in-depth research focussing on HCD projects specifically designed

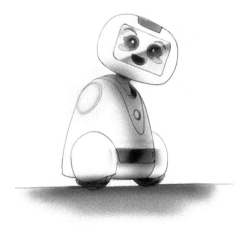

Fig. 1 Sketch of BUDDY, one of the two assistive robots for elderly, developed for ACCRA project

for elderly care and with the implementation of IoT technology. For each project, benefits and methodologies are analyzed and presented based on three different levels: products, services, and systems.

3.1 Product Level—ACCRA

On the product level, one interesting project is ACCRA.[1] ACCRA, an acronym which stands for Agile Co-creation of Robots for Ageing, is a project funded by program Horizon H2020_EU.3.1.4, with an overall budget of 1 999 711,25 € within a timeframe from 1st December 2016 to 31st March 2020.

Contextualized between Europe and Japan, the project is an advanced ICT robot specifically designed to enhance elderly daily routines and to extend autonomous ageing in a safe and healthy way.

Both in Europe and in Japan, seniors prefer to age at home rather than moving to specialized facilities. However, while their stay at home can be seen as a positive factor, because it means that they are autonomous, on the other hand it represents a risky situation for several reasons. One of the most important is that poor health, cognitive impairment, fragility, and social exclusion lead to negative consequences not only for seniors' independence and quality of life, but also for their caregivers, as well as for the sustainability of health care systems.

This is the reason why ACCRA is a promising solution: it focuses on building solutions to support older people in their ordinary daily life. In particular, the project led to the creation of two robots, ASTRO and BUDDY (Fig. 1). While ASTRO was an assistive smart robotic platform dedicated to movement at home and within the residential environment, BUDDY was a small-size robot designed as a home companion.

---

[1] More information at https://www.accra-project.org/en/sample-page/.

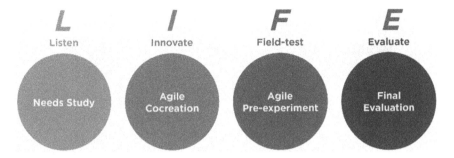

Fig. 2 Graphic representation of LIFE methodology in four steps: listen, innovate, field-test, and evaluate

For both robots, an innovative methodology was adopted. The name of the approach is LIFE (Fig. 2), an acronym that stands for the four phases represented in the picture below: Listen, Innovate, Field-test, and Evaluate.

Listen identifies needs and robotic capabilities through in-depth interviews with older adults and with formal and informal caregivers. Innovate is characterized by an agile co-creative circle made of co-design, testing, development, and quality check. Agile Pre-experiment tests the robotic solutions in a real-life context with a larger group of end users and gathers data to further develop the AI algorithms in the robot. The final phase, Evaluate, is characterized by several sub-steps: an assessment of the robot value both in real-life and in an experimental setup; an investigation of its potential market through a market survey; a sustainable assessment of what is needed for sustainable entry market implementation on multiple domains.

According to Antonio Kung, CEO of Trialog and coordinator of ACCRA project, the basic operations and capabilities are easy to be provided, but the robot's cost remains high for a standard consumer. The project highlighted the need to further develop the range of capabilities of the product and it will pave the way to the creation of future robots for an ageing population. Furthermore, another important outcome of LIFE methodology is that it will enhance the creation of robots not only in the field of ageing population, but also in any kind of future robots with an integrated human factor.

3.2 Service Level—Carr(e)ers Rally Case Study (Autonom' Lab)

"*Carr(e)ers*" Rally[2] is a project that aims to improve the quality of home services delivered to elderly or disabled people. The overall objective of *Carr(e)ers* is an experimental service-event to allow people interested in elderly care professions to discover them through role-playing workshops and discussion with experienced

---

[2] More info at https://87.rallyedelaidealapersonne.fr/accueil.html.

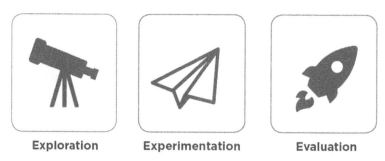

Fig. 3 Graphic representation of living lab methodology phases

professionals. The innovative feature of this project was the use of IoT granted by partners who were involved in the planning of online and offline workshops and presentations about home-help sector.

For the creation of this project, a Human-centered design, FORM IT methodology, was used [15]. This methodology consists of three main phases: Exploration, Experimentation, and Evaluation (Fig. 3).

Exploration analyzes the current context and hypothesizes possible "future states". *Experimentation* involves the decision of a scenario and the development of a testing phase in real-life cases. Finally, *Evaluation* is characterized by the assessment of experiments' impact, with particular focus on the "current state" and "future states".

Several methodologies were integrated into this scheme, such as: Design thinking, Interviews, Visual interviews (Collage), observation/shadowing, Photo journal, User persona, Brainstorming, Usability workshop.

The results of this project were really encouraging because the participation was significant. In total, 220 people took part in the project, with the mobilization of 44 partners, 27 of whom proposed a total of 42 actions all over the month of the rally.

The results were mainly positive, with some margin for improvement. In fact, while participants were really satisfied with the event, employers were not totally satisfied, because of the low quality of the application received.

3.3 System Level—HABITAT

HABITAT[3] is a project financed by Italian region Emilia Romagna POR FESR 2014–2020, aiming to develop an IoT ecosystem to help elderly people who prefer ageing in their own place. The primary goal is to ensure seniors home assistance in their routines to prevent possible issues caused by their frail status (Fig. 4).

Another goal is to transform existing elements of the house (radio furniture, alarm) to keep the house environment safe, help elderly manage their natural cognitive, physical, and social decline, encourage them to take actions and enrich their daily

---

[3] More info at http://www.eng.habitatproject.info/home.

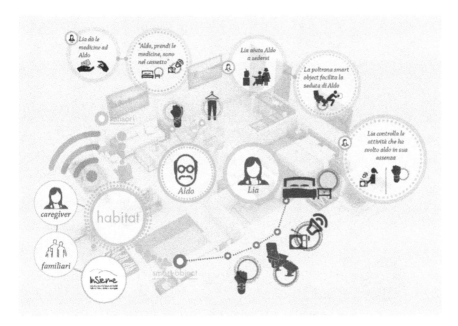

Fig. 4 The System Layout of HABITAT PROJECT

life with all the possibilities offered by cloud computing. To ensure a high level of usability, accessibility, and inclusiveness [16], a User-centered Design (UCD) approach was applied, as shown in the picture below (Fig. 5).

The project consists of five main phases: Research, Definition, Ideation, Design, and Testing. It started with Research, that is the analysis of users' goals, needs, and product features. Afterwards, Definition was implemented to define users' needs and their technical correlation (Quality Function Deployment, QFD), Technical attributes and User satisfaction. Ideation was then accomplished by means of a brief, a co-design workshop, and a concept validation. Finally, a prototype was made in the Design phase and usability and functional tests were conducted in the final Testing phase.

The project had several positive results. One of the most important accomplishments is the realization of a family product that ensures a Technology readiness level (TRL) of 5. A TRL level 5 means that a product should be able to be used and work properly in a controlled real-life environment and not only in laboratory.

Together with the creation of these products, HABITAT also offered several benefits to Emilia Romagna region, such as: the spread of effective knowledge about purposes, activities, and final results; the enhancement of the collaboration between high-technology net laboratories in similar sectors; the improvement of competitive placements with result sharing.

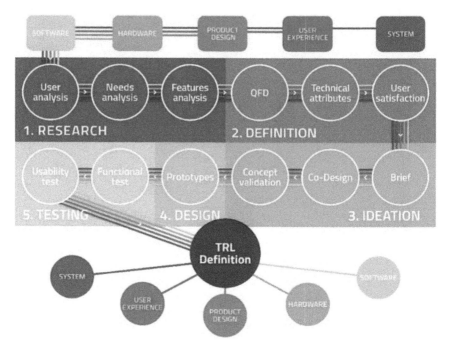

Fig. 5 The HABITAT PROJECT methodology
(image from https://www.researchgate.net/publication/331714340_HABITAT_An_IoT_Solution_for_Independent_Elderly)

4 Discussion

Due to constant increase of ageing society, a consequent raise of interest has spread all over the scientific community, also in Design research. Nevertheless, while the number of projects regarding elderly and elderly care is quite significant, it is not possible to notice the same situation for methodology description. Even in European projects, the methodology is rarely described and only in a few cases it is well presented and described.

Another interesting point to highlight is that only public and European projects present a well-defined methodology, while private projects only show the final results. However, it would be beneficial to have some references from the private sector in the analysis, not only to enhance the discussion, but also to provide a more in-depth view of the current practice of elderly care IoT projects.

Finally, while the digitalization process is a great harbinger of new opportunities, it also comes with high possibilities to exclude fragile people that are not particularly good at technology and changes. This is particularly true in the case of elderly people that suffer, albeit with some exceptions, from a progressive slowing down of mental, physical, hearing, and movement abilities. Human-centered design has proven to be effective to ensure the goals, needs, and behaviors of these fragile people, but in many cases the technological approach is still dominant. A possible future point of investigation could be how to make more feasible HCD projects to promote a more inclusive and senior-friendly society.

5 Conclusions

With the analysis of the current context, a progressively ageing society, digitalization, and the consequent actions by national and international organizations, this contribution has highlighted the possibilities that Human-centered design can offer to facilitate innovation in elderly care sector thanks to IoT technology and based on three levels of implementation. Considering the context and the three cases here presented, it is possible to highlight the following conclusions:

- The case studies above have shown that Human-centered design approach seems to be a promising tool to facilitate the integration of elderly needs into the product, service, and IoT ecosystem.
- HCD is an approach that has the flexibility to be used at all levels: product, service, and system. At all levels, user needs are taken into account, and they are implemented through several techniques, such as co-workshops, usability tests, observations.
- CO-design is a versatile tool that can be effective at all levels: product, service, system. It is widely used in HCD projects, and this is mainly due to the fact that it guarantees the integration of users' feedback at every stage of the project: from the initial research phase to the concept phase (workshop). Furthermore, CO-design fosters an emotional and effective connection between the user and the stakeholder, enhancing the acceptance of the final product.
- All the projects presented aim at leveraging IoT technology to improve elderly care services and, consequently, elderly life routines.
- IoT Technology is mature enough to be effectively applied to products, services, and systems that focus on an elderly care scenario.
- IoT solutions are a promising technology to foster the transition from current elderly care scenario to e-health elderly care, characterized by remote monitoring, prevention, and digital assistance.

In conclusion, HCD can contribute at multiple levels to foster a transition from current health care to remote and digital elderly care. In this shift, HCD can contribute not only to improve current products, services, and IoT systems, but it can also enhance, especially through Co-design, an increased entanglement between users and the services used. Consequently, a win–win situation is generated for stakeholders and users: on the one hand, users and others feel more included into the process, on the other hand, stakeholders are able to reduce the probability of failure. Furthermore, the openness toward new forms of collaboration between stakeholders, companies, and users can be used not only as a significant network to acquire knowledge and test ideas, but also as a form of marketing and advertising.

References

1. Aguiar, B., Macário, R.: The need for an elderly centered mobility policy. Transp. Res. Proced. **25**:4355–4369
2. WHO: Facts about ageing, Retrieved 20 May 2021, from https://www.who.int/ageing/about/facts/en/#:~:text=The%20world%20population%20is%20rapidly,billion%20over%20the%20same%20period (2014)
3. Gartner Information Technology Glossary: Definition of Digitalization, Retrieved 21 May 2021, from https://www.gartner.com/en/information-technology/glossary/digitalization#:~:text=Digitalization%20is%20the%20use%20of,moving%20to%20a%20digital%20business (2021)
4. Global health care outlook the evolution of smart healthcare: digital deloitte (2018)
5. The Aging Population: The Increasing Effects on Health Care. Retrieved 28 January 2021, from https://www.pharmacytimes.com/publications/issue/2016/January2016/The-Aging-Population-The-Increasing-Effects-on-Health-Care (2016)
6. Kohlbacher, F.: The Silver Market Phenomenon: Business Opportunities in an Era of Demographic Change. In: Herstatt, C. (ed.), p. 59 Springer, Berlin (2008)
7. World Health Organization: Global strategy and action plan on ageing and health (2017)
8. AAL Home 2020 - AAL Programme. Retrieved 26 May 2021, from http://www.aal-europe.eu/ (2021)
9. ActiveAdvice: What is Smart Health and How do People Benefit? Retrieved from https://www.activeadvice.eu/news/concept-projects/what-is-smart-healthand-how-do-people-benefit/ (2017)
10. Internet adoption by the elderly: employing IS technology acceptance theories for understanding the age-related digital divide Björn Niehaves & Ralf Plattfaut 2017).
11. Pal, D., Funilkul, S., Charoenkitkarn, N., Kanthamanon, P.: Internet-of-things and smart homes for elderly healthcare: an end user perspective. IEEE Access **6**, 10483–10496 (2018)
12. Steen, M.: Human-centered design as a fragile encounter. Des. Issues **28**(1), 72–80 (2012)
13. Imbesi, S., Mincolelli, G.: Design of smart devices for older people: a user centered approach for the collection of users' needs. In: International Conference on Intelligent Human Systems Integration. Springer, Cham, pp. 860–864 (2020)
14. NN group: Design for Elderly [Image]. Retrieved from https://www.youtube.com/watch?v=uP6IbeggAeo (2021)
15. Ståhlbröst, A.: Forming Future IT—The Living Lab Way of User Involvement. Luleå University of Technology, Luleå (2008)
16. Mincolelli, G., Marchi, M., Chiari, L., Costanzo, A., Borelli, E., Mellone, S., Masotti, D., Paolini, G., Imbesi, S.: Inclusive design of wearable smart objects for older users: design principles for combining technical constraints and human factors. In: International Conference on Applied Human Factors and Ergonomics. Springer, Cham, pp. 324–334 (2018)

Digital Human Modelling: Inclusive Design and the Ageing Population

Russell Marshall, Erik Brolin, Steve Summerskill, and Dan Högberg

Abstract Digital human modelling (DHM) is a tool that allows humans to be modelled in three-dimensional CAD. An almost infinite variety of humans can be modelled and families of so-called manikins can be created to act as virtual user groups, evaluating the interactions between humans and products, workplaces and environments. This chapter introduces the concept of DHM, its use of, and reliance on, anthropometric data from national populations and showcases two exemplar tools in SAMMIE and IPS IMMA. Case studies are presented that highlight the advantages DHM can bring to understanding the requirements of designing for the ageing population; covering designing for the ageing workforce, the exploration of transport accessibility and how users can generate representative manikin families to properly represent the diversity of people. DHM is demonstrated to be a powerful tool for practitioners aiming to understand and design for people, including older people within society.

Keywords Digital human modelling · Ageing · Anthropometry · SAMMIE · IPS IMMA

R. Marshall (✉) · S. Summerskill
School of Design and Creative Arts, Loughborough University, Loughborough, UK
e-mail: R.Marshall@lboro.ac.uk

S. Summerskill
e-mail: S.J.Summerskill2@lboro.ac.uk

E. Brolin · D. Högberg
School of Engineering Science, University of Skövde, Skövde, Sweden
e-mail: erik.brolin@his.se

D. Högberg
e-mail: dan.hogberg@his.se

© The Author(s), under exclusive license to Springer Nature Singapore Pte Ltd. 2022
S. Scataglini et al. (eds.), *Internet of Things for Human-Centered Design*,
Studies in Computational Intelligence 1011,
https://doi.org/10.1007/978-981-16-8488-3_5

1 Introduction

It is widely acknowledged that the global population is ageing. According to the World Health Organization (WHO), the proportion of the global population over 60 years old will increase from 12 to 22% between 2015 and 2050 [1]. Once, this was a phenomenon most readily observed in high income countries such as Japan, who's population is the oldest in the world and where nearly 30% of their population is over 65 years old [2]. However, population ageing is now a significant factor amongst the developing countries [3].

The ageing population is widely reported as a concern for various global socio-economic factors. Amongst those concerns are the impact of the increase in average age on the working population, with the expectation that an ageing population results in many more people working into older age. This will be partly driven by a greater number of people who are older seeking to remain active, and indeed countries such as the UK have made it a legal right to keep working beyond state pension age [4], with similar legislation in the US prohibiting employment discrimination against those over 40 years [5], and elsewhere. In addition, many companies wish to retain the skills and experience of older workers [6], this is also combined with the economic factors of governments raising retirement ages [7] and pension schemes struggling to fund the number of those retired with a shift in the demographic from being weighted from those paying into schemes to those drawing upon them. In the US is it reported that between 2000 and 2016, the number of Americans aged 65 or over in part or full time employment has increased from 4 million (12.8% of those aged 65 or over) to 9 million (18.8%) people.

With an ageing population comes the expectation that older people still have equal access to and ability to use, benefit from and enjoy, products, facilities and services. One of the ongoing challenges, with this, is that many of these products and services are designed by younger people for younger people. It is all too common for those who are older, or who have particular needs or capabilities outside of those considered to be the norm, to not be considered during the design process. The ageing population spotlights this fallacy as increasingly older people become the norm in society. Thankfully, the need to adopt a more holistic approach to the understanding of user capabilities, behaviours, needs and desires is increasingly well recognized and inclusive design, universal design, design for all are now core design approaches. BS 7000–6, (2005) design management systems, the guide to managing inclusive design, define inclusive design as *[the] design of mainstream products and/or services that are accessible to and usable by, people with the widest range of abilities and the widest range of situations without the need for special adaptation or design* [8]. Whilst inclusive design and associated approaches have been inspired by the need to accommodate people with disabilities, it is important to recognize that human diversity is much more complex than a binary definition of those who are disabled and those who are not. Human capability is a spectrum with almost infinite variety across populations in physical and cognitive abilities. Thus, it can be beneficial to not focus on the specifics of an individuals' capabilities but rather to understand the barriers faced and the severity of those barriers in accessing a given design. In research commissioned by Microsoft to explore the impact of accessible computer technology, the population was defined by the prevalence of difficulties with daily tasks that may impact on computer use [9]. Their findings identified that 37% of the population were not likely to encounter difficulties (split between no difficulties and minimal difficulties), 37% were likely to encounter difficulties (mild) and 25% were very likely to encounter difficulties (severe). Within this, it was also clearly identified that ageing plays a significant factor with both the prevalence and severity of difficulties increasing as people get older.

Ageing is not a disability, however, it is well recognized that as people age, they typically develop progressive multiple impairments and a decrease in mobility [10]. Whilst these impairments are often relatively minor, affecting, physical and cognitive capabilities, when combined can become a disabling factor. In addition, it should be recognized that poor design can itself be a disabling factor, if it does not take into account sufficient understanding of human variability in cognitive and physical performance.

Due to the complexity of understanding and designing for this richness of human variability, computer-based tools can play a role in supporting the design process. One particular family of tools has a significant part to play in addressing the challenges in this area. These tools, known broadly as digital human models (DHMs), are now typically three-dimensional (3D) computer simulations of humans that can be placed alongside 3D computer representations of products, workplaces and environments and the interaction between the two explored [11]. These DHM systems offer the ability to explore human variability, to gain some understanding of potential barriers, all whilst a product or environment is in its development phase, where changes can be rapidly iterated and a more accessible solution found prior to implementation.

The aim of this chapter is to introduce DHM technology, outlining how DHM technologies can aid in addressing the needs of the whole population in particular those who are older. To achieve this aim, this chapter has the following objectives: to showcase two exemplar DHM tools; to explore the challenges of modelling humans; to present different approaches to representing representative users in DHM; to present three case studies of the use of DHM in areas relevant to the ageing population and to explore the potential future for this technology.

2 Digital Human Modelling

Digital human modelling and Digital human models, both are abbreviated interchangeably to DHM, typically refers to a specific type of 3D computer aided design (CAD) software [12]. Whilst specific capability of these tools can vary significantly, they all share the common ability to model humans (Fig. 1). These humans are typically able to be varied across various factors to replicate the size, shape and capability of national populations [13]. The human models are highly data driven

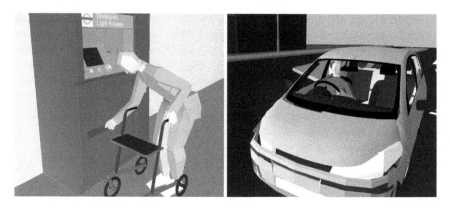

Fig. 1 Examples of DHM

and rely on databases of human characteristics to be able to represent these characteristics, observable in real people, in the digital simulation, in a valid manner. DHM has increasingly become more sophisticated and widespread in its use since its inception in the 1960s [14]. Over these decades, there have been many DHM tools [15], currently, there are a number of popular and more specialized tools available such as Jack, Safework, Ramsis, Santos, SAMMIE, IPS IMMA, Anybody, CASIMIR amongst others [16]. Some of these tools are stand alone, able to import data from other 3D CAD tools, and others are integrated into CAD suites allowing seamless integration with the design of products and workstations. Whilst the use of DHM remains relatively niche in comparison with standard 3D CAD, it still sees significant levels of use in applications such as the automotive and aerospace industries, both related to product design and production. Transport is one area of application where the requirements for a human operator are such that designers are faced with a complex set of requirements, all of which vary across populations of typical users. The challenge for the designer is to ensure that as many people as possible are accommodated across all of this variability. This is what is referred to as multivariate accommodation and often optimizing one variable compromises another [17]. Seated operating conditions, where users need to interact with various aspects of a workstation, from a relatively fixed posture, form a uniquely wicked problem [18]. DHM is ideally suited to exploring the implications of these types of situations on the human operator and how the variability of the desired user population can be accommodated as efficiently as possible.

In most applications, there is a clear focus on physical characteristics of the human and their interactions: fit, posture, reach, vision, etc., are all common features of DHM that can be evaluated. In addition, some tools offer biomechanics tools such that muscle forces can be evaluated to consider whether tasks are possible by human operators, whether there will be ergonomic issues, or possible risks of injury or long term musculoskeletal problems [19, 20]. DHM tools can, therefore, be used both reactively and proactively. Reactively to evaluate an existing design of a product or workstation or proactively to define some of the key design variables to ensure a design is optimized for human use. A major strength of DHM tools is that they enable, in a proactive manner, the evaluation of human-object interaction of designs that only exist as CAD models. This is an essential strength due to the fact that most products and workstations are designed by the use of CAD software. Hence, DHM tools facilitate the integration of human factors matters in contemporary design processes.

Where DHM is currently less well developed is in the non-physical aspects of humans or in the 'softer' physical domain such as comfort and behaviour. These are very desirable capabilities, and DHM researchers and developers are continuously exploring ways in which these aspects can be quantified and simulated. However, they typically pose even greater challenges than the physical variability in human populations, so much so, that some of the characteristics do not even have clearly agreed definitions. For example, comfort is a very desirable characteristic in many designs, however, what might be comfortable for one person may not be for another, in addition something may be comfortable for a finite period of time, after which it becomes uncomfortable. For applications such as seating comfort and modelling approaches have made significant headway but these remain a challenge [21]. This highlights one of the benefits and sometimes limitations of DHM, in that its reliance on data can provide fundamental insights into the needs of users, but equally without the appropriate data, the tools can also become redundant or force the users of DHM into using inappropriate data in lieu of anything more appropriate. One of the main data sources required for DHM tools is body size data or anthropometry [22]. Anthropometric databases underpin the ability for DHM tools to accurately replicate human body dimensions. However, anthropometric data also have their challenges, to make it valid you often need very large samples, and these are typically expensive and very time consuming to collect. As such, suitable anthropometric databases are often not as available as may be desired. This poses specific challenges for the application of DHM to older people and ageing populations where data on the characteristics of older people are rare.

Arguably, all DHM tools exhibit limits to the insight and guidance that can be provided and there is an expectation that the DHM tool user has some fundamental knowledge of ergonomics and human factors. Users should always be familiar with the tasks they are designing for or are evaluating, and preferably drive their modelling from data obtained first-hand from actual users interacting with the same or similar products or workstations and performing the same or similar tasks. These data and associated knowledge should be used to inform posturing and human-object interactions and be used to help interpret human factors results from the tool. It is important to remember that DHM tools will generally only provide insights into what is possible, and potentially, what is likely but will not generally provide insight into what might be. As such, it is easy to construct evaluations that assume all people act in a 'correct' manner, e.g., ergonomic, safe, etc., when in reality, many are driven by other factors such as time, minimal energy expenditure and habit. However, when used appropriately with an understanding of their strengths and weaknesses, DHM tools can offer fundamental advantages over a purely real-world approach.

3 Anthropometry and Anthropometric Data

Anthropometric data can usually be divided into either functional (dynamic) dimensions or structural (static) dimensions. Functional dimensions are, for example, measurements of reach range during an activity. These measurements are generally for special situations and can be difficult to measure but are often valuable in the design of products and workplaces. Structural dimensions are measurements between anatomical (body) landmarks defined for standardized postures at rest. These measurements are relatively easy to measure, but may have limited value in a design context since they can be too artificial to directly use as input in the design process [23]. In large ethnic, age and gender separated populations most body measurements can be considered normally distributed. However, body weight and muscular strength often show a positively skewed distribution curve [23]. An additional fact is that the proportions of the human body vary from person to person, e.g., people of average stature are unlikely to have an average value for all body measurements [23, 24]. The correlation coefficient between different anthropometric measurements can be analyzed to see how strongly they are connected. Length measurements usually have high mutual correlation and the same can be seen when analyzing weight, depth and width measurements. However, in total, body measurements have low correlation dependencies [25, 26]. This fact leads to a reduction in accommodation when multiple measurements are affecting the design and only a few are incorporated in the ergonomics evaluation and analysis [24, 27].

Utilizing anthropometric data are often a fundamental part of the process to achieve good fit between capabilities of humans and design of products or workplaces. However, industry practice for consideration of anthropometric diversity has shown to sometimes be based on the utilization of rough approaches, containing misconceptions of average people and inadequate use of percentile based methods [24, 28–30]. Because humans vary a lot in size and shape, there is a considerable uncertainty whether the expected proportion of the target population is actually covered by the utilization of such rough anthropometric approaches. Robinette [30] gives examples of serious design flaws caused by improper use of anthropometric data. Bertilsson et al. [31] found that DHM tool-based ergonomics evaluations, and analyses are often done with only two or three manikins, because of the time consuming process of creating and performing analyses for each manikin or due to the lack of knowledge or availability of efficient and supportive tools and methods for anthropometric diversity. Hence, it is important to support DHM tool users to consider anthropometric diversity in an efficient and successful manner.

4 Modelling Representative Users

A central theme in DHM is the way the tool is designed to represent variation within targeted user groups, e.g., assembly staff, vehicle drivers, etc. The basic argument is that humans are different, hence the digital manikins need to be able to represent this variability. Most likely, there is a need to use more than two or three manikins in the simulation to ensure good ergonomics and to represent the variety within the targeted user group in a successful way, at least for most design situations. Guidelines for the consideration of anthropometric diversity and for how to select relevant test cases, e.g., manikins for virtual simulation and evaluation, has been presented by Dainoff et al. [32], and Hanson and Högberg [33] in the form of flowcharts where the type of cases depends on the design problem at hand. The objective of these guidelines is to facilitate an appropriate process of handling issues related to anthropometric diversity. In the simplest cases, it can be enough to just consider the smallest and largest possible future users for one specific anthropometric measurement, utilizing what is known as the percentile approach. However, in many cases, multiple measurements are affecting the design and only incorporating a few in the ergonomics evaluation and analysis can lead to a reduction in accommodation [24, 27].

4.1 Multidimensional Consideration of Anthropometric Diversity

Several methods have been developed to facilitate much more sophisticated multidimensional consideration of anthropometric diversity in a design process. Most of these methods are based on one or both of the fundamental methods: *boundary case* and *distributed case* method [32]. These two methods are in many ways similar, which makes it possible to use them simultaneously. The concept is that a confidence region is defined that bounds an area of a scatter graph. Typically, these scatter graphs plot the data from a range of users for two or more relevant characteristics (Fig. 2). Boundary cases are data points located towards the edges of the region, and distributed cases are points spread throughout the region randomly or by some systematic approach. This confidence region is typically an ellipse, in two dimensions (i.e. for two measures), but can become a hyper-ellipsoid when further key dimensions (measures) are added. The hyper-ellipsoid is scaled based on a desired accommodation level, i.e. to cover and encapsulate a certain amount of the population [34]. The same principles apply regardless of the number of selected anthropometric key measurements. The use of boundary cases is based on the same principle as the identification of extreme users in the approach of inclusive design, i.e. that evaluations of boundary cases will be sufficient to meet the demands of the whole population. However, this assumption might be wrong in some cases and distributed cases can, therefore, also be used to decrease the risk of missing key areas when using boundary cases [32].

The statistical treatment and mathematical modelling of confidence hyper-ellipsoids are done under the assumption that the measurement distribution can be approximated with a normal distribution. However, since this approximation is not always completely successful in representing real measurement distributions, especially for certain body measurements in many of today's populations, it is important,

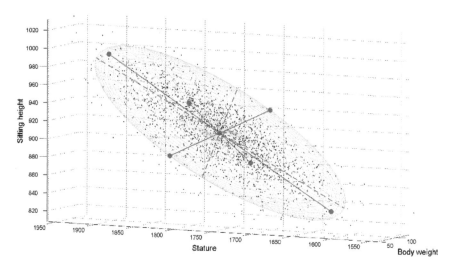

Fig. 2 Depiction of boundary cases and confidence ellipsoid enclosing 90% of the multivariate normal distribution for body weight, stature and sitting height

this can be addressed when seeking to create digital manikins that will represent the anthropometric diversity of the user population. Different types of transformations can be applied when handling skewed data in order to make the data more normally distributed. Transforming skewed distributions when generating confidence ellipses and boundary cases are appropriate to more accurately consider this type of diversity and correctly describe the shape of the actual skewed distribution (Fig. 3). This process is further elaborated by Brolin [35].

4.2 Hadrian

Another approach to representing a diverse range of users is to echo real-world approaches. Designers engaged in development projects often employ personas, to guide the design direction [36]. These can be entirely fictional but often these are data driven, representing typical characteristics observed in the user population. By their definition, they are selective in the characteristics they represent but they are powerful design tools to focus the activity of the design team. Virtual users within DHM can be created to act as equivalents to these personas with characteristics that are both representative but also useful drivers for design activity [37].

In physical data collection or user testing, design teams will sample users based on representative characteristics. However, practical limitations will normally keep the sample sizes to manageable numbers. In a similar way, these specific users, who demonstrate a breadth of diversity on a relevant design characteristic, can be represented in DHM. This may at first appear very similar to using extremes of the

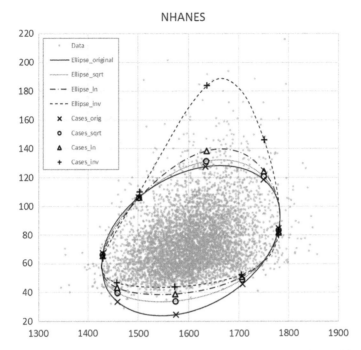

Fig. 3 Confidence ellipses and boundary cases for the original body weight data and for the three transformation methods, data from NHANES [12]. Stature (mm) on *x*-axis and weight (kg) on *y*-axis

population or even boundary manikins. However, the fundamental difference is that these are based upon real people who have not been specifically constructed for the purposes of the modelling. This can be considered as something more than a persona, each digital human is effectively a digital twin of their real counterpart. Whilst this will typically mean the most extreme users are not represented, it does provide a degree of authenticity and the users will be highly diverse as humans are inherently variable as we have seen earlier. One of the significant advantages of this approach is one of empathy. Even in a virtual world, designing for a real person is much more engaging than designing for a statistically derived or by other means fabricated human model.

An example of this digital twin approach is the HADRIAN database [38]. Human anthropometric data requirements investigation and analysis (HADRIAN) was the outcome of research into equality in design and resulted in a rich database of characteristics for more than 100 people, the majority of whom were older or who had some form of disability (see Table 1). These people collectively form a virtual user group that can be used in DHM applications.

Table 1 Data for each individual in the HADRIAN database

Anthropometry (mm)	Stature Weight Arm length Upper arm length Elbow-to-shoulder (link) Wrist-to-elbow (link) Abdominal depth (standing) Abdominal depth (sitting) Thigh depth (standing) Thigh depth (sitting) Knee-to-hip (link) Ankle-to-knee (link) Ankle height Foot length Sitting height Sitting shoulder height	Hip-to-shoulder (link) Chest height Chest depth Head height Eye-to-top-of-head Buttock-knee length Knee height Shoulder breadth Hip breadth Hand length Hand grip length Wheelchair length Wheelchair height Wheelchair width Wheelchair seat height
Joint constraints (deg)	Shoulder extension/flexion Shoulder abduction/adduction Upper arm extension/flexion Upper arm abduction/adduction Upper arm medial/lateral rotation	Elbow extension/flexion Elbow pronation/supination Wrist extension/flexion Wrist abduction/adduction
Reach range (~100 coordinates mm)	Functional reach volume generated by dominant arm/hand	
Somatotype (three digit number)	Somatotype code based on Sheldon [39]	
Task capability (encoded postures for each task plus task videos)	Four pick and place tasks (high shelf, worksurface, oven, low shelf) with three load types (cup, bag, tray) each set to maximum comfortable weight, 1 or 2 hands as appropriate	Seating: two designs - high and hard, low and soft; restricted access to single side (bus), both sides (toilet cubicle), no restriction Ingress/egress: step up/step down from maximum comfortable step height, two handle types, maximum of 4 handle locations
Additional capability	Bending to touch toes Getting up from lying down Reaching to tie shoelaces Twisting upper body to left and right	Peg test (dexterity) Grip strength Vision
Transport questionnaire (question and answer transcripts and videos)	Transport use (frequency, etc.) Issues with transport usage (problems, assistance required, etc.) Issues with lifts, steps and escalators	Issues with environment (personal safety, etc.) Issues with signage and timetables Local issues

(continued)

Table 1 (continued)

Background	Age	Handedness
	Nationality	Disability
	Occupation/work history	Front and side photographs

5 Materials and Method

This section presents two typical DHM tools: SAMMIE and IPS IMMA. The tools are examples of DHM applications in use today, representing a range of capability. As discussed previously, both tools share many similar characteristics but equally they demonstrate very different approaches to many key DHM issues. Both tools are introduced, along with their core capabilities.

5.1 System for Aiding Man–Machine Interaction (SAMMIE)

SAMMIE is a DHM system software tool originally developed at Nottingham University, and later at Loughborough University in the UK. SAMMIE was the outcome from PhD research initiated in 1968 and since that time has been extensively used in research and consultancy at Loughborough University. In addition, as a commercial tool [40], SAMMIE is widely used by universities and businesses around the world. By modern standards, SAMMIE is a relatively simple human model, consisting of an internal structure formed of 49 links representative of the human skeleton [41]. Each link (bone) has a representative joint constrained by joint movement limits [42], and an external flesh form constrained by body shape data [39]. SAMMIE's form and core capabilities are driven by access to the data discussed earlier. A representative human form can be generated based on an inbuilt or otherwise available dataset of nationality and gender and up to eight anthropometric measurements. At its simplest, a human model can be constructed as a proportional human from either a stature measurement (in mm) or a percentile value. Alternatively, every limb can be customized to create individuals using eight core measurements of stature, sitting height, sitting shoulder height, buttock-knee length, knee height, arm length, hand length and shoulder breadth. Thus, models can be created to represent exemplar values within a national population or a collection of individuals measured for a specific application.

SAMMIE provides facilities to manipulate the human model through gross posture, or individual limb movements, constrained to prevent postures that are not possible. When combined with the data in the HADRIAN database, these joint constraints can be limited to represent the impact of ageing or specific disabilities. Through manipulation of the human model and various inbuilt tools, analyses can be performed of fit, posture, reach and vision.

SAMMIE is a standalone tool and is able to import data from the majority of 3D CAD software using the common wavefront.obj file format. It also includes a basic

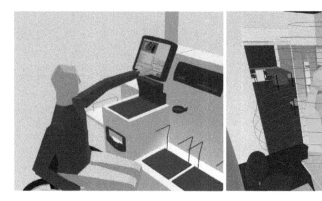

Fig. 4 Different reach assessment tools in SAMMIE. Finger-tip reach assessment to a touch screen (left). Reach volume assessment for identification of working envelopes (right)

built in modeller for the construction of simple geometry. Interactions can, thus, be explored between humans and products or workplaces, largely independently of whatever CAD tool the user has access to or a model has been constructed in. Up to 100 humans can be created within a single model providing a large degree of freedom to explore variation within the desired user population and to evaluate interactions between humans in shared spaces or collaborative tasks.

Once a human model has been created, sized and postured in a representative or possible posture for a task, a combination of direct reach, e.g., SAMMIE attempts to reach a specific reach target using a representative grip type or reach areas/volumes can be generated to understand potential working envelopes (Fig. 4). For visual tasks, SAMMIE can provide a humans' view representing what that human would be able to see form their eye point(s) in a specific posture (Fig. 5 left). In addition, volumetric projections can be produced either unconstrained as vision cones or constrained to

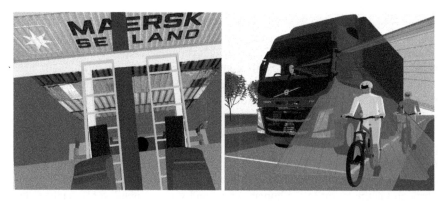

Fig. 5 Visual assessment tools in SAMMIE. Humans view provides a view from the human model's eye (s) (left). Volumetric projections allow the volume of space visible through a window or via a mirror to be visualized (right)

represent the volume of space visible through a window or via a mirror (Fig. 5 right). Through a combination visualization, qualitative and quantitative capabilities and tools, insights can be gained as to the accommodation of a product or workplace.

5.2 Industrial Path Solutions—Intelligent Moving Manikins (IPS IMMA)

IPS IMMA is a DHM tool developed in close cooperation between academia and industry in Sweden. The development of IMMA was initiated from the vehicle industries' need of an effective, efficient, objective and user-friendly software programme for verification of manufacturing ergonomics. Still, the objective is that the tool should be applicable in a wide range of applications when designing and evaluating human-object interactions, e.g., in the health care sector and the tool is continuously developed towards realizing that objective. IPS IMMA was commercialized in 2016, seven years after commencing the first research and development project (Fig. 6).

A key feature of IPS IMMA is the possibility to simulate and evaluate human-object interaction over time, i.e. representing likely motions of humans and objects in the simulation, where these motions are predicted by the DHM tool itself through advanced mathematics, i.e. requiring no collection of human data or need for databases of human motions. Another key feature is that the tool is made to simulate human-object interaction for a family of manikins, where it is enough to instruct one manikin, and the other manikins will perform the same task, but use their own unique motions. This makes it easier and more efficient for the DHM tool user to consider diversity of the user group and to verify that the design is appropriate for a range of users. Hence, aiming to support an inclusive design approach. The anthropometrics module in IPS IMMA enables the definition of manikin families using a range of different approaches, e.g., the boundary case method (see section modelling representative users) (Fig. 7).

The biomechanical model of the IMMA manikin has 82 segments and 162 joints. The spine model consists of five joints (T1/T2, T6/T7, T12/L1, L3/L4, L5/S1), which

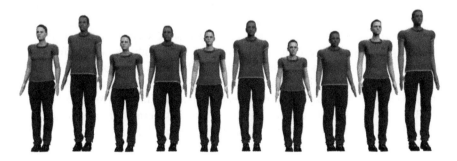

Fig. 6 A family of manikins to support consideration of human diversity in simulations

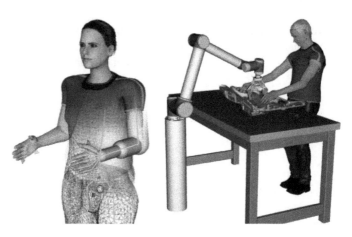

Fig. 7 Skin mesh and appearance of the female manikin in IPS IMMA (left). Simulation of elderly manikin performing work assisted by a collaborative robot (right)

is a compromise between correctness and simplicity, to achieve quick but appropriate simulations and ergonomics assessments. The biomechanical model represents a human adequate for the applications, the tool is mainly created for, i.e. simulation of human-object interaction.

The skin mesh is bound to the biomechanical model. Figure 7 (left) illustrates the skin mesh and the collider model, which are used to identify collisions, both self-collisions and collisions with external objects. Figure 7 (right) shows snapshot of a simulation of a manikin representing an elderly person performing work assisted by a collaborative robot, where range of motion limitations of the human model is considered in the simulation.

Manikin motions are defined as quasi-static, generated by inverse kinematics, where a comfort function seeks to optimize comfort whilst fulfilling present constrains, with the consideration of joint angles, high joint torques, high contact forces and short distances to the vicinity [34]. The manikin avoids collision with external objects and itself.

An alternative way to the mathematical approach for motion prediction, as described above, is to use motions from real humans, either recorded in real time or stored in databases. The first approach requires a motion capture system, and several test persons in order to represent diversity, and likely also a physical mock-up that represents the objects that the manikin interacts with. Drawbacks from such approach are that it takes time and is costly. A challenge of utilizing pre-recorded motions to steer manikins is that the motions may have low conformity for the present simulation case, especially for all members of a manikin family. Hence, by steering manikins by recorded motions, in real time or stored, several of the advantages with virtual design and manufacturing disappear or are reduced. Hence, there are benefits of having motion generators in DHM tools [43], i.e. as implemented in IMMA. Even so, the IMMA manikin can be controlled by the motion capture system Xsens™, e.g., to represent motions that still are hard to predict successfully by the motion generator algorithms.

In the development of IMMA, industry partners highlighted early the need to be able to quickly and easily steer the manikin's actions. The industry also wanted a solution that would lead to good repeatability of simulations, where simulation results would be the same or very similar, regardless of whom uses the DHM tool. This led to the development of a high-level instruction language that allows the tool user to instruct the manikin by the use of high-level commands such as a 'GRASP/HAMMER' [44]. Based on the series of manikin instruction commands entered by the tool user, IMMA automatically defines all the detailed manikin motions needed to fulfil the instructions and for all members in the manikin family. This manner of working saves a lot of time for the IMMA tool user. It also supports objectivity in that simulations are easier to repeat and with less variation in simulation results between tool users.

A central part of DHM tools is the ability to perform ergonomics evaluations of the product-object interaction being simulated. IPS IMMA contains common evaluation methods such as rapid upper limb assessment (RULA) [45] but enables also the addition of bespoke ergonomics evaluation methods, e.g., company specific methods. IPS IMMA also allows measuring and analyzing data such as joint angles and joint torque demands of the manikin.

6 DHM Case Studies

6.1 DHM and the Ageing Workforce

In a study conducted by researchers at Loughborough University in the UK, an evaluation was performed to explore inclusivity in a manufacturing environment [46]. The aim was to explore the implications of ageing on industrial activities such as assembly, where the tasks are largely manual and the demands on physical effort, repetitiveness, speed of work and overall quality are high. Observations at a furniture manufacturing company were used to inform a DHM evaluation of the working postures adopted. The observations captured specific key task related postures from a variety of workers performing the same or similar tasks. These tasks and the relevant postures were replicated in the SAMMIE DHM system. Using data from the HADRIAN database, 31 digital twin manikins were created. The human models created were based on data collected from people who were all older than 40 years and replicated both their anthropometry and their joint range of motion (ROM).

Figure 8 shows three exemplar postures (task postures 1, 2 and 3) for the same task, representing individual operator preference. The differences manifest in a number of ways including tool handling and orientation, the orientation of the item being assembled and their overall body posture. Whilst this exemplar data were collected in the real world, DHM tools have an important role to play in exploring what if scenarios and in exploring the issues for a wider demographic than may be found in

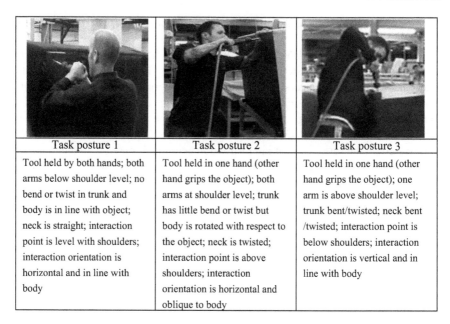

Fig. 8 Three working postures observed for the same manual assembly task

the real-world application. In this case, the use of DHM allowed the researchers to explore the potential implications of these tasks on workers who are older.

To perform the analysis, measurements were collected of the workplace and the workpiece to allow them to be modelled in CAD. The 31 digital twins were created with their representative size and joint ROM. To start, the postures were replicated with normal joint ROM limits to understand where these postures sat within the envelope of typical human capability. Then, for each digital twin, an attempt was made to replicate the observed postures. In total, 93 working postures were evaluated. Figure 9 shows resulting DHM postures for each of the three task example postures.

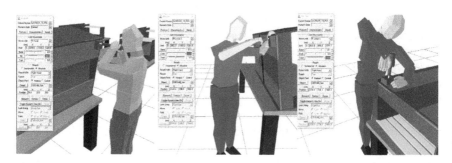

Fig. 9 HADRIAN database workers exploring task inclusion for assembly task postures: 1 (left), 2 (centre) and 3 (right)

The results of the analysis were quite revealing. Task posture 1 proved to be acceptable for 84% of the older workers, task posture 2 was acceptable for 48% and task posture 3 was acceptable for only 19% of the older workers. This resulted in 5 out of 31 older workers being excluded for task posture 1, whereas 16 and 25 were excluded for task postures 2 and 3, respectively. These results demonstrate one of the benefits of using DHM in these types of analyses to inform the understanding of professionals who work in these industries about the task demands of their operations, but also to inform improvements to working practices that can make them more inclusive. The results demonstrate that task posture 1 is the best of those observed and to accommodate older workers can form the basis of task completion training to ensure the task is as accessible and low risk as possible. In addition, DHM can be used to explore whether there are even more inclusive task postures that can be adopted to further improve practice in the real world.

6.2 DHM and Public Transport Safety

In a second study conducted by researchers at Loughborough University in the UK, an evaluation was performed to explore inclusivity on public transport and specifically buses. The evaluation was part of broader research into improving safety for older public transport users [47]. Accident data analysis shows that injury rates for bus passengers are typically low (~3%) but that older people are over represented and that a common accident type is that of standing passengers being injured due to rapid acceleration or deceleration of the vehicle [48].

To explore accident causation and potential design interventions, DHM was used to investigate any challenges faced by passengers stood on a bus or traversing through the bus [49]. A common bus type used in the UK was scanned using a 3D FARO scene scanner and replicated in the DHM system, including seating positions, steps and hand holds. Figure 10 shows the resulting bus model. The bus was populated with passengers to represent any potential obstruction to the aisle or to hand holds for the standing passenger.

A range of variables were explored in the digital environment including the implications for varying anthropometry and particularly reach range, joint ROM, the ability

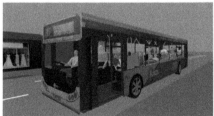 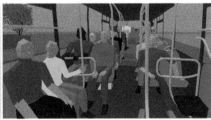

Fig. 10 Bus model reproduced from 3D scanned data for accessibility analysis in DHM

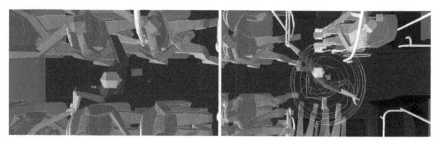

Fig. 11 Postures exploring a passenger traversing through a bus. Consistent hand holds are available up until the frontal area where holding on to brace against sudden movements is problematic

to always have at least one hand on a hand hold, whilst traversing the bus from front to back, and the implications of carrying a bag or a walking stick/cane. DHM proved useful in exploring the challenges potentially faced by passengers across a range of passenger demographic. Figure 11 shows a small (10th percentile UK female) passenger from the HADRIAN database who is 69 years old with a good range of mobility and who lives independently. From the analysis, it became clear that for the majority of the fully seated section of the bus hand holds were plentiful and the passenger could take advantage of the support provided. However, at the more open front section of the bus, near to the doors, hand holds became too infrequent to maintain grip. As such, if the bus performs a sudden manoeuvre whilst the passenger is in this section, they may not be able to sufficiently brace themselves. Furthermore, the modelling showed that if the passenger is in any way encumbered, e.g., holding a bag, using a walking stick/cane, carrying a young child, etc., that this effectively makes them one handed, and only able to use hand holds with their free arm/hand. In such cases, the passenger moving through the bus will have frequent instances where they are not braced against sudden movements of the vehicle and more liable to being involved in an accident. Given the likelihood of a passenger carrying an item, this is a significant implication for safety. A further aspect revealed during the evaluation was that hand hold type also played a role. The bus contains two main types of handle, a vertical pole from the floor to ceiling and a grab handle on the back rest of the seats. Due to potential obstruction from seated passengers, the back rest hand holds were of little use to the standing passenger.

The findings of the analysis highlighted the risks with being stood or attempting to move through the bus when not stationary. This can inform bus policy for standing passengers. In addition, the design and placement of hand holds were able to be explored and established the ground work for the investigation of design solutions to improve passenger safety, particularly in the frontal area of the bus. DHM again proved fundamental in enabling this type of evaluation where the logistical implications of obtaining a bus for a prolonged period of real-world evaluation combined with the challenges of finding appropriate users would likely result in a much too complex or costly exercise. However, in the digital environment, a broad range of variables was able to be explored expediently and design solutions could be both prototyped and tested without the need to create physical mockups.

6.3 DHM with Diverse Anthropometric Data by Cluster Analysis

In a study conducted by researchers at University of Skövde in Sweden, diverse anthropometric data were included in the process of generating data for a group of virtual test persons. The first version of the anthropometric module in the DHM tool IPS IMMA focussed on representing size variability. However, human-system interaction is not only affected by human size variability but also other kinds of variability, e.g., muscle strength and joint ROM variability. Hence, work has been carried out to enhance the functionality of the anthropometric module in IPS IMMA so that more aspects of human variability can be considered in simulations. Due to the low correlation between and in-between different groups of variables, especially for ROM variables, the boundary case method has shown to have limited use when applied on data of body size, strength and ROM [50]. Instead, cluster analysis has shown to be an appropriate alternative as it enables the generation of distributed test cases with different body size, strength and ROM, and indeed also other capability measures when data are available [51]. Cluster analysis is done by grouping a set of objects in subsets called clusters in such a way that objects in the same cluster are similar to each other and objects in different clusters are as dissimilar as possible [52].

Data on body size, strength and ROM were either collected on an individual level or predicted and synthesized which gave a dataset of 46 variables necessary for generating digital manikins in IPS IMMA. The synthesized data, consisting of 266 women and 210 men, were used in cluster analysis where the clustering algorithm was set to give six unique distributed cases, and each case was given by taking the average value of all individuals belonging to a specific cluster. The gender of each case was determined as either female or male, and the age of each case was rounded to the nearest integer.

To evaluate the generated virtual test people, two of them were used as digital manikins in a dynamic simulation in IPS IMMA. Case 4 was a 43 year old male, 1783 mm in stature and 84.6 kg in body weight. His strength was high and ROM medium to low. Case 5 was a 67 year old female, 1535 mm in stature and 77.4 kg in body weight. Her strength was low and ROM varied between high, medium and low. These two virtual test persons were used to demonstrate the difference between the cluster generated cases. In IPS IMMA, the manikins were visualized through a biomechanical model consisting of rigid links and joint centres. Maximum joint torques were calculated based on the joint strength and link length for each body part. Maximum joint torques and angles were then adjusted for each manikin. The simulation in IPS IMMA consisted of a case where the manikins were instructed to lift down a 5 kg oil tray from a truck. During the simulation, extreme joint angles and high joint torques were penalized and minimized through an ergonomic comfort function. When used in simulations, the digital manikins showed differences in movements (Fig. 12) and joint torque actuations (Fig. 13) where the shorter and not so strong manikin was forced to use more of its strength and more extreme joint angles.

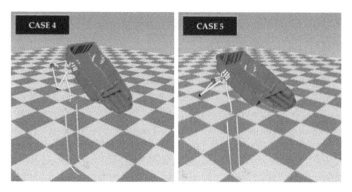

Fig. 12 Visualization and simulation of two virtual test persons as manikins in IPS IMMA

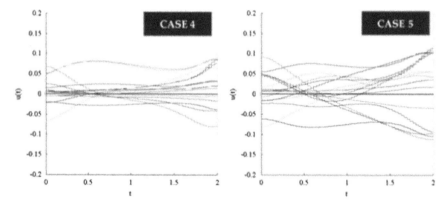

Fig. 13 Visualization of joint torque actuations during the simulation in IPS IMMA

This case study shows that it is possible to achieve more realistic and accurate simulations, as joint motors or muscle models are included into the motion prediction algorithms used to generate motions in IPS IMMA. More accurate simulations with detailed data such as joint torque actuations enable more comprehensive evaluations of the biomechanical load regarding muscle activity and possible fatigue in DHM tools. In parallel to the development of DHM tools, able to produce more advanced simulations and evaluations, systems and sensors for direct measurement of motions and muscle activity have become better, cheaper and easier to use [53–55]. These systems, with small sensors connected using the concept of IoT, give possibilities of more advanced and detailed analysis on an individual level. Similar to DHM tools, which can generate individual simulations and evaluations, easy to use direct measurement systems can help identifying which type of persons that has problems using a product or workplace and are thus excluded by the design solution. Using advanced, DHM tools in parallel with direct measurement systems can enable an improved process for inclusive design.

7 Discussion

It is clear that the ageing population poses many societal challenges. This chapter has made the case that DHM is a tool that can aid in the understanding of human capability as people age and to exploit this improved understanding in the development of more inclusive products, workplaces and environments. However, there are a number of challenges and opportunities for DHM to properly support this ambition.

As with all technologies, the capability of DHM tools continues to grow and become more sophisticated, allowing broader and more in-depth analyses to be performed. However, as discussed earlier, one of the main challenges to the use of DHM is the availability of appropriate data. In the context of being able to appropriately represent the older people within our populations, this means the need for access to high quality data on older people from nationalities across the globe. This is not a new challenge for DHM, and data for users are typically limited, but for underrepresented groups such as older people or people with disabilities, data are very limited at present and the community will need to come together to look to address these shortcomings.

As we start to improve our understanding of human capability, our need for more representative data becomes even more critical. If we follow the understanding that typically as we age, we become less capable, what we also start to observe is that humans are very adaptable. This adaptability manifests as coping strategies that allow people to manage their limitations. To properly understand, model and design for older people, we not only need data on their size, shape and capability but increasingly we also need to understand behaviour. This is one area where DHM still has significant opportunities for further development. In the main, users of DHM tools will often explore interactions and resultant behaviours of humans and products or environments typically informed by the task, the size of the human, the joint ROM and so on. However, there is an opportunity to understand what is likely for a given individual or range of people, not just what is possible. With an understanding of the characteristics of the humans being modelled, DHM has the potential to move to a position where it can offer insights into how people really behave in a given scenario and for these insights to then allow practitioners and users of DHM tools to explore innovative solutions towards a goal of much more inclusive and accommodating products.

8 Conclusion

This chapter has highlighted the challenges of the ageing population, it has also identified 3D modelling software in the form of DHM that can be used to explore some of these challenges. The value of DHM manifests in a number of key ways, the first is in the ability to explore and understand the impact of ageing on users and workers, such that the design of products, workstations and environments can take into account the full variety of human capability to develop truly inclusive solutions. Due to the digital nature of the tools, they can be exploited early in a design or development project to explore the implications of ideas on the intended users. Ideas can then be rapidly iterated to optimize solutions and remove barriers. Two DHM tools have been presented to provide insight into the types of tools that currently exist and their range of capability. In addition, a number of case studies have been presented showing how DHM tools have been used to analyze typical situations covering the workplace and manual assembly, and in the use of public transport, where the implications of being older and having potentially reduced capability may require accommodations, or design changes, to facilitate greater inclusivity. A third case study addresses the accurate modelling of users with diverse characteristics, essential for the modelling of older users. This chapter has also presented some of the challenges for DHM technologies as they continue to develop and become increasingly sophisticated. Whilst there are still many further aspects of development to pursue, DHM has many advantages to offer and can be an asset to all those looking to understand and improve the interactions between the things we make and the people that use, work and live with them.

References

1. United Nations Department of Economic and Social Affairs: World Population Ageing 2017—Highlights. ST/ESA/SER.A/397. United Nations, (2017)
2. European Union: European Parliament Briefing—Japan's Ageing Society. PE 659.419. European Parliamentary Research Service (2020)
3. Shetty, P.: Grey matter: ageing in developing countries. The Lancet. **379**, 1285–1287 (2012)
4. Gov.UK: Default Retirement Age to end this year. Department for Business, Innovation & Skills (2011)
5. USEEOC: Age Discrimination I U.S. Equal Employment Opportunity Commission. U.S. Equal Employment Opportunity Commission (2017)
6. McNair, S.: Older people and skills in a changing economy. UK Commission for Employment and Skills (2011)
7. Oxlade, A.: State pension ages on the rise: when will you retire? (2017)
8. BS 7000–6: Design management systems. Part 6: managing inclusive design—guide. British Standards Institution (2005)
9. Forrester Research Inc.: The Wide Range of Abilities and Its Impact on Computer Technology. Microsoft Corporation (2004)
10. Stubbs, N.B., Fernandez, J.E., Glenn, W.M.: Normative data on joint ranges of motion of 25- to 54-year-old males. Int. J. Ind. Ergon. **12**(4), 265–272 (1993)
11. Scataglini, S., Paul, G. (eds.): DHM and Posturography. Academic Press, (2019)
12. Duffy, V.G.: Handbook of Digital Human Modeling: Research for Applied Ergonomics and Human Factors Engineering. CRC Press, Boca Raton, (20008)
13. Chaffin, D.B.: Digital Human Modeling for Vehicle and Workplace Design. Society of Automotive Engineers Inc., Warrendale, PA (2001)
14. Case, K., Marshall, R., Summerskill, S.: Digital human modelling over four decades. Int. J. Dig. Hum. **1**(2), 112–131 (2016)
15. Bubb, H.: Why do we need digital human models. In: S. Scataglini, G. Paul (eds.) DHM and Posturography, Elsevier, pp.7–32 (2019)

16. Chaffin, D.B.: Digital human modeling for workspace design. Rev. Hum. Factors Ergon. **4**(1), 41–74 (2008)
17. Porter, J.M., Porter, C.S.: Occupant accommodation: an ergonomics approach. In: Happian-Smith, J. (ed.) An Introduction to Modern Vehicle Design, pp. 233–276. Butterworth-Heinemann, Oxford (2001)
18. Dempster, W.T.: Space Requirements of the Seated Operator: Geometrical, Kinematic and Mechanical Aspects of the Body with Special Reference to the Limbs. Wright Air Development Center, Wright Patterson Air Force Base, Ohio (1955)
19. Rasmussen, J.: The AnyBody Modeling System. In: S. Scataglini, G. Paul (eds.) DHM and Posturography, Academic Press, pp. 85–96 (2019)
20. Siefert, A. and Hofmann, J.: CASIMIR—a human body model for the analysis of seat vibrations. In: S. Scataglini, G. Paul (eds.) DHM and Posturography, Academic Press, pp.105–114 (2019)
21. Kolich, M., Taboun, S.: Ergonomics modelling and evaluation of automobile seat comfort. Ergonomics **47**(8), 841–863 (2007)
22. Marshall, R. and Summerskill, S.: Posture and anthropometry. In: S. Scataglini, G. Paul (Eds.), DHM and Posturography, Academic Press, pp. 333–350 (2019)
23. Pheasant, S., Haslegrave, C.M.: Bodyspace: Anthropometry, Ergonomics, and the Design of Work, 2nd edn. Taylor & Francis, London, (2006)
24. Roebuck, J.A., Kroemer, Karl, H.E., Thomson, W.G.: Engineering Anthropometry Methods. Wiley (1975)
25. McConville, J.T., Churchill, E.: Statistical Concepts in Design. Aerospace Medical Research Laboratory, Wright-Patterson air Force Base, Ohio (1976)
26. Greil, H., Jürgens, H.: Variability of dimensions and proportions in adults or how to use classic anthropometry in man modeling. In: K. Landau (ed.), Ergonomic Software Tools in Product and Workplace Design, IfAO Institut für Arbeitsorganisation, Stuttgart (2000)
27. Moroney, W.F., Smith, M.J.: Empirical Reduction in Potential User Population as the Result of Imposed Multivariate Anthropometric Limits. Naval Aerospace Medical Research Laboratory, Pensicola, Florida (1972)
28. Daniels, G.S.: The "Average Man"? Technical Note WCRD 53–7. Wright Air Development Center, Wright Patterson Air Force Base, Ohio, (1952)
29. Ziolek, S.A., Nebel, K.: Human Modeling: Controlling Misuse and Misinterpretation on JSTOR. J. Passeng. Cars Electron. Electr. Syst. **112**(7), 623–628 (2003)
30. Robinette, K.M.: Anthropometry for Product Design. In: G. Salvendy (ed.) Handbook of Human Factors and Ergonomics, 4th edn, John Wiley and Sons, pp. 330–346 (2012)
31. Bertilsson, E., Svensson, E., Högberg, D., and Hanson, L.: Use of digital human modelling and consideration of anthropometric diversity in Swedish industry. In: Proceedings of the 42nd Annual Nordic Ergonomic Society Conference, Stavanger, Norway (2010)
32. Dainoff, M., Gordon, C., Robinette, K.M., and Strauss, M.: Guidelines for using anthropometric data in product design. In: HFES Institute Best Practices Series, Human Factors & Ergonomics Society, Santa Monica, CA (2004)
33. Hanson, L., Högberg, D.: Use of anthropometric measures and digital human modelling tools for product and workplace design. In: Preedy, V.R. (ed.) Handbook of Anthropometry: Physical Measures of Human Form in Health and Disease, pp. 3015–3034. Springer, New York (2012)
34. Brolin, E., Högberg, D., Hanson, L.: Description of boundary case methodology for anthropometric diversity consideration. Int. J. Hum. Factors Model. Simul. **3**(2), 204–223 (2012)
35. Brolin, E., Högberg, D., Hanson, L.: Skewed boundary confidence ellipses for anthropometric data. In: DHM2020: Advances in Transdisciplinary Engineering, IOS Press BV, pp. 18–27 (2020)
36. Marshall, R., Cook, S., Mitchell, V., Summerskill, S., Haines, V., Maguire, M., et al.: Design and evaluation: end users, user datasets and personas. Appl. Ergon. **46**, Part B (2015)
37. Högberg, D., Lundström, D., Hanson, L., and Wårell, M.: Increasing functionality of DHM software by industry specific program features. In: SAE Technical Papers, SAE International (2009)

38. Marshall, R., Case, K., Porter, M., Summerskill, S., Gyi, D., Davis, P., et al.: HADRIAN: A virtual approach to design for all. J. Eng. Des. **21**(2), 253–273 (2010)
39. Sheldon, W.H.: The Varieties of Human Physique: An Introduction to Constitutional Psychology. Harper, New York (1940)
40. SAMMIE: System for aiding Man Machine Interaction Evaluation. SAMMIE CAD Ltd., Loughborough, UK., (n.d.)
41. Summerskill, S.J., Marshall, R.: Digital human modeling in the user-centered design process. In: W. Karwowski, M.M. Soares, N.A. Stanton (eds.) Human Factors and Ergonomics in Consumer Product Design: Methods and Techniques, CRC Press, pp. 293–324 (2011)
42. Barter, J.T., Emmanuel, I., Truett, B.: A Statistical Evaluation of Joint Range Data, WADC Technical Note 57–311. Wright Patterson Air Force Base, Ohio (1957)
43. Chaffin, D.B.: Improving digital human modelling for proactive ergonomics in design. Ergonomics **48**(5), 478–491 (2005)
44. Mårdberg, P., Carlson, J.S., Bohlin, R., Delfs, N., Gustafsson, S., Hanson, L.: Using a formal high-level language to instruct manikins to assemble cables. In: Procedia CIRP, Elsevier B.V., pp. 29–34 (2014)
45. McAtamney, L., Nigel Corlett, E.: RULA: a survey method for the investigation of work-related upper limb disorders. Appl. Ergon. **24**(2), 91–99 (1993)
46. Case, K., Hussain, A., Marshall, R., Summerskill, S., Gyi, D.: Digital human modelling and the ageing workforce. In: Procedia Manufacturing., vol. 3 (2015)
47. Barnes, J., Lawton, C., Morris, A., Marshall, R., Summerskill, S., Kendrick, D., et al.: Improving Safety for Older Public Transport Users (OPTU)-A Feasibility Study. Loughborough University (2013)
48. Barnes, J., Morris, A., Welsh, R., Summerskill, S., Marshall, R., Kendrick, D., et al.: Injuries to older users of buses in the UK. Public Transport. **8**(1), 25–38 (2016)
49. Marshall, R., Summerskill, S., Case, K., Hussain, A., Gyi, D., Sims, R., et al.: Supporting a design driven approach to social inclusion and accessibility in transport. Soc. Incl. **4**(3), 7–23 (2016)
50. Brolin, E., Högberg, D., Hanson, L.: Design of a digital human modelling module for consideration of anthropometric diversity. In: V. Duffy (ed.), Advances in Applied Digital Human Modeling, Proceedings of the 5th International Conference on Applied Human Factors and Ergonomics, AHFE Conference 2014, pp.114–120 (2014)
51. Brolin, E., Högberg, D., Hanson, L., Örtengren, R.: Generation and evaluation of distributed cases by clustering of diverse anthropometric data. Int. J. Hum. Factors Model. Simul. **5**(3), 210–229 (2016)
52. Kaufman, L., Rousseeuw, P.J.: Finding Groups in Data. An Introduction to Cluster Analysis. John Wiley & Sons Inc., Hoboken, NJ, USA (1990)
53. Pascual, A.I., Högberg, D., Kolbeinsson, A., Castro, P.R., Mahdavian, N., Hanson, L.: Proposal of an Intuitive Interface Structure for Ergonomics Evaluation Software. In: S. Bagnara, R. Tartaglia, S. Albolino, T. Alexander, Y. Fujita (eds.) Advances in Intelligent Systems and Computing IEA 2018: Proceedings of the 20th Congress of the International Ergonomics Association, Springer Verlag, pp. 289–300 (2019)
54. Garcia Rivera, F., Brolin, E., Syberfeldt, A., Hogberg, D., Iriondo Pascual, A., Perez Luque, E.: Using Virtual Reality and Smart Textiles to Assess the Design of Workstations. In: K. Säfsten, F. Elgh (eds.) Advances in Transdisciplinary Engineering, SPS2020—Proceedings of the 9th Swedish Production Symposium, IOS Press, pp. 145–154 (2020)
55. Zelck, S., Verwulgen, S., Denteneer, L., Vanden Bossche, H., and Scataglini, S.: Combining a Wearable IMU Mocap System with REBA and RULA for Ergonomic Assessment of Container Lashing Teams. In: N.L. Black, W.P. Neumann, I. Noy (eds.), Lecture Notes in Networks and Ststems, IEA 2021: Proceedings of the 21st Congress of the International Ergonomics Association, Springer, pp. 462–465 (2021)

IoT-Enabled Biomonitoring Solutions for Elderly Health, Care and Well-Being

IoT-Powered Monitoring Systems for Geriatric Healthcare: Overview

Alexey Petrushin, Marco Freddolini, Giacinto Barresi, Matteo Bustreo, Matteo Laffranchi, Alessio Del Bue, and Lorenzo De Michieli

Abstract Older people can be among the primary beneficiaries of Internet of things (IoT) technologies: These are capable of adapting the living environment to individual needs, enabling continuous remote monitoring, increasing social participation, improving the visual and acoustic quality of communication between people, and helping them to conduct an active and independent lifestyle. In the healthcare domain, intelligent environments empower implementation of continuous collection of behavioral information, bio-signals, and other health-related data. They can allow the development of person-centered healthcare systems, which would be capable of reducing disease burden through improved diagnostics, prognostics, personalized therapies, and follow-up solutions based on the smart interplay of long-term continuous monitoring and traditional medical treatments. This chapter provides an overview of various IoT technologies and their application in older persons' healthcare in daily living environments. First, the chapter presents the major building blocks of IoT solutions: sensors, communication protocols and algorithms, and how this technology can be beneficial for older adults. Second, the aspects of people-centered and participatory design as well as confidentiality and user data management are discussed. Lastly, an architecture of IoT-powered monitoring system is presented and design requirements are discussed.

Keywords Sensor technologies · Intelligent home · Older people · Elderly healthcare · Personalized healthcare · IoT

A. Petrushin (✉) · M. Freddolini · G. Barresi · M. Laffranchi · L. De Michieli
Rehab Technologies Lab, Istituto Italiano di Tecnologia, Genoa, Italy
e-mail: alexey.petrushin@iit.it

M. Bustreo · A. Del Bue
Pattern Analysis and Computer Vision (PAVIS), Istituto Italiano di Tecnologia, Genoa, Italy

© The Author(s), under exclusive license to Springer Nature Singapore Pte Ltd. 2022
S. Scataglini et al. (eds.), *Internet of Things for Human-Centered Design*,
Studies in Computational Intelligence 1011,
https://doi.org/10.1007/978-981-16-8488-3_6

1 Introduction

Technological innovation and achievements in medical science have significantly improved life expectancy. According to the United Nations (UN), the percentage of the world population aged 65 years and over will increase from approximately 9% in 2019 to about 16% in 2050. Even though the aging trend affects virtually all countries, it has the highest impact on Europe and Northern America, where one out four people are projected to be over 65 years of age by 2050 [1]. With age, the number of health problems tends to increase, thus osteoarthritis, diabetes, neck and back pain, hearing loss, dementia, depression, and nervous system disorders are common in older adults. In addition, older people typically experience geriatric syndromes such as functional decline, pressure ulcers, falls, incontinence, and delirium. Inevitable decline of functional ability with age calls for solutions capable of coping with the reduction of physical and mental capabilities. A rapidly aging society needs effective solutions for its healthy aging, which would help older adults to remain in good health, maintain their independence, and improve their well-being. The age shift of society is recognized as a global challenge, thus the UN launched an initiative called "decade of healthy aging 2021–2030," which helps the stakeholders to take actions to guarantee that people are able to age well [2].

Increase in population age and the fact that the number of older adults is growing faster compared to other age groups (Fig. 1) and also has implications for the economic system and labor market. Older persons are the main users of the public health system, and as their share grows, the economic pressure on employed individuals will increase. Assistive technologies and their integration with the Internet

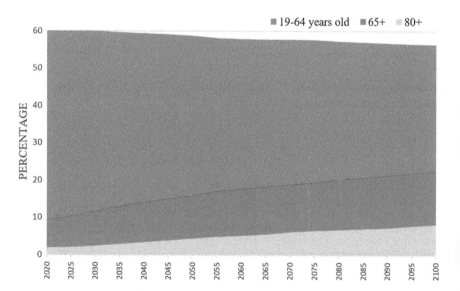

Fig. 1 World total population by age group [1]

of things (IoT) will be key factors in addressing the higher demand for healthcare services and improve the quality of life of older adults.

The IoT is a concept that encompasses a number of objects, called "things," capable of collecting and sharing information over private or public networks. The IoT includes a large range of devices: (i) ambient-based sensors that, for example, can control lighting, detect the activity in the room, and signal an emergency; (ii) wearable devices that measure a person's heart rate, skin conductance, blood pressure, etc.; (iii) smartphones, tablets, security cameras, and virtually any object connected to the network and exchanging data. Now, IoT devices play a significant role in everyday life and it will continue to grow with the evolution of technology. The healthcare industry is one of the very promising domains for IoT solutions, but the use of IoT for healthcare is still in its early developmental phase and mostly consists of limited-scale studies.

IoT technology can enable a paradigm shift from a centralized healthcare system to a pervasive model capable of being older person-centered, preventive, and personalized. Sensors integrated in the living environment and wearable sensors can make health monitoring and healthcare support accessible anywhere, anytime, and by anyone. In order to make such systems truly accepted by the user, the design should focus on the needs and requirements of older adults and heavily involve them in the design and developmental processes.

This chapter is organized as follows. Section 2 presents the available IoT technologies and their exemplary applications with special focus on monitoring functions. Section 3 discusses the aspects of the older person-centered design and challenges of privacy protection. It also presents the key design principles of an IoT-powered monitoring system and shows potential of IoT technology usage during the COVID-19 emergency. Section 4 concludes this chapter.

2 Technological Solutions

IoT has the potential to revolutionize the healthcare system in multiple ways, enabling applications such as continuous monitoring, predictive analysis of disease, interaction of patients with clinicians and relatives online, and early warnings of epidemics and drug management. From a technological perspective, the design of IoT-powered solutions can be based on various architectures and use different sensors, communication protocols, privacy protection mechanisms, and data processing algorithms. In this section, we will discuss the technologies most commonly used in IoT healthcare applications for older adults.

2.1 IoT Technologies

IoT encompasses a multitude of protocols, formats, and standards. Due to its fast development and heterogeneity, IoT technology still lacks unified standardization and does not have a reference architecture [3]. Architecture layouts vary among different industries and can differ from project to project [4]. Analysis of existing IoT architectures is beyond the scope of this chapter; nevertheless, the general data flow for every IoT architecture is roughly the same, and here, we will discuss the four-layer architecture shown in Fig. 2. This architecture provides a good tradeoff between security and simplicity and consists of the sensor layer, the network layer, the processing layer, and the application layer.

2.1.1 Sensor Layer

The sensor layer is the closest tier to the person, and it is where actuators and sensors come into play. It is responsible for gathering data from the environment and people as well as for interaction with them. The portfolio of sensors that can beneficially contribute to the wellness, and healthcare of older people is large and varied. The sensors can be classified according to (a) their proximity to the body: implantable [5, 6], wearable [7–17], and ambient sensors [18–32]; (b) type of sensed data: physiological data [33–36] and behavioral data [37–43]. Figure 3 represents the range of sensors used in IoT-based healthcare applications for older persons.

The implantable and wearable sensors measure a person's state (e.g., accelerometers, EMG, GPS) or their vital signs (e.g., thermometer, ECG, manometer). Ambient sensors are often fixed and serve to sense environmental parameters, collect physiological data, and information about the person's activities. Some ambient sensors are mobile (e.g., smartphone, RFID tag, barcode reader), though companion robots can also fit in this category.

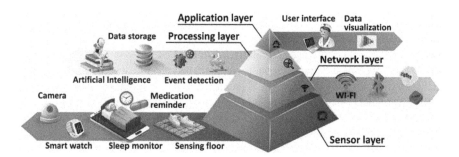

Fig. 2 IoT four-layer architecture made up of sensor layer, network layer, processing layer, and application layer

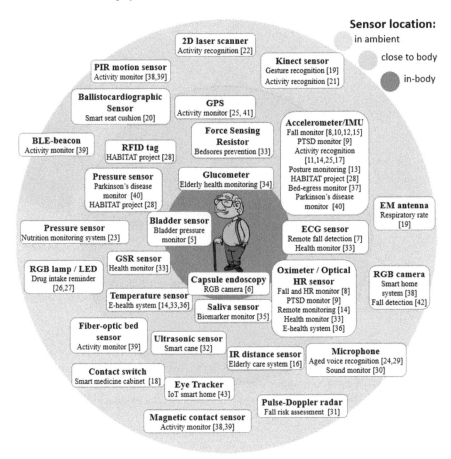

Fig. 3 Sensors used in IoT-powered elderly healthcare arranged according to the distance to the person: in-body, close-to-body, and in-ambient sensors [the numbers in square brackets indicate the reference citations]

2.1.2 Network Layer

The network layer is responsible for data collection from edge devices via wired or wireless communication protocol and their reliable delivery to the processing layer for future analysis. Due to their inherent diversity, IoT-based healthcare applications cannot adopt a single communication protocol for all possible implementations (Fig. 4). Each protocol has its pros and cons and its use should be evaluated for specific applications in terms of power efficiency, coverage, data rate, latency, cost, and security. For networks in close proximity to the person, passive radio frequency identification (RFID) is commonly used for energy-autonomous sensing while Bluetooth low-energy (BLE) is used in battery-powered applications. For home area networks where sensors need to carry a small amount of data, the energy efficient protocols

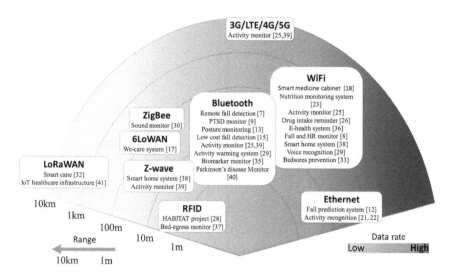

Fig. 4 Communication protocols commonly used in IoT-powered elderly healthcare, arranged according to data rate (left-to-right color gradient axis) and communication distance (radial axis) [the numbers in square brackets indicate the reference citations]

ZigBee, Z-Wave, and 6LoWPAN are most suitable. For sensors where higher transmission rates are required (e.g., RGB and depth cameras), Wi-Fi and Ethernet are good choices. The outdoor applications need long-range protocols: LoRaWAN can be used for low-power applications and cellular networks when a higher bandwidth is required.

2.1.3 Processing Layer

The processing layer is responsible for data analysis and extracting meaningful information. Translation of the collected IoT data into knowledge creates unprecedented opportunities for effective and proactive support of older persons. The use and integration of the complementary data collected by multiple heterogeneous sensors allows for improving system accuracy and reliability by compensating for occasional sensor failures, by improving spatial coverage and by reducing noise and ambiguities [44]. When the sensors have sufficient computational power, part of the processing can be done on the edge device, reducing the amount of data to be transmitted via the network.

The IoT systems can produce large amounts of data from multiple sensors, challenging the human ability for their processing. To improve the ability of data interpretation and decision-making, various artificial intelligence (AI) techniques can be used. Sensor measurements are processed and transformed from raw data to compact and informative features by either using hand-crafted or data-driven AI approaches. Hand-crafted algorithms allow for explicit modeling of important features and are typically used when we want to include prior knowledge of the data structure in the computational pipeline. However, these algorithms can be far from ideal, as they require considerable human effort to manually extract the most relevant features from the raw sensor acquisitions. Data-driven techniques are preferred for features extraction in case of unstructured high-dimensional data, such as images or video streams, but they can also be applied to other data types for reducing noise and redundancy.

In further processing stages, data patterns can be detected using either supervised or unsupervised algorithms. Supervised approaches have provided excellent results in data processing, even surpassing human skills, but their drawback is that large annotated training datasets are typically required. For this reason, a recent trend is fostering approaches that implement unsupervised and self-supervised training procedures that are becoming more reliable without the strong need for data annotation [45].

The features generated from the heterogeneous sensor data can be fused into a multisensory array and processed to extract useful knowledge related to the entire sensor network. Once all processing steps have been computed, the results are passed to the application layer.

2.1.4 Application Layer

The application layer is a top layer that provides interface and data control services for medical personnel, older people, family members, technical support, and other authorized stakeholders for interaction with and control of the IoT system. It includes Website, mobile app, service management, sensor management, health record management, and so on.

2.2 Representative Examples of IoT Applications

Telemedicine and remote monitoring have been used for home monitoring of older adults with chronic conditions, demonstrating that they are capable of reducing unnecessary hospitalizations, while ensuring urgent care when needed [46, 47]. Several studies showed positive effects on patients' health conditions, including increased improvement of quality of life [48], social functioning, general health, improvements in depression, and decreasing the number of hospital re-admissions and emergency room visits [49, 50].

Below are examples of some applications where technological solutions proved to be beneficial for specific age-related conditions.

- Risk of falls has a high impact on the health status and self-confidence of older adults [51]. Approximately, one out of three adults over 65 years old falls at least once a year and about half of them are not able to stand up without assistance [52]. Alert fall monitor [53] and video game-based trainings [54] are examples which demonstrate how technology reduces fall risk in older adults.

- Physical inactivity and social isolation are shown to be very widespread among older persons [55, 56]. Several technologies, including well-established information and communication technologies (ICTs), IoT, and robotic companion pets, have been used to increase social interaction and physical activity, showing positive effects in patients such as stress reduction, improved well-being, and quality of life [57–61].
- Dementia has a negative impact on older adult quality of life [62], safety, and independence. Technological solutions, including basic sensors such as pressure sensors, shake sensors, passive infrared sensors, and smartphones, help caregivers to detect degradation of patient condition early [63], improving care for patients.
- Reduced independence affects older adults' well-being, but technology has proven to be an effective tool for reducing falls, hospitalizations and emergency room visits [64], increasing general independence [65], as in the case of a robotic stride assistance system which improves walking performance, and in turn, decreases dependency of older adults on assistance [66]. Independence is also increased by helping older adults with medication management, which can be very demanding and potentially dangerous, with risk of missed or wrong medical therapy. Smart medication dispensers and mobile applications have been shown to effectively help older people to adhere to their medical prescriptions [26, 27].
- Depression was shown to improve with both robotics, which include robotic pet companions and IoT [67, 68], including social interaction through Internet networking.

As several IoT technologies demonstrated efficacy in improving the health and quality of life of older adults, an integrated system approach started to be developed and implemented [69]. However, most of the presented solutions have been tested in small-scale pilot studies and the process of across-the-board adoption of the technology is still challenging. Below, we will discuss two IoT healthcare projects that have been demonstrated in real-world scenarios and aim for a large-scale implementation.

2.2.1 Renewing Health

The renewing health project is an example of a partially integrated solution that aims to use telemedicine systems for the remote monitoring of older adults discharged after heart failure hospitalization. The primary outcome measured by the study was the combined occurrence of 12-month all-cause mortality or at least one hospitalization for heart failure, while secondary outcomes measured were 12-month all-cause mortality, number of hospitalizations, time of hospitalizations, number of clinical visits, and quality of life survey results [70].

Clinical data about the patients in the interventional group were collected using a digital weight scale and a wearable wrist device, given to the patients after an instruction on the appropriate use of the equipment. Data collected by the patients or with the help of a caregiver included: heart rate, blood pressure, 1-lead ECG, pulse-oximetry, and body weight. On a daily basis, collected data were transmitted to the eHealth center and automatically processed for alarm values identification. At the end of the 12-month follow-up of 339 patients (229 remotely controlled, 110 usual care), significant difference was not found regarding mortality and hospitalization for heart failure between the two groups, while the remote monitoring significantly improved patients' quality of life, showing the usefulness of the approach [70].

2.2.2 City4age

City4age is a framework consisting of different IoT services and tools capable of detecting age-related conditions and risks in the aged population. It aims to promote healthy and positive living and to improve independence and quality of life.

City4age's approach deals with the detection of older adults' behavior during everyday life in different environments such as the home (indoor and outdoor) and at city level using non-invasive technologies. Data are collected and stored in a central repository where they are processed with complex behavioral analysis and risk detection algorithms to implement a customized response for each subject, which can be delivered to the person directly or after an evaluation by a team comprising different types of clinical expertise. Smartphones play a central role in the system and are used to transmit data from the subject and to deliver services from the system to the subject. In addition, the project aims to create a large database of older adults' data, which can be used to understand possible risk factors and behavior changes, improving the quality and the speed of the response to the onset of a certain older adults' condition [25].

A preliminary trial of this system was implemented in a longitudinal cohort study performed in Madrid, where 45 older adult users were involved. Data were collected when users were moving around the city, considering nine point of interest (POIs) regions that represent places where participants usually do their activities. Collected data include activity of the user (number of steps, distance covered, and average walking speed), visiting pattern (type of POI, number of visits per POI, and visit duration), and daily transport usage pattern (number of trips, bus lines used, distance, and time per trip). The system uses a wide set of technologies, including smartphone-embedded GPS and IMU sensors, smart wristband, Bluetooth beacons, public bus networks providing information about bus trips, and the city open data service, to get different environmental information including real-time traffic, pollution, planned events, and weather conditions.

Feasibility of involving older adults in an IoT-based system for activity data collection, which could not be detected by usual assessment tools, was confirmed by this study. Preliminary data also showed the possibility of early detection of activity pattern variation, which may be related to initial functional decline; thus empowering the healthcare system with a tool for effective and preventative intervention [71].

In summary, several IoT solutions targeting older adults have already demonstrated effectiveness and usefulness in healthcare applications, improving quality of life and healthcare services. They seem to be promising to satisfy societal healthcare needs, however, more studies and large-scale implementation are needed to confirm this.

3 IoT Design for Older People

In this section, we will present a set of user-centered design requirements for IoT-powered healthcare systems for older people. The following in particular will be discussed: (i) aspects of the technology acceptance and adaptation of the IoT-powered solutions to specific needs of the user; (ii) issues of privacy violation and possible approaches for privacy protection; (iii) main design principles of an IoT-based healthcare system. Finally, we will discuss the potential of the IoT system during a pandemic emergency.

3.1 User-Centered Perspectives

The pervasive characteristics of IoT systems raise issues that must be faced to appropriately design any technology-enhanced environment for older people. For instance, the distrust of the users toward the sensor systems and the difficulties in usability can severely affect acceptance of the technology and its adoption. In particular, older users can be affected by age-related sensory, motor, or cognitive impairments, which require specific interventions in terms of usability and accessibility in service design [72]. For example, the user interfaces must be visually and acoustically appropriate for reading and listening (considering the sensory senescence) [73] should have high learnability and memorability (countering age-related cognitive decline) [74] and should be controllable through voice-based/gesture-based/touch-based commands (according to motor impairments of the users) [75]. However, the technology's acceptance is not only related to the usability in this domain: IoT solutions in intelligent environments tend to adapt contextual items to the users' conditions and needs even without their explicit commands [76].

Examining the topic of technology acceptance more closely, Tural et al. [77] discuss older people's attitudes and intentions toward smart home systems. The authors highlight that the perceived usefulness of the devices is a key aspect of all technology acceptance models (TAMs) [78] and is critical in predicting if the proposed solutions will be adopted by the users.

According to a set of real needs, the subjects involved in [77] marked the difference between products that can be (i) useful for themselves, (ii) useful for others, and (iii) overall unnecessary. Furthermore, safety was a priority for all subjects for accepting a novel solution that should increase personal security and independence.

Perceived affordability was another critical predictor for system adoption, in particular, when evaluated in terms of "return-on-investment." Privacy and security of personal information were especially relevant because of a certain distrust of technology among older adults. Finally, the requirement of usability made the authors suggest the importance of making the users try the proposed technologies.

The authors also highlighted demographic factors affecting the intention to use home automation systems. For instance, certain factors decrease such an intention: being male, getting older, or living with other people that can provide assistance. On the other hand, homeownership increases the chance of using such systems. Furthermore, the ownership of technologies like smartphones improves the acceptance of smart home systems; this observation suggests that the reluctance to accept new devices will decrease for current and future cohorts of users.

This effort to collect users' observations pragmatically constitutes a methodological premise in all ambient intelligence studies and projects: Analyzing the older user experience and preferences is definitely paramount, even when the main effort seems limited to make the technology just unnoticeable yet all-encompassing. All aspects of the older person's life must be carefully considered, including their rights, within the effort of co-designing technologies for older adults [79]—involving the final users and the stakeholders within the iterative design process. Moreover, novel tools and methodologies to identify user-related issues in IoT systems design must be devised, especially considering the quality of experience and its relationship to the quality of services provided [80]. This approach is quite beneficial to understand the most common user experience issues, with benefits for both research and industry. For instance, an innovative approach in co-design was offered by Ambe et al. [81], who proposed the IoT Un-Kit Experience: An apparently uncompleted and decontextualized set of sensors, actuators, and media components that engage older people in exploring and creating personally meaningful IoT applications. This kind of solution offers an original way to involve the final users and to collect unique information about design issues that directly affect the person/user.

Considering the most common user-centered design issues, Meulendijk et al. [82] discuss how technology acceptance in the home automation field is specifically tied to issues like obtrusiveness and intrusiveness that can derive from [83]: (1) physical discomfort (noise, obstacles impeding perception and action, asthetic incongruence); (2) usability and accessibility problems (lack of user-friendliness, additional demand of time and effort); (3) privacy violations (invasion of personal information and personal space); (4) system reliability and effectiveness (functional issues, inaccurate monitoring and feedback, low perceived usefulness); (5) lack of human interaction (detrimental effects on human relationships, absence of human response in emergencies); (6) self-perception (stigma and signs of loss of independence and related embarrassment); (7) interference with daily activities (issues with their everyday routine); (8) sustainability (affordability, concerns for future changes in abilities and needs). For example, technology acceptance can be affected by simple changes in furniture and ambient design (e.g., redecorating the rooms to adapt the spaces for the equipment) required to implement IoT solutions.

In order to mitigate these issues, Meulendijk et al. present a set of cumulative layers of technology implementation in users' environments [82]. Within these layers [84], appropriate design solutions can be exploited in each context of use.

For instance, physically embedding technologies in environments can make them less visually obtrusive. Furthermore, building context-aware systems that detect and classify the users' characteristics and actions are necessary to implicitly personalize their activity and adapt it to environmental and individual changes. This last feature is especially useful to anticipate and prevent undesirable events from occurring, completing the advantages of customization activities explicitly performed by the user. Such solutions improve technology acceptance and offer design suggestions that can be adopted in most cases.

However, these systems require an intensive and extensive level of data collection that can create further issues related to privacy violation. Indeed, the pervasive and almost invisible presence of environmental and wearable sensors in the daily life of an individual must be appropriately analyzed. This would help to design solutions to protect the users' dignity and privacy, also overcoming their distrust toward useful innovations, and consequently improving the quality of their life. A way to approach such issues is value-sensitive design [85], which is based on conceptual investigations (defining ethical and legal notions and definitions related to values), empirical investigations (studying what occurs in real contexts, primarily behaviors of users and stakeholders), and technical investigations (establishing implementation requirements like user-friendly systems for informed consent collection or state-of-the-art cybersecurity solutions). This kind of approach in user-centered design is becoming a priority in many aspects of technology-based geriatric care, including robotics and intelligent systems [86].

Considering the potential of value-sensitive design of intelligent environments for older people [87], the issues related to privacy will be discussed from a practical perspective in the following sub-section in terms of exemplary implementation approaches and solutions.

3.2 Privacy

According to the value-sensitive design framework, the definition of privacy belongs to the conceptual level and the users' trust can be considered as an empirical consequence of their privacy perception. Such a perception should be improved [88] to make IoT systems acceptable after solving objective flaws in personal data management. Moving from this premise, this sub-section will discuss privacy-related technical improvements of IoT solutions that empower the smart environments for older people.

IoT sensors are non-invasive and non-collaborative, in most cases, which means the monitored person does not need to provide any information or personal data to the intelligent system, which is able to autonomously and precisely collect and aggregate the required information. Security and privacy are, therefore, critical aspects to be taken into account in the design of any intelligent continuous assistive technology [89–91] and they are regulated by strict laws, both at the national and international level.

Usage of different communication protocols, difficulties of patching, the heterogeneity of IoT sensors, and their small storage capacities and computing power make it difficult to define effective and generalizable policies at the sensor level for reducing the risk of hacking and data breaches [92, 93]. However, privacy-preserving protocols can be implemented in data aggregation, transmission, and storage.

Traditional encryption protocols as well as the emerging technologies (e.g., software defined network (SDN) and blockchain) can be employed for mitigating the risks of fraudulent access to the data [94]. The blockchain technology, in particular, is the most efficient one [95] because of its properties such as immutability, irreversibility, and peer-to-peer verifiability of all transactions. The decentralized and distributed structure used by blockchains, along with its cryptographic properties, make it perfectly suited for healthcare applications, where security and confidentiality of the information are the priority of the system. Moreover, the current AI technologies and policies are mature enough to effectively manage the ethical and privacy concerns during data processing stages [96, 97].

The servers where data are collected should be designed so that the possibility of unauthorized data access and accidental data misuse is prevented, in the case of both cyber and physical threats. In order to achieve this goal, strong security policies should be implemented, such as firewall protection, login authentication, data encryption and anti-virus as well as limited and logged access to the data warehouses, and suitable alarming systems.

Computer vision applications (image acquisition devices and image processing software) represent particularly important examples where efficient privacy-preserving methods need to be implemented. In fact, video acquisitions expose sensitive personal information regarding people's identity, health status, property, personal relations, and more which can be fraudulently used without any further algorithmic analysis. The current computer vision technology is capable of effectively managing privacy concerns [97]. For many use cases, it is possible to use a privacy-by-design approach: Smart camera sensors can process on board and before transmitting the acquired sensitive data, discarding all the visual information that is not relevant or needed for the intended purpose. Notable examples of this approach are face masking via blurring or pixelation and object removal via inpainting [98]. Information about body joints and their dynamics is significantly less privacy-invasive than the originally acquired images and videos and still contains a large number of clues that can be further analyzed for assessing a person's health status and their response to therapy.

Nevertheless, focusing only on technological solutions for protecting privacy is not sufficient. Proactive effort should be put into increasing users' awareness [99] of data collection, processing and usage pipeline, and to support them in making better and more informed decisions about opting in or out (especially through informed consent policies) [100]. Both technology-side and user-side interventions constitute impactful value-sensitive strategies that can promote privacy protection within smart environments for older people. The next sub-section will organize the approaches presented above within a wider set of design principles that focus on IoT-powered monitoring.

3.3 Design Principles for IoT-Powered Monitoring

Ubiquitous healthcare solutions differ in terms of employed sensors, communication protocols, and data processing algorithms; nevertheless, they can still share the same framework for people-oriented design and guidelines for high-level technology acceptance among older persons. In this section, we will discuss design requirements for development of a ubiquitous healthcare system for older adults (Fig. 5). Most of these requirements were introduced in the Multiplat Age project, which aims to help geriatricians in identifying frailty conditions in older people and used in this section as a reference project [101].

An older person is located in the center of the proposed elderly healthcare architecture and monitored biomechanically and physically through **unobtrusive** sensing technologies. The system is intended to monitor multiple parameters for long periods

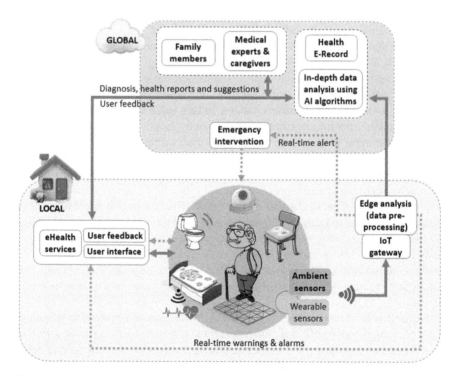

Fig. 5 Proposed architecture of ubiquitous monitoring system for older adults

of time, such as weeks and months, and it should not disturb in any way the activities of daily living (ADL) of the person nor require any training sessions, and ideally, it should be completely transparent for the user. Unobtrusive sensing is prone to human factors that can occur with wearable devices when forgotten to be worn or charged. However, monitoring of some vital parameters demands that the sensor be implanted [5] or positioned on the body [13–15] though usage of such sensors should be minimized.

In the hospital-centered healthcare system, the medical records are based on anecdotal accounts and memories of the patient between the medical visits whereas many chronic diseases require continuous monitoring rather than episodic assessments. The IoT-based monitoring system is capable of closing this gap and has to be designed to provide *continuous* evaluation of the person's health.

In the reference project, a variety of sensors for a person's unobtrusive monitoring is used (Table 1). These include floor sensors that cover the whole area of person's apartment and used for monitoring motility and basic ADL. Arrays of pressure sensors will be used to register duration and weight distribution patterns of people while on their beds or sitting on a chair. In conjunction with the bed pressure mat, a ballistocardiography (BCG) sensor is provided to assess the quality of sleep. The BCG sensor allows for no-contact measurements of heart and respiration rate as well as monitoring of bed activity. Smart toilet seat registers toileting ADL and monitors weight and heart rate during every bathroom stop. RGB cameras will be used to collect behavior data.

The sensor system must be *reliable* to produce high confidence data for medical diagnoses and prescriptions. In the proposed sensing system, the uncertainty in the data acquisition is mitigated by using more sensors to measure the same parameter. Thus, for example: (a) bed-egress event is registered by both BCG and bed pressure sensors (b) person's location and movements are monitored by RGB cameras as well as by the sensorized floor. This multimode detection approach pays back in terms of system reliability, which is particularly important in emergencies (e.g., fall detection).

Table 1 Sensors network designed for the reference project

Sensor type	Monitored geriatric factor
Floor sensor	Moving around the rooms, in-home transitions, fall detection, gate analysis
Chair pressure mat	Chair occupancy, posture, sit-to-stand/stand-to-sit transition monitoring
Bed pressure mat	Weight distribution, position monitoring, bed occupancy, bed movement activities, bedsores alarm, falling off from bed alarm, postural transition
BCG sensor	Heart rate, respiratory rate, heart rate variability, bed occupancy, bed movement activities
Toilet seat sensor	Postural position, frequency, duration, weight monitor, heart rate
RGB camera	Moving around the rooms, in-home transitions, bed/chair occupancy, fall detection

The gateway acquires data from the sensor network and aggregates them for future transmission and analysis. Collected data are processed in two steps. First, *real-time* data analysis that takes place at the edge node before being transmitted to the cloud. Edge processing provides support in situations when immediate reaction is critical (e.g., fall event, sudden cardiac arrest, falling off the bed) and it helps to reduce the amount of data that have to travel over the network. Second, data stored on the server are used for in-depth analysis, which does not require immediate feedback but can assess the trend in physical and mental states of the person and forecast the frailty conditions and illness before the symptoms become irreversible.

Results of the data analysis are stored in the database that can be queried by authorized stakeholders (e.g., medical caretakers, specialists, family members). Older adults should not rely on the assistance of the medical personnel to access their electronic health record and they should be able to consult the collected data at any time through their smartphone or tablet. The interaction system should have low usability barriers and require minimal technical skills. The older people can track their health status, communicate with doctors, seek services/support, provide feedback and receive notifications, warnings and alerts through a simple, and clear user interface (UI). Each person has specific requirements for the system (e.g., based on their habits, diseases, capabilities) which also evolve over time. To cope with these changes in requirements, the system should be *customizable* (the user can adapt the system for their needs) and *personalized* (the system is capable of self-adapting to the needs of the user).

The interaction between the system developer and the older person should already be established from the early stages of the design process. Participatory design with high involvement of older people helps designers to define and translate the user needs and requirements into the system design. Continuous *co-design* and designing-in-use [102] permit older adults to participate in the design not only during the product development, but also contribute to the characteristics of the system during its usage.

When design choices are made, particular attention should be paid to ability of the system to adapt for large-scale implementation. *Scalability* is a crucial characteristic of the design and numerous aspects can influence the ability of a system to grow. The network protocols and encryption methods should be capable of accommodating communication with an increased number of sensors; storage resources and processing algorithms should be effective in dealing with large amounts of data; implementation of access control should permit a secure interaction with the system for an increased number of stakeholders and level of decentralization. In addition, in full-scale system energy efficiency, provision chain capability, computational complexity, and cost become singular challenges and should be considered in the early design stages.

Continuous health monitoring involves collection of multiple privacy-sensitive data, therefore, methods and techniques for personal data security and *privacy* must be implemented. Ideally, the protection of a person's information should be guaranteed by design [103]. Effective privacy-preservation measures also help to build trust in the technology and improve its acceptance. In the reference project, a high level of privacy and security is achieved by depersonalization of data collected from sensors, applying privacy-preservation filters on the RGB camera images, using a 128-bit encryption key for network data transmission, and implementing identity management, where only authorized personnel have access to the system.

3.4 The Potential of IoT During the COVID-19 Emergency

The recent emergency of the COVID-19 pandemic has stimulated the development of solutions that can take advantage of IoT systems. For instance, Yassine et al. [104] discussed how the high impact of the pandemic spread on older people pushed healthcare institutions, industries, and academics to innovate policies, methods, and technologies to protect older people in long-term geriatric care homes in Canada. In particular, the authors observed the risks deriving from: (i) a lack of infection measurement, detection, monitoring, and alert systems; (ii) a lack of connected devices to detect and measure signs and symptoms of illness and to continuously track the well-being of older people; (iii) a lack of appropriate communication solutions for enabling quick interventions by caregivers, emergency units, analysis laboratories, and patient's relatives when a positive case of COVID-19 is discovered. Worldwide, these kinds of observations triggered growing global attention toward intelligent health monitoring systems. The technologies discussed in this chapter are capable of coping with the issues raised by employing minimally obtrusive, network-connected smart devices (e.g., wearable systems, actuators, sensors) to continuously track actions and conditions of older residents.

These solutions empowered through telemedicine services supported by IoT systems are obviously also valid for older adults living in their own homes. In particular, the pandemic exacerbated [105] a well-known issue affecting older people: loneliness. The COVID-19 emergency forced the authorities to establish restrictions of contact between people for stopping the spread of the disease, especially for protecting older people. This solution created further challenges in engaging them physically and mentally through social interactions, worsening their individual loneliness. Digital systems [106] (e.g., video games) [107] can help to counter such a problem by reducing social distancing and isolation through computer mediated communication solutions based on psychosocial models that guided the design of interventions. Indeed, all these solutions find in IoT several key solutions to empower and extend their effectiveness in addressing the problem of loneliness of older people, especially when the older person must cope in quarantine with the health-related consequences of a disease [108]. Thus, IoT-empowered home Gerontechnologies demonstrate that they are not only a solution for long-term issues of aging but also an effective response to a current emergency that dramatically hit older adults.

4 Conclusions

The world's aging population brings new challenges for the healthcare system, and the rapid adoption of IoT technology in the medical sector offers great potential to overcome these challenges. In recent years, a number of implanted, wearable, and ambient sensing technologies were developed for remote monitoring of behavioral and physiological parameters of human beings. These devices can be connected through IoT networks to enable older people to live an independent lifestyle for longer. These solutions could additionally improve the quality of the healthcare system by making it more proactive and cost-effective. Such an IoT-based healthcare system can be further enhanced by using efficient communication protocols, AI-powered data analysis for transforming sensor data into knowledge, and blockchain technology for secure data exchange and storage.

Implementation of IoT technology for healthcare may be prone to security and privacy threats due to unauthorized access to health records, attacks during the data transmission between the network layers, vulnerability in the device design that can allow an attacker to access the device remotely, difficulty of implementing the security patches for the devices, and inadequate data encryption. An effective defensive mechanism against the security loopholes and respect of the privacy choices of the people is a fundamental pillar of IoT technology acceptance in the healthcare domain.

In addition to an overview of IoT technologies for geriatric cares and health monitoring, in this chapter, we also provided discussion on several aspects related with technology acceptance. First, we introduced the four-layer IoT architecture which is typically used in this context and presented sensor types, communication protocols, and data processing algorithms recently proposed for monitoring older people. Second, we covered the solutions proposed in the literature and discussed in detail two projects that have had greater adoption among the healthcare community. Third, the aspects of older person-centered design and privacy were discussed. Finally, we have presented a possible model architecture of the IoT-powered healthcare system and identified main design requirements that it should satisfy, namely to be: unobtrusive, continuous, real-time, reliable, person-centered, co-created, customizable, personalizable, scalable, and privacy-aware.

We believe that this chapter can be a useful point of reference for anyone interested in technological advances in IoT-based medical care for older people.

References

1. World Population Prospects 2019: Department of Economic and Social Affairs Population Dynamics. United Nations, New York (NY) (2019). https://population.un.org/wpp/Publications/Files/WPP2019_Highlights.pdf. Accessed 30 Apr 2021
2. UN Decade of Healthy Ageing: World Health Organization (2019). https://cdn.who.int/media/docs/default-source/decade-of-healthy-ageing/final-decade-proposal/decade-proposal-final-apr2020-en.pdf?sfvrsn=b4b75ebc_25&download=true. Accessed 10 June 2021

3. Lombardi, M., Pascale, F., Santaniello, D.: Internet of Things: a general overview between architectures protocols and applications. Information **12**(2), 87 (2021)
4. Da Xu, L., He, W., Li, S.: Internet of things in industries: a survey. IEEE Trans. Ind. Inf. **10**(4), 2233–2243 (2014)
5. Dakurah, M.N., Koo, C., Choi, W., Joung, Y.-H.: Implantable bladder sensors: a methodological review. Int. Neurourol. J. **19**(3), 133 (2015)
6. Alam, M.W., Sohag, M.H.A., Khan, A.H., Sultana, T., Wahid, K.A.: Chapter 1—IoT-Based intelligent capsule endoscopy system: a technical review. In: Hemanth, D.J., Gupta, D., Emilia Balas, V. (eds.) Intelligent Data Analysis for Biomedical Applications. Academic Press, pp. 1–20. https://doi.org/10.1016/B978-0-12-815553-0.00001-X
7. Boukhennoufa, I., Amira, A., Bensaali, F., Anagnostopoulos, D., Nikolaidou, M., Kotronis, C., Politis, E., Dimitrakopoulos, G.: An IoT-Based framework for elderly remote monitoring. In: Paper Presented at the 2019 22nd Euromicro Conference on Digital System Design (DSD) (2019)
8. Bernadus, T.F., Subekti, L.B., Bandung, Y.: IoT-Based fall detection and heart rate monitoring system for elderly care. In: Paper Presented at the 2019 International Conference on ICT for Smart Society (ICISS) (2019)
9. McWhorter, J., Brown, L., Khansa, L.: A wearable health monitoring system for posttraumatic stress disorder. Biologically Inspired Cognitive Architectures **22**, 44–50
10. Bet, P., Castro, P.C., Ponti, M.A.: Foreseeing future falls with accelerometer features in active community-dwelling older persons with no recent history of falls. Exp. Gerontol. **143**, 111139. https://doi.org/10.1016/j.exger.2020.111139
11. Chen, W.-L., Chen, L.-B., Chang, W.-J., Tang, J.-J.: An IoT-based elderly behavioral difference warning system. In: Paper Presented at the 2018 IEEE International Conference on Applied System Invention (ICASI) (2018)
12. Buisseret, F., Catinus, L., Grenard, R., Jojczyk, L., Fievez, D., Barvaux, V., Dierick, F.: Timed Up and go and six-minute walking tests with wearable inertial sensor: one step further for the prediction of the risk of fall in elderly nursing home people. Sensors (Basel) **20**(11), (2020). https://doi.org/10.3390/s20113207
13. Cajamarca, G., Rodríguez, I., Herskovic, V., Campos, M., Riofrío, J.C.: StraightenUp+: monitoring of posture during daily activities for older persons using wearable sensors. Sensors (Basel) **18**(10), (2018). https://doi.org/10.3390/s18103409
14. Duran-Vega, L.A., Santana-Mancilla, P.C., Buenrostro-Mariscal, R., Contreras-Castillo, J., Anido-Rifon, L.E., Garcia-Ruiz, M.A., Montesinos-Lopez, O.A., Estrada-Gonzalez, F.: An IoT system for remote health monitoring in elderly adults through a wearable device and mobile application. Geriatrics (Basel) **4**(2), (2019). https://doi.org/10.3390/geriatrics4020034
15. Filgueiras, T.P., Torres, C.R.P., Filho, P.B.: Low Cost system for fall detection in the elderly. In: Paper presented at the 2020 IEEE 20th International Conference on Bioinformatics and Bioengineering (BIBE) (2020)
16. Al Hossain, M.N., Pal, A., Hossain, S.K.A.: A wearable sensor based elderly home care system in a smart environment. In: Paper Presented at the 2015 18th International Conference on Computer and Information Technology (ICCIT) (2015)
17. Pinto, S., Cabral, J., Gomes, T.: We-care: an IoT-based health care system for elderly people. In: Paper Presented at the 2017 IEEE International Conference on Industrial Technology (ICIT) (2017)
18. Ishak, S.A., Abidin, H.Z., Muhamad, M.: Improving medical adherence using smart medicine cabinet monitoring system. Indonesian J. Electr. Eng. Comput. Sci. **9**(1), (2018). https://doi.org/10.11591/ijeecs.v9.i1.pp164-169
19. Frontoni, E., Pollini, R., Russo, P., Zingaretti, P., Cerri, G.: HDOMO: smart sensor integration for an active and independent longevity of the elderly. Sensors (Basel) **17**(11). https://doi.org/10.3390/s17112610
20. Malik, A.R., Pilon, L., Boger, J.: Development of a smart seat cushion for heart rate monitoring using ballistocardiography. In: Paper presented at the 2019 IEEE International Conference on Computational Science and Engineering (CSE) and IEEE International Conference on Embedded and Ubiquitous Computing (EUC) (2019)

21. Cebanov, E., Dobre, C., Gradinaru, A., Ciobanu, R.-I., Stanciu, V.-D.: Activity recognition for ambient assisted living using off-the-shelf motion sensing input devices. In: Paper Presented at the 2019 Global IoT Summit (GIoTS) (2019)
22. Hu, X., Chu, D., Li, Z., Dai, R., Cui, Y., Zhou, Z., An, B., Han, Y., Jiang, C., Ding, D.: Coarse-to-Fine activity annotation and recognition algorithm for solitary older adults. IEEE Access **8**, 4051–4064 (2020). https://doi.org/10.1109/access.2019.2962843
23. Sundaravadivel, P., Kesavan, K., Kesavan, L., Mohanty, S.P., Kougianos, E.: Smart-log: A deep-learning based automated nutrition monitoring system in the iot. IEEE Trans. Consum. Electron. **64**(3), 390–398 (2018)
24. Aman, F., Vacher, M., Rossato, S., Portet, F.: Speech recognition of aged voice in the AAL context: detection of distress sentences. In: Paper Presented at the 2013 7th Conference on Speech Technology and Human—Computer Dialogue (SpeD) (2013)
25. Abril-Jiménez, P., Rojo Lacal, J., de Los Ríos Pérez, S., Páramo, M., Montalvá Colomer, J.B., Arredondo Waldmeyer, M.T.: Ageing-friendly cities for assessing older adults' decline: IoT-based system for continuous monitoring of frailty risks using smart city infrastructure. Aging. Clin. Exp. Res. **32**(4), 663-671.https://doi.org/10.1007/s40520-019-01238-y
26. Baranyi, R., Rainer, S., Schlossarek, S., Lederer, N., Grechenig, T.: Visual health reminder: a reminder for medication intake and measuring blood pressure to support elderly people. In: Paper Presented at the 2016 IEEE International Conference on Healthcare Informatics (ICHI) (2016)
27. Casciaro, S., Massa, L., Sergi, I., Patrono, L.: A Smart pill dispenser to support elderly people in medication adherence. In: Paper Presented at the 2020 5th International Conference on Smart and Sustainable Technologies (SpliTech) (2020)
28. Borelli, E., Paolini, G., Antoniazzi, F., Barbiroli, M., Benassi, F., Chesani, F., Chiari, L., Fantini, M., Fuschini, F., Galassi, A., Giacobone, G.A., Imbesi, S., Licciardello, M., Loreti, D., Marchi, M., Masotti, D., Mello, P., Mellone, S., Mincolelli, G., Raffaelli, C., Roffia, L., Salmon Cinotti, T., Tacconi, C., Tamburini, P., Zoli, M., Costanzo, A.: HABITAT: An IoT solution for independent elderly. Sensors (Basel) **19**(5), (2019). https://doi.org/10.3390/s19051258
29. Francese, R., Risi, M.: Supporting Elderly People by Ad Hoc Generated Mobile Applications Based on Vocal Interaction. Future Internet **8**(3), (2016). https://doi.org/10.3390/fi8030042
30. Griffiths, N., Chin, J.: Towards unobtrusive ambient sound monitoring for smart and assisted environments. In: Paper Presented at the 2016 8th Computer Science and Electronic Engineering (CEEC) (2016)
31. Rantz, M., Skubic, M., Abbott, C., Galambos, C., Popescu, M., Keller, J., Stone, E., Back, J., Miller, S.J., Petroski, G.F.: Automated in-home fall risk assessment and detection sensor system for elders. Gerontologist **55**(Suppl_1), S78-S87 (2015)
32. Wang, T., Grobler, R., Monacelli, E.: EVAL Cane: an IoT based smart cane for the evaluation of walking gait and environment. In: Paper Presented at the 2020 IEEE International Symposium on Broadband Multimedia Systems and Broadcasting (BMSB) (2020)
33. Ganesh, D., Seshadri, G., Sokkanarayanan, S., Rajan, S., Sathiyanarayanan, M.: IoT-based google duplex artificial intelligence solution for elderly care. In: Paper presented at the 2019 International Conference on contemporary Computing and Informatics (IC3I) (2019)
34. Imran, Iqbal, N., Ahmad, S., Kim, D.H.: Health monitoring system for elderly patients using intelligent task mapping mechanism in closed loop healthcare environment. Symmetry **13**(2), (2021). https://doi.org/10.3390/sym13020357
35. Pataranutaporn, P., Jain, A., Johnson, C.M., Shah, P., Maes, P.: Wearable lab on body: combining sensing of biochemical and digital markers in a wearable device. In: 2019 41st Annual International Conference of the IEEE Engineering in Medicine and Biology Society (EMBC), pp 3327–3332. IEEE (2019)
36. Ben Hassen, H., Dghais, W., Hamdi, B.: An E-health system for monitoring elderly health based on Internet of Things and Fog computing. Health Inf Sci Syst **7**(1), 24 (2019). https://doi.org/10.1007/s13755-019-0087-z

37. Awais, M., Raza, M., Ali, K., Ali, Z., Irfan, M., Chughtai, O., Khan, I., Kim, S., Ur Rehman, M.: An Internet of Things based bed-egress alerting paradigm using wearable sensors in elderly care environment. Sensors (Basel) **19**(11), (2019). doi:https://doi.org/10.3390/s19112498
38. Choi, Y.K., Thompson, H.J., Demiris, G.: Use of an Internet-of-Things smart home system for healthy aging in older adults in residential settings: pilot feasibility study. JMIR Aging **3**(2), e21964 (2020). https://doi.org/10.2196/21964
39. Aloulou, H., Mokhtari, M., Abdulrazak, B.: Pilot site deployment of an IoT solution for older adults' early behavior change detection. Sensors (Basel) **20**(7), (2020). https://doi.org/10.3390/s20071888
40. Chiuchisan, I., Geman, O.: An approach of a decision support and home monitoring system for patients with neurological disorders using internet of things concepts. WSEAS Trans. Syst. **13**(1), 460–469 (2014)
41. Della Mea, V., Popescu, M.H., Gonano, D., Petaros, T., Emili, I., Fattori, M.G.: A communication infrastructure for the health and social care Internet of Things: proof-of-concept study. JMIR Med Inform **8**(2), e14583. https://doi.org/10.2196/14583
42. Ezatzadeh, S., Keyvanpour, M.R.: Fall detection for elderly in assisted environments: Video surveillance systems and challenges. In: Paper Presented at the 2017 9th International Conference on Information and Knowledge Technology (IKT) (2017)
43. Klaib, A.F., Alsrehin, N.O., Melhem, W.Y., Bashtawi, H.O.: IoT smart home using eye tracking and voice interfaces for elderly and special needs people. J. Commun. 614–621 (2019). https://doi.org/10.12720/jcm.14.7.614-621
44. Gravina, R., Alinia, P., Ghasemzadeh, H., Fortino, G.: Multi-sensor fusion in body sensor networks: state-of-the-art and research challenges. Inf. Fusion **35**, 68–80 (2017)
45. Jing, L., Tian, Y.: Self-supervised visual feature learning with deep neural networks: a survey. IEEE Trans. Pattern Anal. Mach. Intell. (2020)
46. Khosravi, P., Ghapanchi, A.H.: Investigating the effectiveness of technologies applied to assist seniors: A systematic literature review. Int. J. Med. Informatics **85**(1), 17–26 (2016)
47. Ekeland, A.G., Bowes, A., Flottorp, S.: Effectiveness of telemedicine: A systematic review of reviews. Int. J. Med. Informatics **79**(11), 736–771 (2010). https://doi.org/10.1016/j.ijmedinf.2010.08.006
48. Sicotte, C., Pare, G., Morin, S., Potvin, J., Moreault, M.-P.: Effects of home telemonitoring to support improved care for chronic obstructive pulmonary diseases. Telemedicine e-Health **17**(2), 95–103 (2011)
49. Pinto, A., Almeida, J.P., Pinto, S., Pereira, J., Oliveira, A.G., de Carvalho, M.: Home telemonitoring of non-invasive ventilation decreases healthcare utilisation in a prospective controlled trial of patients with amyotrophic lateral sclerosis. J. Neurol. Neurosurg. Psychiatry **81**(11), 1238–1242 (2010). https://doi.org/10.1136/jnnp.2010.206680
50. Giordano, A., Scalvini, S., Zanelli, E., Corrà, U., Longobardi, G.L., Ricci, V.A., Baiardi, P., Glisenti, F.: Multicenter randomised trial on home-based telemanagement to prevent hospital readmission of patients with chronic heart failure. Int. J. Cardiology **131**(2), 192–199 (2009). https://doi.org/10.1016/j.ijcard.2007.10.027
51. Spoelstra, S.L., Given, B.A., Given, C.W.: Fall prevention in hospitals: an integrative review. Clin. Nurs. Res. **21**(1), 92–112 (2012). https://doi.org/10.1177/1054773811418106
52. Ambrose, A.F., Paul, G., Hausdorff, J.M.: Risk factors for falls among older adults: a review of the literature. Maturitas **75**(1), 51–61 (2013)
53. Diduszyn, J., Hofmann, M.T., Naglak, M., Smith, D.G.: Use of a wireless nurse alert fall monitor to prevent inpatient falls. JCOM-WAYNE PA **15**(6), 293 (2008)
54. Schoene, D., Lord, S.R., Delbaere K, Severino C, Davies TA, Smith ST (2013) A randomized controlled pilot study of home-based step training in older people using videogame technology. PloS One **8**(3), e57734
55. Ballantyne, A., Trenwith, L., Zubrinich, S., Corlis, M.: 'I feel less lonely': what older people say about participating in a social networking website. Qual. Ageing Older Adults **11**(3), 25–35 (2010). https://doi.org/10.5042/qiaoa.2010.0526

56. Blažun, H., Saranto, K., Rissanen, S.: Impact of computer training courses on reduction of loneliness of older people in Finland and Slovenia. Comput. Hum. Behav. **28**(4), 1202–1212 (2012). https://doi.org/10.1016/j.chb.2012.02.004
57. Bradley, N., Poppen, W.: Assistive technology, computers and Internet may decrease sense of isolation for homebound elderly and disabled persons. Technol. Disabil. **15**(1), 19–25 (2003)
58. Kanamori, M., Suzuki, M., Tanaka, M.: Maintenance and improvement of quality of life among elderly patients using a pet-type robot. Nihon Ronen Igakkai Zasshi Jpn. J. Geriatr **39**(2), 214–218 (2002)
59. Karavidas, M., Lim, N.K., Katsikas, S.L.: The effects of computers on older adult users. Comput. Hum. Behav. **21**(5), 697–711 (2005). https://doi.org/10.1016/j.chb.2004.03.012
60. Shapira, N., Barak, A., Gal, I.: Promoting older adults' well-being through Internet training and use. Aging Ment. Health **11**(5), 477–484 (2007). https://doi.org/10.1080/13607860601086546
61. Wada, K., Shibata, T.: Living with seal robots—its sociopsychological and physiological influences on the elderly at a care house. IEEE Trans. Rob. **23**(5), 972–980 (2007)
62. Moyle, W., Venturto, L., Griffiths, S., Grimbeek, P., McAllister, M., Oxlade, D., Murfield, J.: Factors influencing quality of life for people with dementia: a qualitative perspective. Aging Ment. Health **15**(8), 970–977 (2011). https://doi.org/10.1080/13607863.2011.583620
63. Aloulou, H., Mokhtari, M., Tiberghien, T., Biswas, J., Phua, C., Lin, J.H.K., Yap, P.: Deployment of assistive living technology in a nursing home environment: methods and lessons learned. BMC Med. Inform. Decis. Mak. **13**(1), 1–17 (2013)
64. Rantz, M.J., Skubic, M., Miller, S.J., Galambos, C., Alexander, G., Keller, J., Popescu, M.: Sensor technology to support aging in place. J. Am. Med. Dir. Assoc. **14**(6), 386–391 (2013)
65. van Hoof, J., Kort, H.S.M., Rutten, P.G.S., Duijnstee, M.S.H.: Ageing-in-place with the use of ambient intelligence technology: perspectives of older users. Int. J. Med. Informatics **80**(5), 310–331 (2011). https://doi.org/10.1016/j.ijmedinf.2011.02.010
66. Shimada, H., Hirata, T., Kimura, Y., Naka, T., Kikuchi, K., Oda, K., Ishii, K., Ishiwata, K., Suzuki, T.: Effects of a robotic walking exercise on walking performance in community-dwelling elderly adults. Geriatr. Gerontol. Int. **9**(4), 372–381 (2009)
67. Cotten, S.R., Ford, G., Ford, S., Hale, T.M.: Internet use and depression among older adults. Comput. Hum. Behav. **28**(2), 496–499 (2012). https://doi.org/10.1016/j.chb.2011.10.021
68. Wada, K., Shibata, T., Saito, T., Tanie, K.: Effects of robot assisted activity to elderly people who stay at a health service facility for the aged. In: Proceedings 2003 IEEE/RSJ International Conference on Intelligent Robots and Systems (IROS 2003) (Cat. No. 03CH37453), pp 2847–2852. IEEE (2003)
69. Tun, S.Y.Y., Madanian, S., Mirza, F.: Internet of things (IoT) applications for elderly care: a reflective review. Aging clinical and experimental research:1–13
70. Olivari, Z., Giacomelli, S., Gubian, L., Mancin, S., Visentin, E., Di Francesco, V., Iliceto, S., Penzo, M., Zanocco, A., Marcon, C.: The effectiveness of remote monitoring of elderly patients after hospitalisation for heart failure: the renewing health European project. Int. J. Cardiol. **257**, 137–142 (2018)
71. Almeida, A., Fiore, A., Mainetti, L., Mulero, R., Patrono, L., Rametta, P.: An IoT-aware architecture for collecting and managing data related to elderly behavior. Wireless Commun. Mobile Comput. (2017)
72. Petrie, H.: Accessibility and usability requirements for ICTs for disabled and elderly people: a functional classification approach. Taylor and Francis, London, UK (2001)
73. Morris, J.M.: User interface design for older adults. Interact. Comput. **6**(4), 373–393 (1994)
74. Alsswey, A., Al-Samarraie, H.: Elderly users' acceptance of mHealth user interface (UI) design-based culture: the moderator role of age. J Multimodal User Interfaces **14**(1), 49–59 (2020)
75. Awada, I.A., Mocanu, I., Florea, A.M., Cramariuc, B.: Multimodal interface for elderly people. In: 2017 21st International Conference on Control Systems and Computer Science (CSCS), pp 536–541. IEEE (2017)

76. Capodieci, A., Budner, P., Eirich, J., Gloor, P., Mainetti, L.: Dynamically adapting the environment for elderly people through smartwatch-based mood detection. In: Collaborative Innovation Networks, pp. 65–73. Springer (2018)
77. Tural, E., Lu, D., Austin Cole, D.: Safely and actively aging in place: older adults' attitudes and intentions toward smart home technologies. Gerontol. Geriatr Med **7**, 23337214211017340 (2021)
78. Klimova, B., Poulova, P.: Older people and technology acceptance. In: International Conference on Human Aspects of IT for the Aged Population, pp. 85–94. Springer (2018)
79. Sumner, J., Chong, L.S., Bundele, A., Lim, Y.W.: Co-designing technology for ageing in place: a systematic review. The Gerontologist (2020)
80. Shin, D.-H.: Conceptualizing and measuring quality of experience of the internet of things: exploring how quality is perceived by users. Inf. Manage. **54**(8), 998–1011 (2017)
81. Ambe, A.H., Brereton, M., Soro, A., Chai, M.Z., Buys, L., Roe, P.: Older people inventing their personal internet of things with the IoT un-kit experience. In: Proceedings of the 2019 CHI Conference on Human Factors in Computing Systems, pp. 1–15. (2019)
82. Meulendijk, M., Van De Wijngaert, L., Brinkkemper, S., Leenstra, H.: Am I in good care? Developing design principles for ambient intelligent domotics for elderly. Inform. Health Soc. Care **36**(2), 75–88 (2011)
83. Hensel, B.K., Demiris, G., Courtney, K.L.: Defining obtrusiveness in home telehealth technologies: a conceptual framework. J. Am. Med. Inform. Assoc. **13**(4), 428–431 (2006)
84. Aarts, E., Marzano, S.: The new everyday: views on ambient intelligence. 010 Publishers (2013)
85. Friedman B, Kahn P, Borning A (2002) Value sensitive design: Theory and methods. University of Washington technical report (2–12)
86. Umbrello, S., Capasso, M., Balistreri, M., Pirni, A., Merenda, F.: Value sensitive design to achieve the UN SDGs with AI: a case of elderly care robots. Minds Mach. 1–25 (2021)
87. Bhattacharya, S., Wainwright, D., Whalley, J.: Internet of Things (IoT) enabled assistive care services: designing for value and trust. Procedia Comput. Sci. **113**, 659–664 (2017)
88. Schulz, T., Tjøstheim, I.: Increasing trust perceptions in the internet of things. In: International Conference on Human Aspects of Information Security, Privacy, and Trust, pp. 167–175. Springer (2013)
89. Tun, S.Y.Y., Madanian, S., Parry, D.: Clinical perspective on Internet of Things applications for care of the elderly. Electronics **9**(11), (2020). https://doi.org/10.3390/electronics9111925
90. Alaba, F.A., Othman, M., Hashem, I.A.T., Alotaibi, F.: Internet of Things security: a survey. J. Netw. Comput. Appl. **88**, 10–28 (2017)
91. Conti, M., Dehghantanha, A., Franke, K., Watson, S.: Internet of Things security and forensics: challenges and opportunities. Elsevier (2018)
92. Hussain, M.I.: Internet of Things: challenges and research opportunities. CSI Trans. ICT **5**(1), 87–95 (2017)
93. Yu, T.-J., Sekar, V., Seshan, S., Agarwal, Y., Xu, C.: Handling a trillion (unfixable) flaws on a billion devices: rethinking network security for the Internet-of-Things. In: Proceedings of the 14th ACM Workshop on Hot Topics in Networks (2015)
94. Alkhatib, S., Waycott, J., Buchanan, G., Bosua, R.: Privacy and the Internet of Things (IoT) monitoring solutions for older adults: a review. Stud. Health Technol. Inform. **252**, 8–14 (2018)
95. Patil, P., Sangeetha, M., Bhaskar, V.: Blockchain for IoT access control, security and privacy: a review. Wireless Pers. Commun. 1–20
96. Stahl, B.C., Wright, D.: Ethics and privacy in AI and big data: Implementing responsible research and innovation. IEEE Secur. Priv. **16**(3), 26–33 (2018)
97. Cristani, M., Del Bue, A., Murino, V., Setti, F., Vinciarelli, A.: The visual social distancing problem. IEEE Access **8**, 126876–126886 (2020)
98. Liu, G., Reda, F.A., Shih, K.J., Wang, T.-C., Tao, A.: Catanzaro B Image in painting for irregular holes using partial convolutions. In: Proceedings of the European Conference on Computer Vision (ECCV), pp. 85–100. (2018)

99. O'Connor, Y., Rowan, W., Lynch, L., Heavin, C.: Privacy by design: informed consent and internet of things for smart health. Procedia Comput. Sci. **113**, 653–658 (2017)
100. Pardo, R., Métayer, D.L.: Analysis of privacy policies to enhance informed consent (extended version) (2019). arXiv preprint arXiv:190306068
101. MultiplatAge project: E.O. Ospedali Galliera—department geriatric care, OrthoGeriatrics and rehabilitation (2019). https://www.galliera.it/20/56/unita-di-ricerca-di-progettazione-e-di-attivita/multiplat-age. Accessed 22 May 2021
102. Maceli, M., Atwood, M.E.: "Human Crafters" once again: supporting users as designers in continuous co-design. In: International Symposium on end User Development, pp. 9–24. Springer (2013)
103. Regulation, G.D.P.: Regulation EU 2016/679 of the European Parliament and of the Council of 27 April 2016. Official J. Eur. Union (2016). Available at: http://ec europa eu/justice/data-protection/reform/files/regulation_oj_en.pdf. Accessed 20 Sept 2017
104. Yassine, A.: Health monitoring systems for the elderly during COVID-19 pandemic: measurement requirements and challenges. IEEE Instrum. Meas. Mag. **24**(2), 6–12 (2021)
105. Stuart, A., Katz, D., Stevenson, C., Gooch, D., Harkin, L., Bennasar, M., Sanderson, L., Liddle, J., Bennaceur, A., Levine, M.: Loneliness in older people and COVID-19: applying the social identity approach to digital intervention design. (2021)
106. Riva, G., Mantovani, F., Wiederhold, B.K.: Positive technology and COVID-19. Cyberpsychol. Behav. Soc. Netw. **23**(9), 581–587 (2020)
107. Marston, H.R., Kowert, R.: What role can videogames play in the COVID-19 pandemic? Emerald Open Res. **2**, (2020)
108. Chen, K.: Use of gerontechnology to assist older adults to cope with the COVID-19 pandemic. J. Am. Med. Dir. Assoc. **21**(7), 983–984 (2020)

Neuro-Gerontechnologies: Applications and Opportunities

Giacinto Barresi, Jacopo Zenzeri, Jacopo Tessadori, Matteo Laffranchi, Marianna Semprini, and Lorenzo De Michieli

Abstract A positive aging requires placing human changes due to healthy or pathological senescence at the center of gerontechnology design. A set of key solutions for accomplishing this goal is offered by neurotechnologies. These systems can monitor and interpret data related to the central and peripheral nervous systems for understanding the individual conditions, enabling the control and the adaptation of assistive and rehabilitative devices, influencing the nervous system itself and empowering mental processes. Focusing on non-invasive approaches (closer to real-world applications), this chapter describes how adopting these solutions can improve the daily life of seniors and help the translational study of the aging brain in real settings through approaches like the one of neuroergonomics. This manuscript also highlights the potential of neuro-gerontechnologies within emerging frameworks that could enable digital biomarker-based assessment and personalization features. In particular, pervasive solutions of Internet of Things and Minds (IoTM) can make everyday devices truly human-centered (and, in this case, senior-centered). Indeed, a network of systems interpreting a person's will and needs defines a step-change to properly serve human beings according to their fragilities.

Keywords Neurotechnology · Gerontechnology · Human-Centered Design · Personalization · Internet of Things · Digital Health

---

Marianna Semprini and Lorenzo De Michieli equally contributed to this work.

G. Barresi (✉) · M. Laffranchi · M. Semprini · L. De Michieli
Rehab Technologies Lab, Istituto Italiano di Tecnologia, Genoa, Italy
e-mail: giacinto.barresi@iit.it

J. Zenzeri
Robotics, Brain and Cognitive Sciences, Istituto Italiano di Tecnologia, Genoa, Italy

J. Tessadori
Visual Geometry and Modelling, Istituto Italiano di Tecnologia, Genoa, Italy

© The Author(s), under exclusive license to Springer Nature Singapore Pte Ltd. 2022
S. Scataglini et al. (eds.), *Internet of Things for Human-Centered Design*,
Studies in Computational Intelligence 1011,
https://doi.org/10.1007/978-981-16-8488-3_7

1 Introduction

Elderly people typically show age-specific mild-to-severe progressive impairments to cognitive, sensory, and motor skills because of multiple health conditions [1]. Such conditions span from chronic metabolic illnesses like diabetes [2] to neurodegenerative processes in dementia syndromes [3], with potential co-morbidities [4]. In this context, enabling a positive aging depends on carefully considering the human changes due to healthy or pathological senescence. According to skills, limitations, and needs of older adults, gerontechnologies [5, 6] (here labeled as gerontech) are conceived for improving the quality of their life in daily contexts.

Gerontech can exploit various technological advances targeting the different needs of seniors. Among the systems that can improve the quality of elder people's life, neurotechnologies [7] (or neurotech) offer a rich set of versatile and groundbreaking key solutions.[1] In this manuscript, we will consider neurotech [8] as a class of solutions designed according to neurophysiological principles (e.g., the relationship of cognitive and motor activity with the neural plasticity) or devices processing data related to the (central or peripheral) nervous system.

Accordingly, neurotech can (i) infer or map the state of the individual nervous system, (ii) control other technologies according to physiological and motor data on a person's activity, (iii) act on the nervous system anatomo-physiology through direct (e.g., electromagnetically eliciting the brain cortex) or indirect (e.g., guiding and perturbing a limb motion according to neurorehabilitation protocols) stimulations. These general features are certainly useful to maintain and restore elderly's well-being and autonomy in many ways.

This chapter introduces sample applications of what such heterogeneous solutions can offer to improve the quality of seniors' life across activities of daily living (ADLs) and clinical procedures. The adoption of neurotech in this context, intended as devices or as accessories for solutions like assistive systems, leads us to the definition of "neuro-gerontechnologies" (or neuro-gerontech) for referring to senior-oriented devices with neurotech features. Furthermore, we will propose the potential of synergies between these technologies and recent advances in Digital Health and Internet of Things (IoT), offering personalization features definitely useful for older adults.

Before introducing these applications and opportunities, the next section will introduce general aspects of aging processes affecting the nervous system and the related individual skills.

2 The Aging Nervous System

The border between healthy and pathological senescence [9, 10] can be quite fuzzy [11]. However, a healthy aging of the brain is characterized by diversified anatomical

---

[1] https://www.ft.com/content/9792bb60-b794-11e9-8a88-aa6628ac896c

and functional changes that can lead to deficits in attention, emotions, sleep, language, speech, decision-making, and working memory [12]. On the other hand, such changes [13] increase the risk for pathological conditions to occur.

Thus, even in typical senescence, we may find alterations that can lead to multiple difficulties in the individual adaptation to everyday life, including sensory [14], motor [15], and cognitive [16] impairments, and abnormalities (caused by medications too) in autonomic functions [17] that affect older people's capability to cope with everyday stressors and accidents.

Pathological conditions can derive from events like ischemic stroke [18] or from etiologically various forms of neurodegeneration [9], e.g., Alzheimer's disease (AD), Parkinson's disease (PD). Certain neurodegenerative conditions tend to occur frequently in older people. They can be initially difficult to detect, as in the differential diagnosis of mild cognitive impairment (MCI) [19] with AD and elderly depression [20]. This occurs for rare diseases too, like the amyotrophic lateral sclerosis (ALS) [21], considering related severe motor impairments [22].

Furthermore, systemic conditions [23] like hypertension and atherosclerosis can lead to neural damage (e.g., stroke, vascular dementia) [24]. Moreover, the variety of morphological and physiological alterations in the aging brain [23] can increase the difficulty of initially distinguishing the intrinsic senescence effects from the consequences of cumulative environmental insult, ingravescent chronic diseases (like diabetes or rheumatoid arthritis), and their psychological impact [25].

Particular attention must be paid to events like falls, which may cause the transition from healthy to pathological aging with a sudden decrease in autonomy. The risk for an older adult to fall can depend on multiple age-related factors as visual, vestibular, somatosensory, proprioceptive, balance, and motor coordination deficits [26–28]. Such impairments can be caused by a large range of medical conditions (e.g., stroke, diabetic peripheral neuropathies). Furthermore, an old age or age-related syndromes of frailty [29] can obstacle the spontaneous recovery and rehabilitation outcome after an accident. They can also deteriorate the elderly conditions, leading to loss of independence, institutionalization, and death.

This section shortly introduced a set of general issues in nervous system aging: constraints and targets for neuro-gerontech, which must be based on aging neuroscience discoveries. For instance, brain plasticity persists in older people [30], especially if they maintain an active lifestyle or perform clinical training tasks [31–33]. The examples of neurotech presented in next section are based on this kind of neuroscientific concepts.

3 Neurotech Applications

Different kinds of neurotech can be successfully exploited as sub-components of neuro-gerontech for improving the conditions of older adults. Considering the introductory scope of this chapter, we will mainly consider non-invasive solutions, more affordable and acceptable for a large population, as seniors not necessarily characterized by severe pathological conditions.

In each sub-section, we will present as neurotech any system based on live processing of data directly or indirectly related to the (central or peripheral) nervous system. According to neural principles, neurotech can be designed to monitor and analyze the physiological states of a person (Sect. 3.1), enable the control of assistive technologies (Sect. 3.2), restore neuromotor functions (Sect. 3.3), regulate, train, enhance, or vicariate mental processes (Sect. 3.4). The list of applications in this section is certainly non-exhaustive: it shows sample neurotech domains with potential benefits for elderly.

3.1 Physiological Monitoring as a Neurotech Foundation

Since the transition to pathological conditions is usually unpredictable, physiological monitoring is a priority for promoting healthy aging. For instance, severe forms of dementia are typically preceded by MCI, whose timely diagnosis allows the prevention or delay of the more advanced stages [34]. In order to find early biomarkers of MCI onset, portable solutions which enable at-home monitoring of physiological indices are preferable, because they allow the collection of health-relevant data, without the need for the person to physically meet a clinician.

While systems to measure physiological parameters such as blood pressure or oxygenation level are routinely used to constantly check on the patient, nowadays, portable neurotechnologies relying on brain signals are also available. Brain activity can indeed be measured with non-invasive techniques, such as electroencephalography (EEG). EEG [35] reflects the sum of neuronal activity within the brain and is used in clinic to diagnose and/or monitor physiological processes (like sleep) and neurological conditions (like epilepsy). Portable EEG systems (even at reasonable prices) comprise: (i) caps that can be customized (in terms of number and location of electrodes) in order to adhere to the specific need; (ii) user-friendly interfaces to allow recording of brain data. Another non-invasive solution (and a promising candidate for extra-laboratory applications) is the functional near-infrared spectroscopy (fNIRS), which allows the monitoring of oxygenation level to perform the functional analysis of brain activity [36].

EEG [37], fNIRS [38], and other (more expensive and hardly portable) solutions like magnetoencephalography (MEG) [39] have been employed in several studies to identify relevant biomarkers of MCI or AD. The proposed methods are relatively easy to replicate and rather effective in assessing sensory and cognitive processes. However, there are, at present, no clinically accepted protocols to provide a definitive dementia diagnosis from EEG, fNIRS, or MEG signals alone. One of the main limitations in the translation from experimental methods to clinical application is the lack of longitudinal studies: the possibility of long-term neuropsychological testing would allow the collection of data critical for the development of new clinical protocols.

It must also be noted how peripheral biosignals (e.g., electromyography, EMG; galvanic skin response, GSR; heart rate variability, HRV) or highly specific motor activities (e.g., at ocular level: the gaze movements and the pupillometry) can be used to monitor cognitive and affective processes, especially "in the wild" [40–43]. They are employed as indices of the nervous system activity without being neural signals themselves. Particularly, their collection is entrusted to highly portable devices that are typically included in low-cost wearable systems. Without being obnoxious to wear like most EEG or fNIRS systems, these solutions are used in daily life to monitor physiological changes that could be used to infer sleep quality [44], stress level [45], or cognitive load [46]. Overall, they can work as "peripheral neurotech." Such approach discloses the opportunity of inserting neurotech within a sensor network including smart objects [47].

In general, monitoring systems constitute the foundations for other types of neurotech based on interactive features sustained by the live processing of physiological data. This is the case of neurointerfaces, exploiting neural signals for enabling human–machine interactions. They mostly refer to central nervous signals under the label of brain–computer interfaces (BCIs). This term leads to the topic of next sub-section, focused on BCIs controlling assistive systems.

3.2 Brain–Computer Interfaces for Assistive Technology Control

BCIs are designed to directly translate brain activity into commands to allow the control of external devices [48–50]. Such technologies can be broadly divided into invasive BCIs, with access to the exposed human brain, or non-invasive BCIs, which does not physically cross the scalp.

The most widely adopted invasive BCIs [51] are based on electrical recordings, with electrodes placed either on the surface of the brain (electrocorticography, ECoG) or within the brain itself (intracranial electroencephalography, iEEG). When compared to their non-invasive counterparts, invasive technologies guarantee a vastly superior signal quality, both in terms of signal-to-noise ratio (snr) and in terms of concurrently controllable degrees of freedom. The obvious drawbacks are the increased costs and risks, complex maintenance, and ethical concerns, which strongly limit the widespread adoption of these BCIs outside laboratories.

The opposite is true for non-invasive, EEG-based BCIs [52]: the required equipment is relatively simple, with user-friendly and portable or wearable solutions already commercially available at different prices and different options for customization (e.g., InterAxon Muse,[2] OpenBCI,[3] Emotiv Insight/Epoc/Flex,[4] g.tec

---

[2] https://choosemuse.com/
[3] https://openbci.com/
[4] https://www.emotiv.com/

Fig. 1 Emotiv EPOC X, a low-cost EEG-BCI used in studies like [54]

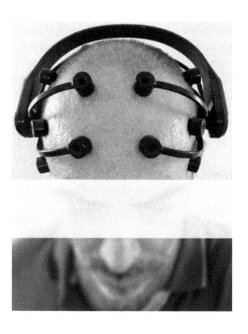

Nautilus Pro,[5] g.tec Unicorn[6]). Their disadvantage is low SNR and the ability to control a small number of degrees of freedom, which, in turn, result in a low information transfer rate (ITR): during active control, in a laboratory setting, the highest claimed ITR is 175 bit/min [53]. Figure 1 shows an example of consumer-level EEG-BCI. These systems can hardly offer the reliability of those for clinical and laboratory use. However, they are useful for fast initial prototyping and for preliminarily testing the neurotech acceptance and user experience in basic settings if their performance is sustained by appropriate signal analysis solutions. Obviously, the system limitations must be considered before implementing any assistive or clinical solution for people with severe impairments as in case of ALS.

Several non-invasive, non-EEG alternative technologies can also provide signals useful to control BCIs: MEG [55], functional magnetic resonance imaging (fMRI) [56], functional transcranial Doppler ultrasonography [57] and fNIRS [58]. While deployable in a laboratory setting, most of these techniques rely on devices that have been, so far, impossible to reduce to a relatively portable size. The only exception regards fNIRS: indeed, in the last few years, a growing number of wearable devices for fNIRS have been introduced [59], paving the way for their use in healthcare solutions.

Overall, the most direct contribution of BCI technologies to quality of life in elderly people is the possibility of reducing the impact of motor control impairments (as the ones occurring after a stroke or during the progression of ALS): one of the most promising developments, in this field, is the introduction of BCI control schemes for

---

[5] https://www.gtec.at/product/gnautilus-pro/

[6] https://www.unicorn-bi.com/

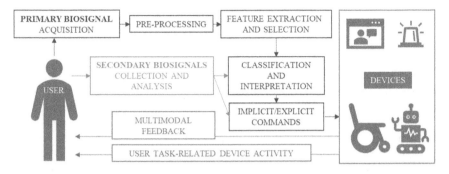

Fig. 2 A sample hybrid BCI setup

assistive devices like wheelchairs [60], robotic devices (e.g., exoskeletons) [61], and smart home technologies [62].

Further innovations come from the integration of multiple information sources to empower BCIs. For instance, hybrid BCIs (Fig. 2) exploits different types of signals (at least one derived from the brain activity) [63], combining them to obtain improvements in understanding the user's commands. Such an approach can be useful, for instance, to enable adaptive processes of self-calibration and personalization according to EEG signals related to voluntary control (e.g., sensorimotor rhythms in motor imagery) and to spontaneous reactions (e.g., error-related potentials) [64, 65]. A typical supplementary source of information in hybrid BCIs is constituted by gaze motion [66]. Eye-trackers are generally more usable than BCIs to control a graphic user interface. Such an advantage is highlighted in hybrid (oculo-cerebral) BCIs for improving the flexibility of communication systems like spellers [67].

Figure 2 shows an example of a generic hybrid BCI [68] concept, where 2 (or more) different types of signals are used to empower the detection of user intentions and conditions. This can increase the adaptability of the technological environment to the individual explicit goals and implicit needs (based on spontaneous reactions related to stress and emotions, for example). Accordingly, we can foresee solutions for both voluntary alarm calls and automated support calls, especially using autonomic nervous system-related signals (like HRV and other physiological indices related to stress, mood and emotion changes, or conditions like drowsiness) [69, 70].

Expanding the topic to hybrid systems that do not include brain signals (thus, body–machine interfaces instead of neurointerfaces) for enabling the user to control other systems, insightful opportunities can come from oculo-physiological interfaces like the one in [71]. That solution is based on GSR-biofeedback and eye-tracking to implement an accessible game design solution for people with severe motor impairments. Such systems offer interesting opportunities for further combinations with BCI solutions.

Overall, the assistive technologies based on BCIs are oriented to restore individual autonomy in performing ADLs. However, neurotechnologies can also be used to assist clinical activities like neurorehabilitation, as the next sub-section will discuss with focus on motor functions recovery.

3.3 Neuromotor Rehabilitation Technologies

Elderly people frequently suffer from brain injuries or neurological disorders (e.g., stroke) that result on motor dysfunctions and, consequently, affect their quality of life and the possibility to perform even simple activities. Extended reality (XR—the set of different combinations of reality and virtuality within the same setting) [72] offers a large set of game-based solutions for supporting the neurorehabilitation activities. The taxonomy of XR (e.g., virtual reality, augmented reality, mixed reality) is furtherly discussed in this book—see the chapter titled "Video Games for Positive Aging: Playfully Engaging Older Adults." Mainly, virtual and augmented environments increase patients' engagement (also at neural level) [73] and, consequently, their clinical adherence. Low-cost XR technologies offer digital tools for neurotraining and neurorehabilitation of elderly [74] as described in the next subsection about cognitive processes too. In general, XR-based solutions like interactive neurorehabilitation (INR) [75] systems enrich the therapeutic protocols with the possibility to assess the patient's movements and deliver an automated and, possibly, adaptive feedback, guiding the motor learning and re-learning too.

However, general XR solutions are based on multimodal feedback usually lacking a kinesthetic physical guidance of the impaired limbs. This kind of activity would be quite effective in engaging all physio-motor functions in any ordinary action. Robotic systems can perform such a process for enhancing neurorehabilitation [76], optimizing and speeding up the recovery of the patients, possibly in synergy with XR systems [77], BCIs [78], and other solutions from neurofeedback [79] to neuromodulation [80] (discussed in next sub-section).

These intelligent mechatronic systems work as neurotechnologies because they assist exercises that actually shape the nervous system of the patient to restore its functions interactively, according to the live processing of motor data and to training protocols based on neural principles (e.g., plasticity) [81]. Rehabilitation robots can be classified as exoskeletons or end-effectors.

Exoskeletons are designed for coupling and aligning the mechanical joints to the human ones. They influence the limb motion through the control of the position and the orientation of each joint. Examples of upper limb exoskeletons are: ARMEO Power [82], UL-EXO7 [83], Pneu-Wrex [84]. On the other hand, examples of lower limb exoskeletons are: Lokomat [85], Ekso [86], Twin [76, 87].

End-effectors are robotic devices designed to mechanically constrain the distal part of the human limb (e.g., the hand), which adapts to robot motion. Examples of upper limb end-effectors are MIT Manus [88], Braccio di Ferro [89], Wristbot [76, 90]. Furthermore, examples of lower limb end-effectors are Haptic Walker [91], G-EO Systems [92], hunova (depicted in Fig. 3) [93].

The clinician can choose between the two types of robotic technologies (exoskeletons or end-effectors) depending on the severity and specific features of the neurological impairment. For instance, if the residual functionalities of the patient are extremely low, exoskeletons could be more appropriate to apply forces to each joint.

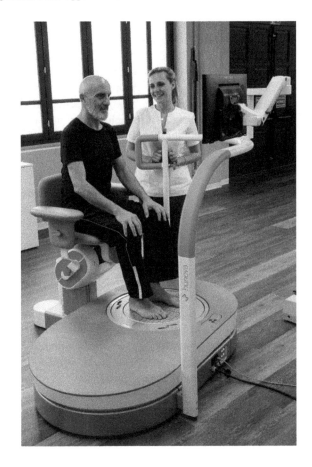

Fig. 3 Features of the hunova robotic platform include valuable solutions for neuromotor rehabilitation (especially effective for elderly) with diagnostic-prognostic functions too (e.g., predicting the risk of fall). Photograph: a patient on hunova. Courtesy of Movendo Technology. www.movendo.technology

Conversely, end-effectors could be more effective to deliver patterns of forces able to exploit the redundancy of the human body, and thus speeding up the recovery.

Overall, these robots have key capabilities in assessment and training. Indeed, rehabilitative robots enable a reliable quantitative functional assessment of the human neurological conditions in order to optimize the patient's chance of recovery [94, 95]. Thus, they offer objective and repeatable outcome measures on the progress of the recovery [96] for increasing the efficiency of patients' care. Furthermore, these robotic systems effectively promote the patients' recovery, according to their residual abilities, through different control strategies [97] based on the latest findings on neuroplasticity too. Training modalities can be robot-driven or patient-driven. Especially useful are the active assistive training modalities, helping the participants to move their impaired limbs according to the desired postures during grasping, reaching, or walking, reflecting the strategies of physical and occupational therapy. Specifically, the assistance-as-needed is widely employed because it reduces the patient risk of relying only on the robot to accomplish the rehabilitative task.

Recent randomized controlled trials aim at demonstrating the effectiveness of robotic technologies in elderly neurorehabilitation programs [98–102] that can also employ EEG and NIRS solutions [103]. However, most examples presented so far tended to show cases of neurotechnological aids oriented to help conditions that typically affect heterogenous groups of people, without specifically targeting older adults. On the other hand, the next sub-section will present another set of system that can be advantageous for people of any age, even if, frequently, the literature specifically focus on their benefits for seniors.

3.4 Neurotech for Supporting and Improving Mental Well-Being and Functions

The different kinds of frailty in seniors impair their psychosocial balance and their possibility and desire to be active, facilitating the emergence of different types of mental issues. Thus, the need of caring for older adults' mental well-being is a priority for the healthcare system. Accordingly, neurotech can contribute in monitoring and stimulating fundamental aspects of the individual life like positive affective states.

For instance, we can talk about biofeedback when live biosignals visualization is designed to be observed by the subject within a closed-loop, enabling the self-regulation of biological variations [104]. Biofeedback is traditionally adopted to display cardiovascular and respiratory indices for training a person in their control, mitigating stress, easing relaxation or emotion regulation, with impact on autonomic nervous functions like sleep. Biofeedback can be empowered by advanced visualization systems like virtual and augmented reality [105, 106]. They can also be based on wearable and mobile low-cost equipment for detecting and displaying (through different sensory modalities) biosignals [107, 108].

Considering age-specific issues, a HRV biofeedback-based sleep improvement (BBSI) [109] was used to help elderly Korean women with overactive bladder syndrome (OAB), mitigating the effects of urinary symptoms and sleep issues. Biofeedback solutions were also implemented for improving the balance of elderly [110] through a smartphone used as a sway sensor. Accordingly, feedback on the tilt of the torso was provided by a screen and a haptic device.

However, biofeedback systems typically target autonomic nervous functions regulation through peripheral biosignals display. When neural signals are directly used, we refer to neurofeedback, implemented through techniques like EEG [111] or fNIRS [112] to empower cognitive (especially attentional) processing through training. Neurofeedback constitutes an example of neurointerface system connecting neural signals to (display) devices.

Overall, biofeedback can support therapeutic activities in mental health domain, as in cases of anxiety and depression of elderly [113]. Particular attention must be paid to design engaging and meaningful solutions—musical neurofeedback has been used to treat depression in older adults [114]. Such systems enable both activities of prevention and treatment of psychological issues.

In particular, they can target the improvement of the cognitive skills during healthy senescence for maintaining the individual autonomy, self-efficacy, and well-being. This can even compensate the general sensorimotor impairments caused by aging and delay the impact of mild or severe mental decline. According to the same principles, these systems can also contribute to elderly cognitive neurorehabilitation, especially through XR and game-based settings [115, 116]. These settings can engage the individual (even in terms of specific mental processes) in meaningful tasks that can simulate different real-life activities (usually targeted by occupational therapy) in a safe and ecologically valid environment [117]. Furthermore, literature suggests how it is possible to shape the nervous system through cognitively challenging training solutions that elicit brain plasticity in VR settings with clinically relevant improvements [118].

Similarly, a certain degree of neurocognitive changes could also happen through low-cost engaging video games (even on commercial portable platforms) like exergames that can work as mental and social stimulation methods while they promote physical activity [119–121]. They can enhance the cognitive processing speed and (executive functions, attention, and working memory) performance in healthy and pathological senescence [122–125]. This approach can also be empowered by solutions that directly access biosignals in closed-loop setups for neurofeedback [126] and other types of BCI [127], possibly based on low-cost equipment [62] and on engaging virtual environments [128].

In any case, the effectiveness of brain trainings is still debated [129], even if it could depend on issues in senior-centered game design, as pondered in this book within the chapter titled "Video Games for Positive Aging: Playfully Engaging Older Adults." Engagement requires an appropriate design, especially based on challenging tasks in meaningful settings [130] instead of non-entertaining patterns.

Interestingly, the effects of neurotraining are not limited to the cognitive processing: they can also holistically involve the psychophysiological health of the older person. For instance, the Healthy Brain Ageing Cognitive Training (HBA-CT) program [131] improved the cognitive functions, the mood, and the sleep functions in seniors at risk of dementia. This suggests the adoption of such a system as secondary prevention strategy.

Considering the most recent advances in neurotech, we need to discuss the opportunity of a more direct approach to assist the nervous system, optimizing neurotraining too. Neuromodulation [132] techniques offer such a solution. They are based on reversible, adjustable, and non-destructive procedures of electrical, mechanical, or chemical modification, inhibition, stimulation, regulation, and therapeutic alteration of the nervous system. It can be used for managing problems like chronic pain, movement disorders, psychiatric disorders, epilepsy, dysmotility disorders, disorders of pacing, spasticity. Among these techniques, transcranial magnetic stimulation (TMS), transcranial direct current stimulation (tDCS), and transcranial alternating current stimulation (tACS) are based on devices altering the electrical activity of the brain by means of applied magnetic field or electric current delivered non-invasively. Importantly, tDCS and tACS can be designed as portable devices [133].

The variety of neuromodulation applications potentially useful for elderly—from improving stroke rehabilitation [134] to promoting brain plasticity through neuromarker-driven neuromodulation [135]—highlights how fertile this approach can be. Indeed, neuromodulation systems can be developed for: managing drug-resistant chronic pain in elderly [136] and other disorders that could be resistant or dangerous to treat pharmacologically, as in some cases of geriatric depression [137], coping with autonomic issues in urinary functions [138], treating geriatric mood and cognitive disorders [139], predicting the progression of mild cognitive impairments to dementia [80]. The potential of neuromodulation in mitigating the cognitive decline in healthy senescence is still debated and investigated [140].

Interestingly, neuromodulation systems also include widespread solutions like cochlear implants [141], which are the most typical example of neuroprosthetic systems [142] for elderly because of their capability to augment and substitute the functions of a neurosensory apparatus. Overall, neuroprosthetics [143] embrace devices that can restore or replace a damaged motor, sensory, or cognitive system. In the last case, they are considered advanced examples of cognitive prostheses, which can also be solutions without any biosignal collection feature: for instance, they can stimulate the memory of older people through experiences like the visual exposure of salient stimuli [144] or the assistance of a robot companion [145].

Neuroprosthetic systems can be non-invasive like EEG-BCIs [146] or invasive like the deep brain stimulation (DBS) neuromodulation systems [147]. Such advances are developed within domains like cognitive neuroengineering, neurobionics, and human augmentation [148–151]. Overall, neuroprostheses can target both people with neurological conditions and healthy individual that aim at performance enhancements. In particular, neuroenhancement technologies [152] can already provide elderly with promising and safe instruments for assisting their independence through the improvement of their capability to acquire novel skills. Overall, the promise of restoring, replacing, or enhancing lost cognitive skills depends on research and development. However, "futuristic" applications of neurotech, potentially shifting to neuro-gerontech, are moving outside the laboratories, for instance as consumer-level tDCS systems [153].

This section presented examples of potential and actual neurotech for elderly. The next section will describe possible routes for innovation in this field, considering the fertile crossing with recent human-centered trends.

4 Perspectives on Neuro-Gerontech Design

Neuro-gerontech design and development must match the elderly needs in real contexts [154] for assisting seniors in daily and clinical activities. Such processes should follow the approach of translational research, especially in clinical domains [155]. Indeed, translational research can ignite the transfer of the laboratory results to real-world applications [156]. Furthermore, translational studies should adopt ecologically valid settings [157] for reaching a high technology readiness level (TRL)—an estimation of a solution maturity (e.g., about smart homes for elderly) [158]. This approach is favored by technology transfer activities, supporting researchers to make their investigations outcome become a real product, especially for a growing market of users like seniors. Such a process is extremely valuable, and it requires an appropriate educational path for scientists [159]. However, the needs of people with fragilities should guide and drive the technological research from its very early stage in laboratory. This effort keeps the balance between the bravest research explorations (generating innovative concepts) and the market access perspective (maintaining the guidance of user needs).

Interestingly, neurotech can become a senior-centered innovation factor to improve the usability and accessibility of other devices [160]. Indeed, they can enable people with impairments to control daily use technology through alternative and augmentative options based on the detection of their will and spontaneous reactions. Considering these peculiarities, neurotech-empowered devices should be considered as neurotechnologies too.

The upcoming sub-section will discuss senior-centered design perspectives. Subsequently, the last sub-section will present opportunities offered by Digital Health and IoT in this context.

4.1 Toward Senior-Centered Design

The collection and analysis of user requirements are necessary to guide the user-centered design and the acceptance of any device, possibly within a co-design [161] based on the contribution of all stakeholders. In particular, user experience (UX) experts [162] are key figures in this process, considering the expectations and the reactions of the users to characterize and predict the behaviors that will occur during the interaction with a device. This is a premise to interaction design, which shapes the user activity through affordances and constraints.

Such a perspective helps the developers to create technologies that will be employed by the users as expected by the clinician or the researcher who planned a certain task for them. For instance, the design of a rehabilitative exercise mediated by a technological device should also include solutions to holistically engage the patients and their skills to improve the clinical (and experimental) compliance. These skills do not include only the ones targeted by the treatment, defined by the experts who planned the tasks: the processes of perception, cognition, and action that sustain any activity must be considered to design the interaction required in those tasks (a duty of user-centered design experts).

Furthermore, this approach is advantageous during all phases of the iterative and participatory processes of usability engineering [163] based on international standards for products like medical devices. Accordingly, it is advisable to intertwine the tracks of translational research in academic, clinical, and industrial contexts to allow the user needs to guide technological design. Disciplines like neuroergonomics offer great opportunities in this convergence.

Indeed, neuroergonomics [8] investigates the human nervous system in daily life contexts to improve the user-centered design of interaction technologies. Thus, it offers a set of methodologies for adjusting neurotech to elderly needs and, simultaneously, to study the aging brain through ecologically valid data collected, for example, by means of wearables and environmental sensors.

This approach can reveal, for instance, how horticultural leisure activities (e.g., washing leaves, sowing seeds, transplanting plants) in ecologically valid settings improve the neurophysiological processes (evaluated through a portable EEG headset) and the emotional stability of elderly people [164]. This observation can suggest to implement horticultural simulated scenarios for cognitive stimulation or rehabilitation, or automated reminders that propose certain activities when wearable sensors reveal a fall in mood. Overall, this study highlights the importance of including exercises similar to meaningful and engaging activities in (often tiresome and demotivating) procedures (e.g., laboratory experiments, training and rehabilitation protocols, device calibrations) in order to collect consistent data.

Feedback design is another aspect that should be cared for: as example, VR neurofeedback can trigger positive reactions in healthy seniors, while the same system can raise both positive and negative consequences in neurological old patients experience [165]. Thus, it is difficult to find a unique solution for this heterogenous population: the increasing number and variety of impairments require appropriate design choices.

However, a starting point is compulsory, and it should be the investigation of healthy older adults' needs for appropriately designing interaction technology (e.g., they constitute an under-represented category in AR studies, and commercial AR systems are typically not designed for them) [166] in general, and neurotech in particular. Unfocused design of neurotech can lead to issues like BCI illiteracy.

BCI illiteracy [167]—about 10–25% of users are unable to achieve an effective control of a neurointerface—is a challenge that must be faced in case of elderly users too. Seniors are typically annoyed by flickering lights used during the calibration of certain types of EEG-BCIs like the ones based on steady-state visual evoked potentials (SSVEP). They are also sensitive to difficulties in gaze shifting. Another EEG-BCI paradigm, based on the detection of motor imagery (MI), can be complex for elderly because of an age-related decrease in lateralization of the hand motion cortical representation, which summons an excessively widespread brain activation in terms of both spatial distribution and frequency domain.

In this case [168], solutions like using motor execution of a limb to generate a classifier of MI is an effective strategy, especially when the motion of a paralyzed limb can be passively generated through the assistance of a robot. A "robot-assisted" BCI is a solution that can provide kinesthetic feedback (possibly based on meaningful everyday actions like pressing a mouse button actually controlled by the BCI instead of a finger) that reinforces the gap between imagery and execution, as explored in laboratory studies [169].

Neurotech (BCIs in previous examples) literacy in general is a factor that must be pondered within the wider problem of technology acceptance in case of senior users [170, 171]. For instance, wearable devices acceptance in elderly [172] can be predicted according to performance expectancy, functional congruence, self-actualization, hedonic motivation, and the influence of social context. Thus, we could expect that these factors can become relevant in neurotech acceptance too, overall. Further investigations specifically on neuro-gerontech acceptance should be performed, taking also account of design concepts that can enrich neurotechnology itself, like game features [173] or tangible user interfaces (TUIs) [174], which can improve the engagement and the acceptance of elderly. In this case, haptic feedback can also enhance the effectiveness of neurointerfaces [175], especially considering the role of bodily representations in their control [176] and the senior-specific changes in embodiment processes [177].

These suggestions should be adjusted to the large variety of elderly patients with mild-to-severe conditions: as highlighted above, each specific impairment requires an appropriate set of interaction design choices.

Finally, neurotech ethical issues [178] cross the ones raised by gerontech [179], including topics like the relationship with a machine that can "crack minds" [180] and the pragmatical concerns for privacy and data management. Most guidelines and recommendations on a value-sensitive design (VSD) [181] of interaction technologies and, specifically, on a responsible development (and commercialization) of neurotech [182] can be extended to neuro-gerontech. However, further investigations are necessary to catch the specificities of the senior-centered systems based on neuro-data. Special attention should be paid to neuromodulatory systems, including the invasive ones like DBS, which could be considered a totally invisible factor influencing one's agency (affected by non-invasive brain stimulation techniques) [183] or personality [184].

However, the potential of neuromodulation for helping people with neurodegenerative diseases [185] needs appropriate research policies [186] to counter the skepticism on these techniques. "Neurorights" were proposed [187] for data privacy, security, and consent to enable the users' control on the information collected by neurotech. Interestingly, ethical investigations also proceed in (possibly) futuristic scenarios analysis, as in [188]: the authors discuss if neurotech-based augmentation can include the "diminishment" of a skill or function, like altering our capability to feel pain or discomfort. This is acceptable to manage specific illnesses, yet debatable when in absence of a medical need.

Considering such general issues, next sub-section will depict the opportunities offered by potentially disruptive innovations that could empower neuro-gerontech.

4.2 Personalization, Digital Biomarkers, Internet of Things and Minds

Personalization [189] can be a precious feature for all gerontech in order to match the individual needs of any specific older person. Neuro-gerontech can push forward such a function through the interpretation of the user's will and conditions according to big data managed by Digital Health technologies [190]. Digital Health solutions (resulting from the convergence of platforms aiming at the improvement of health and healthcare services) [191] improve the efficiency, quality, safety, and costs of elderly cares [192].

Within Digital Health, Digital Therapeutics (DTx) [193] software systems constitute a set of evidence-based interventions on medical conditions preventions and management. The "digital active ingredient" (a diagnostic or therapeutic activity) and the "digital excipient" (the technological instruments that engage the users, enhancing their clinical compliance) of DTx low-cost solutions can be implemented in systems like mobile apps or video games. Such systems can target the management of conditions like dementia [194] or diabetes [195] even by means of remote monitoring and interventions of the caregivers [196] or of virtual agents designed to work as health coaches for elderly [197].

In particular, through the connection with wearable and environmental sensors, DTx can enable both diagnostic-prognostic and personalized therapeutic processes alongside translational research activities. This mirrors the medical approach of theranostics [198], based on the simultaneous or coordinated use of methodologies for assess and treat a pathological condition. For instance, recent studies [199] used AR perturbations and EEG recordings to find the contribution of inefficient central modulation to the risk of fall in older adults without neurological issues.

This outcome can be considered an example of digital biomarker [200]. Digital biomarkers are constituted by quantifiable medical signs generated during the interaction between user and device. They are exploited as indices of healthy and pathological processes or of therapeutic outcome, enabling predictive and personalized medical strategies. For instance, digital biomarkers on the nervous system conditions (digital neuromarkers) can be used to identify and distinguish (via artificial intelligence systems) dementia conditions and MCI [201, 202]. Another example can be based on the usage of neuroimaging data for evaluating the outcome of VR trainings [203]. They can also derive from peripheral biosignals analysis for detecting and predicting the mood changes in telemedicine settings [204] or the results of neuromotor tests through robotic platforms of rehabilitation to predict the risk of falls [205]—making such a robot a theranostic machine with dual (therapeutic and diagnostic) functional value.

This approach leads to personalized medicine interventions, which also are the goal of rehabilomics [206], a discipline that aims at translating biomarker research to healthcare according to the analysis of multidimensional data for selecting and adjusting rehabilitative procedures to each patient. Technology-based measures (as the ones collected by rehabilitation robots) can also contribute to this process [76]. Such an observation makes us envision the potential role of digital biomarkers in rehabilomics, suggesting further developments not only in terms of their investigation during technology-assisted neurorehabilitation, but also during the usage of any assistive device. We can call this approach "assistomics" (focusing on the assistive role of technology in clinical and daily activities).

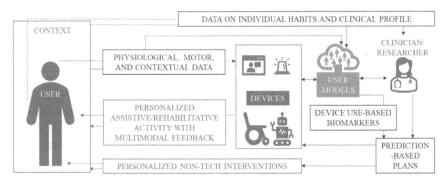

Fig. 4 Example of data-driven infrastructure for BCIs within a distributed personalization ecosystem designed for assistive/rehabilitative technology users

This is also suggested by studies that show how the progression of a medical condition can impair the usage of systems like a neurointerface [207]. This way, any device used by a person can become a source of predictive information on the individual in order to improve: the system capability to respond to user's commands and needs, the medical understanding of the progression of health conditions, the personalized care plans (Fig. 4). In this scenario, neuro-gerontech can become a key element to collect, interpret, and exploit such information.

Accordingly, the example in Fig. 4 highlights the possibility of a cloud platform of BCI user models designed to interpret biosignals for controlling devices and for predicting potential changes in individual conditions. These models could be updated according to the data from different users and different controlled technologies. Such data would be used to improve the capability of each BCI to interpret the information provided by any user in any context, providing features of generalization and personalization. Then, these models could update the resulting software of each BCI within a network. This vision needs the potential of IoT as source of ecologically valid and rich information for neurotech.

Overall, IoT connects different devices within an environment or remotely. Such devices are able to act for the benefits of an individual, especially in case of older adults in smart home contexts to personalize the elderly monitoring and care [208–210]. IoT solutions are quite versatile in connecting different technological solutions—for example: environmental, mobile, and wearable sensors [211] in ambient assisted living (AAL) settings, XR systems [212] for serious game-based telerehabilitation [213], Digital Twin models for context-aware IoT healthcare systems [214]. Nanotechnology-empowered IoT systems (Internet of NanoThings, IoNT) are envisioned too within the Internet of Everything (IoE) general framework [215]. Recently, the advantages of IoT in distance cares for seniors were highlighted during the boost of tele-health and telemedicine advances caused by the distancing policies due to the COVID-19 emergency [216, 217].

IoT, and especially the Internet of Medical Things (IoMT) [218, 219], is highly compatible with wearable neurotechnologies [220]. This domain embraced studies on various topics like: the use of systems for emotion recognition [221], the debate on ethically critical issues on data protection and "Cognitive Privacy" [222], the predictions on their joint impact on the market in terms of Neurotech-enabled IoT (NIoT) [223]. Pervasive and invisible (thus, ethically critical) systems based on both neurotech and IoT processes enable, for instance, ubiquitous biofeedback for relaxation [224], brain training games [225], assistive neurointerfaces to control home devices [226]. Further progress [220] in this domain will require the development of low-cost, energy-efficient, privacy-aware, and pervasive wearable neurotech that should be designed for the benefit of elder people, also exploiting the recent advances in 5G wireless systems.

Interestingly, all potential advances in neurotech-based IoT constitute multiple opportunities for enabling a true "human-centeredness" (and, in our case, the senior-centeredness) of everyday devices and systems spread in our environment.

Indeed, a neurotech-based IoT can make daily use devices truly human-centered: a pervasive network of intelligent systems adaptively interpreting a person's commands, reactions, and needs can constitute a step-change to properly serve human beings according to their fragilities with personalized aids.

Such a perspective makes us adopt the term of "Internet of Things and Minds" (IoTM) to highlight how the devices become "aware" of the current individual mental states according to psychomotor and psychophysiological indices in a certain context. Such continuously collected information can also be used as digital biomarkers for assistomics and as data for longitudinal neuroscientific studies in ecologically valid settings.

In the hypothetical scenario of Fig. 5, IoTM learns how to interpret and anticipate a user's will and feelings according to a day-long data collection and analysis. This personalization process is enhanced by a central cloud platform like the one in Fig. 4. Such a system learns how to shape general IoTM models based on big data collected

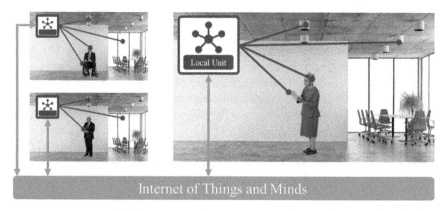

Fig. 5 Contextual elements (e.g., lights, activation of distractors) adapt to the explicit commands and the implicit reactions and conditions (e.g., mood changes) of the user of almost invisible wearable neurotechnologies (e.g., biosensors in a couple of earbuds and in a headband under the hair). The remote central models learn from data on different people

from different individuals in possibly similar tasks and contexts. This would improve the robustness of generalization and personalization capabilities in the neurotech-based IoT solutions. Nevertheless, not all people in this scenario must wear neurotech: the system would also rely on heterogenous indices that will be correlated anyway with the ones of neurotech users.

The approach we depicted needs further investigations for being properly adjusted to the needs of elder people, but it can be extended to help any person with impairments or disabilities. However, it constitutes a potential set of new ways to handle their difficulties, especially considering how the IoTM framework can collect clinically relevant and ecologically valid data from any assistive devices as part of a Digital Health platform, help to identify digital biomarkers, and provide systems for personalized assistance and treatments.

5 Discussion

The chapter described actual and potential neuro-gerontech. We suggested how novel trends in interaction technology, especially in personalized medicine domains, can offer fertile opportunities to improve the impact of neuro-gerontech. Exemplary trends encompass Digital Health and IoT with a focus on collecting and analyzing data. Such data enable the identification of digital biomarkers and the personalization of the device functions alongside the assistance and the treatments for older adults. The interaction of elderly with solutions for technology-assisted rehabilitation and with assistive devices can become a source of ecologically valid diagnostic and prognostic information to personalize the device activity while they enhance our understanding of the current conditions of the elderly user and of any user of assistive solutions (what we labeled as assistomics).

We foresee how the personalization features in IoT frameworks for elderly cares can be revolutionized by the introduction of neurotech. A neurotech-based IoT can detect the commands and the cognitive and affective reactions and conditions of elder people for adapting and adjusting the surrounding technological ecosystem to the individual needs. This solution can drive a true human-centered (and senior-centered) step-change thanks to pervasive neurotech that can establish a continuity with the human nervous system, making an IoTM emerge.

Such an observation becomes even more important if we consider how certain problems can be pervasive too in the daily experience of an elder person. We certainly think about the difficulties in performing activities of daily living or therapeutic exercises, but this is also the case of restless conditions with drug-resistant chronic pain, which are among the targets of neurotech research. Thus, IoTM offers a pervasive (and versatile) approach to handle pervasive (and diversified) problems.

IoTM can feed diagnostic and prognostic systems with ecologically valid data, according to the perspective of neuroergonomics. This would be advantageous for translational research on the aging brain in real-world settings, contributing to define senior-centered design principles. It must also be noticed that, even if in this chapter we mainly focused on health-related issues, this digital ecosystem should also embrace solutions designed for the self-expression of each older person through meaningful activities, possibly in inclusive settings (which, on the other hand, have a positive impact on health itself).

Overall, an IoTM can become a beacon for connecting heterogenous tools that should help people according to their difficulties and disabilities. This is especially true for older adults, whose needs require an appropriate participatory design of neurotech, making it become efficient and acceptable as neuro-gerontech. Obviously, the progress in interaction technologies will create further opportunities alongside ethical issues that must be faced for making neuro-gerontech a key advance for the well-being of each person along the life cycle, toward a positive aging.

6 Conclusion

This chapter presented sample applications of neurotechnologies to the needs of older adults for improving the quality of their life. The exploitation of their potential on this specific (and heterogenous) category of people makes us label the described neurotech-empowered systems with the term neuro-gerontech. This term was defined to emphasize how such solutions must be primarily designed for matching the requirements of aging people when they target the improvement of seniors' conditions and activities.

We also proposed innovation opportunities for neuro-gerontech development within the data-based frameworks of Digital Health and Internet of Things. Such approaches can lead to personalization in device functions, cares, and services for seniors and, in general, for any person with fragilities that require an appropriate adjustment of settings and devices to deal with multiple difficulties.

Simultaneously, they can become a bridge between research laboratories and the seniors' contexts. These connections would generate a continuous flow of information that can improve our understanding of the neural aging processes, both healthy and pathological, while we improve the quality of older people's life.

References

1. Hof, P.R., Mobbs, C.V.: Handbook of the Neuroscience of Aging. Academic Press (2010)
2. Kalra, S., Sharma, S.K.: Diabetes in the elderly. Diab. Ther. **9**(2), 493–500 (2018)
3. Arvanitakis, Z., Shah, R.C., Bennett, D.A.: Diagnosis and management of dementia. JAMA **322**(16), 1589–1599 (2019)
4. Lee, J.E., Shin, D.W., Han, K., Kim, D., Yoo, J.E., Lee, J., Kim, S., Son, K.Y., Cho, B., Kim, M.J.: Changes in metabolic syndrome status and risk of dementia. J. Clin. Med. **9**(1), 122 (2020)
5. Burdick, D.C., Kwon, S.: Gerotechnology: Research and Practice in Technology and Aging. Springer Publishing Company (2004)
6. Graafmans, J., Fozard, J., Rietsema, J., Van Berlo, A., Bouma, H.: Gerontechnology: matching the technological environment to the needs and capacities of the elderly. Aging Hum. Factors 19–30 (1996)

7. Vázquez-Guardado, A., Yang, Y., Bandodkar, A.J., Rogers, J.A.: Recent advances in neurotechnologies with broad potential for neuroscience research. Nat. Neurosci. **23**(12), 1522–1536 (2020)
8. Fairclough, S.H., Lotte, F.: Grand challenges in neurotechnology and system neuroergonomics. Front. Neuroergonomics **1**, 2 (2020)
9. Rajput, R., Kaur, R., Chadha, R., Mani, S, Rachana, R., Kaur, H., Singh, M.: The aging brain: from physiology to neurodegeneration. In: Handbook of Research on Critical Examinations of Neurodegenerative Disorders, pp. 1–23. IGI Global (2019)
10. Huseyn, E.: Examining neurological and neurodegenerative disorders related to aging and elderly. Int. Trends Sci. Technol. **27** (2021)
11. Lo, R.Y.: The borderland between normal aging and dementia. Tzu-Chi Med. J. **29**(2), 65 (2017)
12. Howard, J.H., Jr., Howard, D.V.: Aging mind and brain: is implicit learning spared in healthy aging? Front. Psychol. **4**, 817 (2013)
13. MacNee, W., Rabinovich, R.A., Choudhury, G.: Ageing and the border between health and disease. Eur. Respir. J. **44**(5), 1332–1352 (2014)
14. Crews, J.E., Campbell, V.A.: Vision impairment and hearing loss among community-dwelling older Americans: implications for health and functioning. Am. J. Public Health **94**(5), 823–829 (2004)
15. Seidler, R.D., Bernard, J.A., Burutolu, T.B., Fling, B.W., Gordon, M.T., Gwin, J.T., Kwak, Y., Lipps, D.B.: Motor control and aging: links to age-related brain structural, functional, and biochemical effects. Neurosci. Biobehav. Rev. **34**(5), 721–733 (2010)
16. Votruba, K.L., Persad, C., Giordani, B.: Cognitive deficits in healthy elderly population with "normal" scores on the Mini-Mental State Examination. J. Geriatr. Psychiatry Neurol. **29**(3), 126–132 (2016)
17. Lipsitz, L.A., Novak, V.: Aging and the autonomic nervous system. In: Primer on the Autonomic Nervous System, pp. 271–273. Elsevier (2012)
18. Chen, R.-L., Balami, J.S., Esiri, M.M., Chen, L.-K., Buchan, A.M.: Ischemic stroke in the elderly: an overview of evidence. Nat. Rev. Neurol. **6**(5), 256–265 (2010)
19. Knopman, D.S., Petersen, R.C.: Mild cognitive impairment and mild dementia: a clinical perspective. Mayo Clin. Proc. **10**, 1452–1459 (2014)
20. Kaszniak, A.W., Christenson, G.D.: Differential diagnosis of dementia and depression. In: Neuropsychological Assessment of Dementia and Depression in Older Adults: A Clinician's Guide, pp. 81–117 (1994)
21. Logroscino, G., Traynor, B., Hardiman, O., Couratier, P., Mitchell, J., Swingler, R., Beghi, E.: Descriptive epidemiology of amyotrophic lateral sclerosis: new evidence and unsolved issues. J. Neurol. Neurosurg. Psychiatry **79**(1), 6–11 (2008)
22. Broussalis, E., Grinzinger, S., Kunz, A., Killer-Oberpfalzer, M., Haschke-Becher, E., Hartung, H.P., Kraus, J.: Late age onset of amyotrophic lateral sclerosis is often not considered in elderly people. Acta Neurol. Scand. **137**(3), 329–334 (2018)
23. Mrak, R.E., Griffin, W.S.T., Graham, D.I.: Aging-associated changes in human brain. J. Neuropathol. Exp. Neurol. **56**(12), 1269–1275 (1997)
24. Lis, C., Gaviria, M.: Vascular dementia, hypertension, and the brain. Neurol. Res. **19**(5), 471–480 (1997)
25. Penninx, B.W., Beekman, A.T., Ormel, J., Kriegsman, D.M., Boeke, A.J.P., Van Eijk, J.T.M., Deeg, D.J.: Psychological status among elderly people with chronic diseases: does type of disease play a part? J. Psychosom. Res. **40**(5), 521–534 (1996)
26. Ambrose, A.F., Paul, G., Hausdorff, J.M.: Risk factors for falls among older adults: a review of the literature. Maturitas **75**(1), 51–61 (2013)
27. Lipsitz, L.A., Manor, B., Habtemariam, D., Iloputaife, I., Zhou, J., Travison, T.G.: The pace and prognosis of peripheral sensory loss in advanced age: association with gait speed and falls. BMC Geriatr. **18**(1), 1–8 (2018)
28. Chau, R.M., Ng, T.K., Kwan, R.L., Choi, C.-H., Cheing, G.L.: Risk of fall for people with diabetes. Disabil. Rehabil. **35**(23), 1975–1980 (2013)
29. Kirkland, J.L.: Translating advances from the basic biology of aging into clinical application. Exp. Gerontol. **48**(1), 1–5 (2013)

30. Boyke, J., Driemeyer, J., Gaser, C., Büchel, C., May, A.: Training-induced brain structure changes in the elderly. J. Neurosci. **28**(28), 7031–7035 (2008)
31. Kattenstroth, J.-C., Kolankowska, I., Kalisch, T., Dinse, H.R.: Superior sensory, motor, and cognitive performance in elderly individuals with multi-year dancing activities. Front. Aging Neurosci. **2**, 31 (2010)
32. Maier, M., Ballester, B.R., Verschure, P.F.: Principles of neurorehabilitation after stroke based on motor learning and brain plasticity mechanisms. Front. Syst. Neurosci. **13**, 74 (2019)
33. Tardif, S., Simard, M.: Cognitive stimulation programs in healthy elderly: a review. Int. J. Alzheimer's Dis. (2011)
34. Petersen, R.C., Doody, R., Kurz, A., Mohs, R.C., Morris, J.C., Rabins, P.V., Ritchie, K., Rossor, M., Thal, L., Winblad, B.: Current concepts in mild cognitive impairment. Arch. Neurol. **58**(12), 1985–1992 (2001)
35. Piccini, L., Parini, S., Maggi, L., Andreoni, G.A.: wearable home BCI system: preliminary results with SSVEP protocol. In: 2005 IEEE Engineering in Medicine and Biology 27th Annual Conference, pp. 5384–5387. IEEE (2006)
36. Doi, T., Makizako, H., Shimada, H., Park, H., Tsutsumimoto, K., Uemura, K., Suzuki, T.: Brain activation during dual-task walking and executive function among older adults with mild cognitive impairment: a fNIRS study. Aging Clin. Exp. Res. **25** (5), 539–544 (2013)
37. Huang, C., Wahlund, L.-O., Dierks, T., Julin, P., Winblad, B., Jelic, V.: Discrimination of Alzheimer's disease and mild cognitive impairment by equivalent EEG sources: a cross-sectional and longitudinal study. Clin. Neurophysiol. **111**(11), 1961–1967 (2000)
38. Yang, D., Hong, K.-S., Yoo, S.-H., Kim, C.-S.: Evaluation of neural degeneration biomarkers in the prefrontal cortex for early identification of patients with mild cognitive impairment: an fNIRS study. Front. Hum. Neurosci. **13**, 317 (2019)
39. Zamrini, E., Maestu, F., Pekkonen, E., Funke, M., Makela, J., Riley, M., Bajo, R., Sudre, G., Fernandez, A., Castellanos, N.: Magnetoencephalography as a putative biomarker for Alzheimer's disease. Int. J. Alzheimer's Dis. (2011)
40. Larradet, F., Niewiadomski, R., Barresi, G., Caldwell, D.G., Mattos, L.S.: Toward emotion recognition from physiological signals in the wild: approaching the methodological issues in real-life data collection. Front. Psychol. **11**, 1111 (2020)
41. Raj, A., Roberts, B., Hollingshead, K., McDonald, N., Poquette, M., Soussou, W.A.: Wearable multisensory, multiagent approach for detection and mitigation of acute cognitive strain. In: International Conference on Augmented Cognition, pp. 180–200. Springer (2018)
42. Allanson, J., Fairclough, S.H.: A research agenda for physiological computing. Interact. Comput. **16**(5), 857–878 (2004)
43. Maranesi, E., Fioretti, S., Ghetti, G., Rabini, R., Burattini, L., Mercante, O., Di Nardo, F.: The surface electromyographic evaluation of the functional reach in elderly subjects. J. Electromyogr. Kinesiol. **26**, 102–110 (2016)
44. Shustak, S., Inzelberg, L., Steinberg, S., Rand, D., Pur, M.D., Hillel, I., Katzav, S., Fahoum, F., De Vos, M., Mirelman, A.: Home monitoring of sleep with a temporary-tattoo EEG, EOG and EMG electrode array: a feasibility study. J. Neural Eng. **16**(2), 026024 (2019)
45. Das, D., Datta, S., Bhattacharjee, T., Choudhury, A.D., Pal, A.: Eliminating individual bias to improve stress detection from multimodal physiological data. In: 2018 40th Annual International Conference of the IEEE Engineering in Medicine and Biology Society (EMBC), pp. 5753–5758. IEEE (2018)
46. Johannessen, E.: Measuring Cognitive Load in a Clinical Setting: Medical Learning and Practice. Queen's University, Canada (2019)
47. Papetti, A., Iualé, M., Ceccacci, S., Bevilacqua, R., Germani, M., Mengoni, M.: Smart objects: an evaluation of the present state based on user needs. In: International Conference on Distributed, Ambient, and Pervasive Interactions, pp. 359–368. Springer (2014)
48. Wolpaw, J.R., Birbaumer, N., Heetderks, W.J., McFarland, D.J., Peckham, P.H., Schalk, G., Donchin, E., Quatrano, L.A., Robinson, C.J., Vaughan, T.M.: Brain-computer interface technology: a review of the first international meeting. IEEE Trans. Rehabil. Eng. **8**(2), 164–173 (2000)

49. Chaudhary, P., Agrawal, R.: Brain computer interface: a new pathway to human brain. In: Cognitive Computing in Human Cognition, pp. 99–125. Springer (2020)
50. Saha, S., Mamun, K.A., Ahmed, K., Mostafa, R., Naik, G.R., Darvishi, S., Khandoker, A.H., Baumert, M.: Progress in brain computer interface: challenges and opportunities. Front. Syst. Neurosci. **15**(4) (2021). https://doi.org/10.3389/fnsys.2021.578875
51. Chan, A.T., Quiroz, J.C., Dascalu, S., Harris, F.C.: An overview of brain computer interfaces. In: Proceedings of the 30th International Conference on Computers and Their Applications (2015)
52. Zhuang, M., Wu, Q., Wan, F., Hu, Y.: State-of-the-art non-invasive brain–computer interface for neural rehabilitation: a review. J. Neurorestoratology **8**(1), 4 (2020)
53. Nagel, S., Spüler, M.: World's fastest brain-computer interface: combining EEG2Code with deep learning. PloS One **14**(9), e0221909 (2019)
54. Garg, N., Garg, R., Parrivesh, N., Anand, A., Abhinav, V., Baths, V.: Decoding the neural signatures of valence and arousal from portable EEG headset. bioRxiv (2021)
55. Fukuma, R., Yanagisawa, T., Saitoh, Y., Hosomi, K., Kishima, H., Shimizu, T., Sugata, H., Yokoi, H., Hirata, M., Kamitani, Y.: Real-time control of a neuroprosthetic hand by magnetoencephalographic signals from paralysed patients. Sci. Rep. **6**(1), 1–14 (2016)
56. Kaas, A., Goebel, R., Valente, G., Sorger, B.: Topographic somatosensory imagery for real-time fMRI brain-computer interfacing. Front. Hum. Neurosci. **13**, 427 (2019)
57. Khalaf, A., Sejdic, E., Akcakaya, M.: A novel motor imagery hybrid brain computer interface using EEG and functional transcranial Doppler ultrasound. J. Neurosci. Methods **313**, 44–53 (2019)
58. Wyser, D.G., Lambercy, O., Scholkmann, F., Wolf, M., Gassert, R.: Wearable and modular functional near-infrared spectroscopy instrument with multidistance measurements at four wavelengths. Neurophotonics **4**(4), 041413 (2017)
59. Yaqub, M.A., Woo, S.-W., Hong, K.-S.: Compact, portable, high-density functional near-infrared spectroscopy system for brain imaging. IEEE Access **8**, 128224–128238 (2020)
60. Herweg, A., Gutzeit, J., Kleih, S., Kübler, A.: Wheelchair control by elderly participants in a virtual environment with a brain-computer interface (BCI) and tactile stimulation. Biol. Psychol. **121**, 117–124 (2016)
61. Villa-Parra, A., Delisle-Rodríguez, D., López-Delis, A., Bastos-Filho, T., Sagaró, R., Frizera-Neto, A.: Towards a robotic knee exoskeleton control based on human motion intention through EEG and sEMGsignals. Procedia Manufact. **3**, 1379–1386 (2015)
62. Chai, X., Zhang, Z., Guan, K., Lu, Y., Liu, G., Zhang, T., Niu, H.: A hybrid BCI-controlled smart home system combining SSVEP and EMG for individuals with paralysis. Biomed. Signal Process. Control **56**, 101687 (2020)
63. Pfurtscheller, G., Allison, B.Z., Bauernfeind, G., Brunner, C., Solis Escalante, T., Scherer, R., Zander, T.O., Mueller-Putz, G., Neuper, C., Birbaumer, N.: The hybrid BCI. Front. Neurosci. **4**, 3 (2010)
64. Yousefi, R., Sereshkeh, A.R., Chau, T.: Exploiting error-related potentials in cognitive task based BCI. Biomed. Phys. Eng. Express **5**(1), 015023 (2018)
65. Schiatti, L., Barresi, G., Tessadori, J., King, L.C., Mattos, L.S.: The effect of vibrotactile feedback on ErrP-based adaptive classification of motor imagery. In: 2019 41st Annual International Conference of the IEEE Engineering in Medicine and Biology Society (EMBC), pp. 6750–6753. IEEE (2019)
66. Pasqualotto, E., Matuz, T., Federici, S., Ruf, C.A., Bartl, M., Olivetti Belardinelli, M., Birbaumer, N., Halder, S.: Usability and workload of access technology for people with severe motor impairment: a comparison of brain-computer interfacing and eye tracking. Neurorehabil. Neural Repair **29**(10), 950–957 (2015)
67. Barresi, G., Tessadori, J., Schiatti, L., Mazzanti, D., Caldwell, D.G., Mattos, L.S.: Focus-sensitive dwell time in EyeBCI: pilot study. In: 2016 8th Computer Science and Electronic Engineering (CEEC), pp. 54–59. IEEE (2016)
68. Müller-Putz, G.R., Breitwieser, C., Cincotti, F., Leeb, R., Schreuder, M., Leotta, F., Tavella, M., Bianchi, L., Kreilinger, A., Ramsay, A.: Tools for brain-computer interaction: a general concept for a hybrid BCI. Front. Neuroinform. **5**, 30 (2011)

69. Misbhauddin, M.: Smartwatch-based wearable and usable system for driver drowsiness detection. In: The Proceedings of the Third International Conference on Smart City Applications, pp. 906–920. Springer (2019)
70. Aricò, P., Borghini, G., Di Flumeri, G., Sciaraffa, N., Babiloni, F.: Passive BCI beyond the lab: current trends and future directions. Physiol. Meas. **39**(8), 08TR02 (2018)
71. Larradet, F., Barresi, G., Mattos, L.S.: Effects of galvanic skin response feedback on user experience in gaze-controlled gaming: a pilot study. In: 39th Annual International Conference of the IEEE Engineering in Medicine and Biology Society (EMBC), pp. 2458–2461. IEEE (2017)
72. Parsons, T.D., Gaggioli, A., Riva, G.: Extended reality for the clinical, affective, and social neurosciences. Brain Sci. **10**(12), 922 (2020)
73. Georgiev, D.D., Georgieva, I., Gong, Z., Nanjappan, V., Georgiev, G.V.: Virtual reality for neurorehabilitation and cognitive enhancement. Brain Sci. **11**(2), 221 (2021)
74. Sokolov, A.A., Collignon, A., Bieler-Aeschlimann, M.: Serious video games and virtual reality for prevention and neurorehabilitation of cognitive decline because of aging and neurodegeneration. Curr. Opin. Neurol. **33**(2), 239–248 (2020)
75. Baran, M., Lehrer, N., Duff, M., Venkataraman, V., Turaga, P., Ingalls, T., Rymer, W.Z., Wolf, S.L., Rikakis, T.: Interdisciplinary concepts for design and implementation of mixed reality interactive neurorehabilitation systems for stroke. Phys. Ther. **95**(3), 449–460 (2015)
76. Iandolo, R., Marini, F., Semprini, M., Laffranchi, M., Mugnosso, M., Cherif, A., De Michieli, L., Chiappalone, M., Zenzeri, J.: Perspectives and challenges in robotic neurorehabilitation. Appl. Sci. **9**(15), 3183 (2019)
77. Wenk, N., Buetler, K.A., Marchal-Crespo, L.: Virtual reality in robotic neurorehabilitation. In: Virtual Reality in Health and Rehabilitation, pp. 41–60. CRC Press (2020)
78. Casey, A., Azhar, H., Grzes, M., Sakel, M.: BCI controlled robotic arm as assistance to the rehabilitation of neurologically disabled patients. Disabil. Rehabil. Assist. Technol. **16**(5), 525–537 (2021)
79. Guggenberger, R., Heringhaus, M., Gharabaghi, A.: Brain-machine neurofeedback: robotics or electrical stimulation? Front. Bioeng. Biotechnol. **8**, 639 (2020)
80. Naro, A., Billeri, L., Manuli, A., Balletta, T., Cannavò, A., Portaro, S., Lauria, P., Ciappina, F., Calabrò, R.S.: Breaking the ice to improve motor outcomes in patients with chronic stroke: a retrospective clinical study on neuromodulation plus robotics. Neurol. Sci. 1–9 (2020)
81. Reinkensmeyer, D.J., Kahn, L.E., Averbuch, M., McKenna-Cole, A., Schmit, B.D., Rymer, W.Z.: Understanding and treating arm movement impairment after chronic brain injury: progress with the ARM guide. J. Rehabil. Res. Dev. **37**(6), 653–662 (2014)
82. Calabrò, R.S., Russo, M., Naro, A., Milardi, D., Balletta, T., Leo, A., Filoni, S., Bramanti, P.: Who may benefit from armeo power treatment? A neurophysiological approach to predict neurorehabilitation outcomes. PM&R **8**(10), 971–978 (2016)
83. Perry, J.C., Rosen, J., Burns, S.: Upper-limb powered exoskeleton design. IEEE/ASME Trans. Mechatron. **12**(4), 408–417 (2007)
84. Reinkensmeyer, D.J., Wolbrecht, E.T., Chan, V., Chou, C., Cramer, S.C., Bobrow, J.E.: Comparison of 3D, assist-as-needed robotic arm/hand movement training provided with Pneu-WREX to conventional table top therapy following chronic stroke. Am. J. Phys. Med. Rehabil./Assoc. Acad. Physiatrists **91**(11 0 3), S232 (2012)
85. Jezernik, S., Colombo, G., Keller, T., Frueh, H., Morari, M.: Robotic orthosis lokomat: a rehabilitation and research tool. Neuromodulation: Technol. Neural Interface **6**(2), 108–115 (2003)
86. Kolakowsky-Hayner, S.A., Crew, J., Moran, S., Shah, A.: Safety and feasibility of using the EksoTM bionic exoskeleton to aid ambulation after spinal cord injury. J Spine **4**(003), 1–8 (2013)
87. Vassallo, C., De Giuseppe, S., Piezzo, C., Maludrottu, S., Cerruti, G., D'Angelo, M.L., Gruppioni, E., Marchese, C., Castellano, S., Guanziroli, E.: Gait patterns generation based on basis functions interpolation for the TWIN lower-limb exoskeleton. In: 2020 IEEE International Conference on Robotics and Automation (ICRA), pp. 1778–1784. IEEE (2020)

88. Krebs, H.I., Ferraro, M., Buerger, S.P., Newbery, M.J., Makiyama, A., Sandmann, M., Lynch, D., Volpe, B.T., Hogan, N.: Rehabilitation robotics: pilot trial of a spatial extension for MIT-Manus. J. Neuroeng. Rehabil. **1**(1), 1–15 (2004)
89. Casadio, M., Sanguineti, V., Morasso, P.G., Arrichiello, V.: Braccio di Ferro: a new haptic workstation for neuromotor rehabilitation. Technol. Health Care **14**(3), 123–142 (2006)
90. Masia, L., Casadio, M., Giannoni, P., Sandini, G., Morasso, P.: Performance adaptive training control strategy for recovering wrist movements in stroke patients: a preliminary, feasibility study. J. Neuroeng. Rehabil. **6**(1), 1–11 (2009)
91. Schmidt, H., Hesse, S., Bernhardt, R., Krüger, J.: HapticWalker—a novel haptic foot device. ACM Trans. Appl. Percept. (TAP) **2**(2), 166–180 (2005)
92. Hesse, S., Waldner, A., Tomelleri, C.: Innovative gait robot for the repetitive practice of floor walking and stair climbing up and down in stroke patients. J. Neuroeng. Rehabil. **7**(1), 1–10 (2010)
93. Squeri, V., De Luca, A., Cella, A., Vallone, F., Siri, G., Zigoura, E., Giorgeschi, A., Tavella, E., Puntoni, M., Avella, M.: Robotic evaluation of fall risk in older people: results on trunk parameters in static and dynamic balance conditions by hunova robot. Ann. Phys. Rehabil. Med. **61**, e339 (2018)
94. D'Antonio, E., Galofaro, E., Zenzeri, J., Patané, F., Konczak, J., Casadio, M., Masia, L.: Robotic assessment of wrist proprioception during kinaesthetic perturbations: a neuroergonomic approach. Front. Neurorobot. **15**, 19 (2021)
95. Maggioni, S., Melendez-Calderon, A., Van Asseldonk, E., Klamroth-Marganska, V., Lünenburger, L., Riener, R., Van Der Kooij, H.: Robot-aided assessment of lower extremity functions: a review. J. Neuroeng. Rehabil. **13**(1), 1–25 (2016)
96. Debert, C.T., Herter, T.M., Scott, S.H., Dukelow, S.: Robotic assessment of sensorimotor deficits after traumatic brain injury. J. Neurol. Phys. Ther. **36**(2), 58–67 (2012)
97. Marchal-Crespo, L., Reinkensmeyer, D.J.: Review of control strategies for robotic movement training after neurologic injury. J. Neuroeng. Rehabil. **6**(1), 1–15 (2009)
98. Iwamoto, Y., Imura, T., Suzukawa, T., Fukuyama, H., Ishii, T., Taki, S., Imada, N., Shibukawa, M., Inagawa, T., Araki, H.: Combination of exoskeletal upper limb robot and occupational therapy improve activities of daily living function in acute stroke patients. J. Stroke Cerebrovasc. Dis. **28**(7), 2018–2025 (2019)
99. Dehem, S., Gilliaux, M., Stoquart, G., Detrembleur, C., Jacquemin, G., Palumbo, S., Frederick, A., Lejeune, T.: Effectiveness of upper-limb robotic-assisted therapy in the early rehabilitation phase after stroke: a single-blind, randomised, controlled trial. Ann. Phys. Rehabil. Med. **62**(5), 313–320 (2019)
100. Kim, M.-S., Kim, S.H., Noh, S.-E., Bang, H.J., Lee, K.-M.: Robotic-assisted shoulder rehabilitation therapy effectively improved poststroke hemiplegic shoulder pain: a randomized controlled trial. Arch. Phys. Med. Rehabil. **100**(6), 1015–1022 (2019)
101. Aprile, I., Germanotta, M., Cruciani, A., Loreti, S., Pecchioli, C., Cecchi, F., Montesano, A., Galeri, S., Diverio, M., Falsini, C.: Upper limb robotic rehabilitation after stroke: a multicenter, randomized clinical trial. J. Neurol. Phys. Ther. **44**(1), 3–14 (2020)
102. Maranesi, E., Riccardi, G.R., Di Donna, V., Di Rosa, M., Fabbietti, P., Luzi, R., Pranno, L., Lattanzio, F., Bevilacqua, R.: Effectiveness of intervention based on end-effector gait trainer in older patients with stroke: a systematic review. J. Am. Med. Dir. Assoc. **21**(8), 1036–1044 (2020)
103. Berger, A., Horst, F., Müller, S., Steinberg, F., Doppelmayr, M.: Current state and future prospects of EEG and fNIRS in robot-assisted gait rehabilitation: a brief review. Front. Hum. Neurosci. **13**, 172 (2019)
104. Frank, D.L., Khorshid, L., Kiffer, J.F., Moravec, C.S., McKee, M.G.: Biofeedback in medicine: who, when, why and how? Ment. Health Fam. Med. **7**(2), 85 (2010)
105. Karatsidis, A., Richards, R.E., Konrath, J.M., Van Den Noort, J.C., Schepers, H.M., Bellusci, G., Harlaar, J., Veltink, P.H.: Validation of wearable visual feedback for retraining foot progression angle using inertial sensors and an augmented reality headset. J. Neuroeng. Rehabil. **15**(1), 1–12 (2018)

106. de Zambotti, M., Sizintsev, M., Claudatos, S., Barresi, G., Colrain, I.M., Baker, F.C.: Reducing bedtime physiological arousal levels using immersive audio-visual respiratory bio-feedback: a pilot study in women with insomnia symptoms. J. Behav. Med. **42**(5), 973–983 (2019)
107. Garbarino, M., Lai, M., Bender, D., Picard, R.W., Tognetti, S.: Empatica E3—a wearable wireless multi-sensor device for real-time computerized biofeedback and data acquisition. In: 2014 4th International Conference on Wireless Mobile Communication and Healthcare-Transforming Healthcare Through Innovations in Mobile and Wireless Technologies (MOBI-HEALTH), pp. 39–42. IEEE (2014)
108. Pereira, O., Caldeira, J.M., Rodrigues, J.J.: Body sensor network mobile solutions for biofeedback monitoring. Mob. Netw. Appl. **16**(6), 713–732 (2011)
109. Park, J., Park, C.H., Jun, S.-E., Lee, E.-J., Kang, S.W., Kim, N.: Effects of biofeedback-based sleep improvement program on urinary symptoms and sleep patterns of elderly Korean women with overactive bladder syndrome. BMC Urol. **19**(1), 1–10 (2019)
110. Afzal, M.R., Oh, M.-K., Choi, H.Y., Yoon, J.: A novel balance training system using multimodal biofeedback. Biomed. Eng. Online **15**(1), 1–11 (2016)
111. Mayer, K., Blume, F., Wyckoff, S.N., Brokmeier, L.L., Strehl, U.: Neurofeedback of slow cortical potentials as a treatment for adults with attention deficit-/hyperactivity disorder. Clin. Neurophysiol. **127**(2), 1374–1386 (2016)
112. Mayer, K., Wyckoff, S.N., Fallgatter, A.J., Ehlis, A.-C., Strehl, U.: Neurofeedback as a nonpharmacological treatment for adults with attention-deficit/hyperactivity disorder (ADHD): study protocol for a randomized controlled trial. Trials **16**(1), 1–14 (2015)
113. Kamranmehr, F., Farsi, A., Kavyani, M.: The effectiveness of mindfulness and biofeedback-relaxation training on anxiety, depression and dynamic and static balance in the elderly women with mild anxiety and depression. Aging Psychol. **6**(3), 248–253 (2020)
114. Ramirez, R., Palencia-Lefler, M., Giraldo, S., Vamvakousis, Z.: Musical neurofeedback for treating depression in elderly people. Front. Neurosci. **9**, 354 (2015)
115. Jirayucharoensak, S., Israsena, P., Pan-Ngum, S., Hemrungrojn, S., Maes, M.: A game-based neurofeedback training system to enhance cognitive performance in healthy elderly subjects and in patients with amnestic mild cognitive impairment. Clin. Interv. Aging **14**, 347 (2019)
116. Bevilacqua, R., Maranesi, E., Riccardi, G.R., Di Donna, V., Pelliccioni, P., Luzi, R., Lattanzio, F., Pelliccioni, G.: Non-immersive virtual reality for rehabilitation of the older people: a systematic review into efficacy and effectiveness. J. Clin. Med. **8**(11), 1882 (2019)
117. Golisz, K.: Occupational therapy interventions to improve driving performance in older adults: a systematic review. Am. J. Occup. Ther. **68**(6), 662–669 (2014)
118. Hao, J., Xie, H., Harp, K., Chen, Z., Siu, K.-C.: Effects of virtual reality intervention on neural plasticity in stroke rehabilitation: a systematic review. Arch. Phys. Med. Rehabil. (2021)
119. Loos, E., Kaufman, D.: Positive impact of exergaming on older adults' mental and social well-being: in search of evidence. In: International Conference on Human Aspects of IT for the Aged Population, pp. 101–112. Springer (2018)
120. Anderson-Hanley, C., Maloney, M., Barcelos, N., Striegnitz, K., Kramer, A.: Neuropsychological benefits of neuro-exergaming for older adults: a pilot study of an interactive physical and cognitive exercise system (iPACES). J. Aging Phys. Act. **25**(1), 73–83 (2017)
121. Barcelos, N., Shah, N., Cohen, K., Hogan, M.J., Mulkerrin, E., Arciero, P.J., Cohen, B.D., Kramer, A.F., Anderson-Hanley, C.: Aerobic and cognitive exercise (ACE) pilot study for older adults: executive function improves with cognitive challenge while exergaming. J. Int. Neuropsychol. Soc. **21**(10), 768–779 (2015)
122. Bonnechère, B., Klass, M., Langley, C., Sahakian, B.J.: Brain training using cognitive apps can improve cognitive performance and processing speed in older adults. Sci. Rep. **11**(1), 1–11 (2021)
123. Ballesteros, S., Prieto, A., Mayas, J., Toril, P., Pita, C., Ponce de León, L., Reales, J.M., Waterworth, J.: Brain training with non-action video games enhances aspects of cognition in older adults: a randomized controlled trial. Front. Aging Neurosci. **6**, 277 (2014)
124. Nouchi, R., Taki, Y., Takeuchi, H., Hashizume, H., Nozawa, T., Kambara, T., Sekiguchi, A., Miyauchi, C.M., Kotozaki, Y., Nouchi, H.: Brain training game boosts executive functions,

working memory and processing speed in the young adults: a randomized controlled trial. PloS One **8**(2), e55518 (2013)
125. Li, X., Zhang, J., Li, X.-D., Cui, W., Su, R.: Neurofeedback training for brain functional connectivity improvement in mild cognitive impairment. J. Med. Biol. Eng. **40**, 484–495 (2020)
126. Sitaram, R., Ros, T., Stoeckel, L., Haller, S., Scharnowski, F., Lewis-Peacock, J., Weiskopf, N., Blefari, M.L., Rana, M., Oblak, E.: Closed-loop brain training: the science of neurofeedback. Nat. Rev. Neurosci. **18**(2), 86–100 (2017)
127. Lee, T.-S., Goh, S.J.A., Quek, S.Y., Phillips, R., Guan, C., Cheung, Y.B., Feng, L., Teng, S.S.W., Wang, C.C., Chin, Z.Y.: A brain-computer interface based cognitive training system for healthy elderly: a randomized control pilot study for usability and preliminary efficacy. PloS One **8**(11), e79419 (2013)
128. Paszkiel, S.: Using BCI and VR technology in neurogaming. In: Analysis and Classification of EEG Signals for Brain–Computer Interfaces, pp. 93–99. Springer (2020)
129. Stojan, R., Voelcker-Rehage, C.: A systematic review on the cognitive benefits and neurophysiological correlates of exergaming in healthy older adults. J. Clin. Med. **8**(5), 734 (2019)
130. Temprado, J.-J.: Can exergames be improved to better enhance behavioral adaptability in older adults? An ecological dynamics perspective. Front. Aging Neurosci. **13**, 242 (2021)
131. Diamond, K., Mowszowski, L., Cockayne, N., Norrie, L., Paradise, M., Hermens, D.F., Lewis, S.J., Hickie, I.B., Naismith, S.L.: Randomized controlled trial of a healthy brain ageing cognitive training program: effects on memory, mood, and sleep. J. Alzheimers Dis. **44**(4), 1181–1191 (2015)
132. Krames, E.S., Peckham, P.H., Rezai, A., Aboelsaad, F.: What is neuromodulation? In: Neuromodulation, pp. 3–8. Elsevier (2009)
133. Solomons, C.D., Shanmugasundaram, V.: A review of transcranial electrical stimulation methods in stroke rehabilitation. Neurol. India **67**(2), 417 (2019)
134. Calderón, M.A.F., Jiménez, L.O., Ledesma, M.J.S.: Transcranial magnetic stimulation versus transcranial direct current stimulation as neuromodulatory techniques in stroke rehabilitation. In: Proceedings of the Sixth International Conference on Technological Ecosystems for Enhancing Multiculturality, pp. 422–427 (2018)
135. DeFina, P.A., Halper, J.P., Fellus, J.L., Machado, C., Chinchilla, M., Prestigiacomo, C.J.: Neuroplasticity and neuromarker driven neuromodulation: the future path to normalizing brain function. Funct. Neurol. Rehabil. Ergon. **6**(1), 27 (2016)
136. Waqar, M.A., Conright, K., Currie, D.R., Cate, J.C.: Technological advancements in pain management in the elderly population. Using Technol. Improve Care Older Adults **124** (2017)
137. Rangarajan, S.K., Suhas, S., Reddy, M.S.S., Sreeraj, V.S., Sivakumar, P.T., Venkatasubramanian, G.: Domiciliary tDCS in geriatric psychiatric disorders: opportunities and challenges. Indian J. Psychol. Med. 02537176211003666 (2021)
138. McACHRAN, S.E., Daneshgari, F.: Sacral neuromodulation in the older woman. Clin. Obstet. Gynecol. **50**(3), 735–744 (2007)
139. McDonald, W.M.: Neuromodulation treatments for geriatric mood and cognitive disorders. Am. J. Geriatr. Psychiatry **24**(12), 1130–1141 (2016)
140. Martins, A.R., Fregni, F., Simis, M., Almeida, J.: Neuromodulation as a cognitive enhancement strategy in healthy older adults: promises and pitfalls. Aging Neuropsychol. Cogn. **24**(2), 158–185 (2017)
141. Luan, S., Williams, I., Nikolic, K., Constandinou, T.G.: Neuromodulation: present and emerging methods. Front. Neuroengineering **7**, 27 (2014)
142. Ceresa, M., Mangado, N., Andrews, R.J., Ballester, M.A.G.: Computational models for predicting outcomes of neuroprosthesis implantation: the case of cochlear implants. Mol. Neurobiol. **52**(2), 934–941 (2015)
143. Warwick, K.: Neuroengineering and neuroprosthetics. Brain Neurosc. Adv. **2**, 2398212818817499 (2018)

144. Alm, N., Arnott, J.L., Dobinson, L., Massie, P., Hewines, I.: Cognitive prostheses for elderly people. In: IEEE International Conference on Systems, Man and Cybernetics. e-Systems and e-Man for Cybernetics in Cyberspace (Cat. No. 01CH37236), pp. 806–810. IEEE (2001)
145. Encarnação, P.: Episodic memory visualization in robot companions providing a memory prosthesis for elderly users. In: Assistive Technology: From Research to Practice, vol. 33, p. 120. AAATE (2013)
146. Belkacem, A.N., Jamil, N., Palmer, J.A., Ouhbi, S., Chen, C.: Brain computer interfaces for improving the quality of life of older adults and elderly patients. Front. Neurosci. **14**, 692 (2020)
147. Panuccio, G., Semprini, M., Natale, L., Buccelli, S., Colombi, I., Chiappalone, M.: Progress in neuroengineering for brain repair: new challenges and open issues. Brain Neurosci. Adv. **2**, 2398212818776475 (2018)
148. Lebedev, M.A., Opris, I., Casanova, M.F.: Augmentation of brain function: facts, fiction and controversy. Front. Syst. Neurosci. **12**, 45 (2018)
149. Rosenfeld, J.V., Wong, Y.T.: Neurobionics and the brain–computer interface: current applications and future horizons. Med. J. Aust. **206**(8), 363–368 (2017)
150. Moxon, K., Saez, I., Ditterich, J.: Mind over matter: cognitive neuroengineering. In: Cerebrum: the Dana Forum on Brain Science. Dana Foundation (2019)
151. Rao, R.P.: Brain Co-Processors: Using AI to Restore and Augment Brain Function (2020). arXiv:201203378
152. Zimerman, M., Nitsch, M., Giraux, P., Gerloff, C., Cohen, L.G., Hummel, F.C.: Neuroenhancement of the aging brain: restoring skill acquisition in old subjects. Ann. Neurol. **73**(1), 10 (2013)
153. Wexler, A.: Who uses direct-to-consumer brain stimulation products, and why? A study of home users of tDCS devices. J. Cogn. Enhancement **2**(1), 114–134 (2018)
154. Bevilacqua, R., Felici, E., Marcellini, F., Glende, S., Klemcke, S., Conrad, I., Esposito, R., Cavallo, F., Dario, P.: Robot-era project: preliminary results on the system usability. In: International Conference of Design, User Experience, and Usability, pp. 553–561. Springer (2015)
155. White, S.W., Richey, J.A., Gracanin, D., Bell, M.A., LaConte, S., Coffman, M., Trubanova, A., Kim, I.: The promise of neurotechnology in clinical translational science. Clin. Psychol. Sci. **3**(5), 797–815 (2015)
156. Callahan, C.M., Foroud, T., Saykin, A.J., Shekhar, A., Hendrie, H.C.: Translational research on aging: clinical epidemiology as a bridge between the sciences. Transl. Res. **163**(5), 439–445 (2014)
157. McDowell, K., Ries, A.A.: Translational approach to neurotechnology development. In: International Conference on Augmented Cognition, pp. 353–360. Springer (2013)
158. Liu, L., Stroulia, E., Nikolaidis, I., Miguel-Cruz, A., Rincon, A.R.: Smart homes and home health monitoring technologies for older adults: a systematic review. Int. J. Med. Informatics **91**, 44–59 (2016)
159. Duval-Couetil, N., Ladisch, M., Yi, S.: Addressing academic researcher priorities through science and technology entrepreneurship education. J. Technol. Transf. **46**(2), 288–318 (2021)
160. Gómez-López, P., Montero, F., López, M.T.: Empowering UX of elderly people with Parkinson's disease via BCI touch. In: International Work-Conference on the Interplay Between Natural and Artificial Computation, pp. 161–170. Springer (2019)
161. Carroll, S., Kobayashi, K., Cervantes, M.N., Freeman, S., Saini, M., Tracey, S.: Supporting healthy aging through the scale-up, spread, and sustainability of assistive technology implementation: a rapid realist review of participatory co-design for assistive technology with older adults. Gerontol. Geriatr. Med. **7**, 23337214211023268 (2021)
162. Vermeeren, A.P., Roto, V., Väänänen, K.: Design-inclusive UX research: design as a part of doing user experience research. Behav. Inf. Technol. **35**(1), 21–37 (2016)
163. Privitera, M.B., Evans, M., Southee, D.: Human factors in the design of medical devices–approaches to meeting international standards in the European Union and USA. Appl. Ergon. **59**, 251–263 (2017)

164. Kim, S.-O., Pyun, S.-B., Park, S.-A.: Improved cognitive function and emotional condition measured using electroencephalography in the elderly during horticultural activities. HortScience **1**(aop), 1–10 (2021)
165. Kober, S.E., Reichert, J.L., Schweiger, D., Neuper, C., Wood, G.: Does feedback design matter? A neurofeedback study comparing immersive virtual reality and traditional training screens in elderly. Int. J. Serious Games **4**(3) (2017)
166. Williams, T.J., Jones, S.L., Lutteroth, C., Dekoninck, E.: Boyd HC augmented reality and older adults: a comparison of prompting types. In: Proceedings of the 2021 CHI Conference on Human Factors in Computing Systems, pp. 1–13 (2021)
167. Allison, B., Luth, T., Valbuena, D., Teymourian, A., Volosyak, I., Graser, A.: BCI demographics: how many (and what kinds of) people can use an SSVEP BCI? IEEE Trans. Neural Syst. Rehabil. Eng. **18**(2), 107–116 (2010)
168. Kaiser, V., Kreilinger, A., Müller-Putz, G.R., Neuper, C.: First steps toward a motor imagery based stroke BCI: new strategy to set up a classifier. Front. Neurosci. **5**, 86 (2011)
169. Petrushin, A., Tessadori, J., Barresi, G., Mattos, L.S.: Effect of a click-like feedback on motor imagery in EEG-BCI and eye-tracking hybrid control for telepresence. In: IEEE/ASME International Conference on Advanced Intelligent Mechatronics (AIM), pp. 628–633. IEEE (2021)
170. Renaud, K., Van Biljon, J.: Predicting technology acceptance and adoption by the elderly: a qualitative study. In: Proceedings of the 2008 Annual Research Conference of the South African Institute of Computer Scientists and Information Technologists on IT Research in Developing Countries: Riding the Wave of Technology, pp. 210–219 (2008)
171. Chen, K., Chan, A.H.S.: Gerontechnology acceptance by elderly Hong Kong Chinese: a senior technology acceptance model (STAM). Ergonomics **57**(5), 635–652 (2014)
172. Talukder, M.S., Sorwar, G., Bao, Y., Ahmed, J.U., Palash, M.A.S.: Predicting antecedents of wearable healthcare technology acceptance by elderly: a combined SEM-Neural Network approach. Technol. Forecast. Soc. Change **150**, 119793 (2020)
173. Oh, S.-J., Ryu, J.-N.: The effect of brain-computer interface-based cognitive training in patients with dementia. J. Korean Soc. Phys. Med. **13**(4), 59–65 (2018)
174. Spreicer, W.: Tangible interfaces as a chance for higher technology acceptance by the elderly. In: Proceedings of the 12th International Conference on Computer Systems and Technologies, pp. 311–316 (2011)
175. Fleury, M., Lioi, G., Barillot, C., Lécuyer, A.: A survey on the use of haptic feedback for brain-computer interfaces and neurofeedback. Front. Neurosci. **14**, 528 (2020)
176. Škola, F., Liarokapis, F.: Embodied VR environment facilitates motor imagery brain–computer interface training. Comput. Graph. **75**, 59–71 (2018)
177. Kuehn, E., Perez-Lopez, M.B., Diersch, N., Döhler, J., Wolbers, T., Riemer, M.: Embodiment in the aging mind. Neurosci. Biobehav. Rev. **86**, 207–225 (2018)
178. Müller, O., Rotter, S.: Neurotechnology: current developments and ethical issues. Front. Syst. Neurosci. **11**, 93 (2017)
179. Sundgren, S., Stolt, M., Suhonen, R.: Ethical issues related to the use of gerontechnology in older people care: a scoping review. Nurs. Ethics **27**(1), 88–103 (2020)
180. Eijkholt, M.: Clinical neuroethics: cracking brains and healthcare systems. J. Hosp. Ethics **6**(1), 74–75 (2019)
181. Friedman, B., Kahn, P., Borning, A.: Value sensitive design: theory and methods. University of Washington Technical Report, pp. 2–12 (2002)
182. Yuste, R., Goering, S., Bi, G., Carmena, J.M., Carter, A., Fins, J.J., Friesen, P., Gallant, J., Huggins, J.E., Illes, J.: Four ethical priorities for neurotechnologies and AI. Nature News **551**(7679), 159 (2017)
183. Crivelli, D., Balconi, M.: The agent brain: a review of non-invasive brain stimulation studies on sensing agency. Front. Behav. Neurosci. **11**, 229 (2017)
184. Bührle, C.P.: Changes in personality: possible hazards arising from chronic implantation of electrostimulation devices such as deep brain stimulation systems (DBS) or advanced electronic neuroprostheses. In: Implanted Minds. Transcript-Verlag, pp. 183–222 (2014)

185. Marson, F., Lasaponara, S., Cavallo, M.: A scoping review of neuromodulation techniques in neurodegenerative diseases: a useful tool for clinical practice? Medicina **57**(3), 215 (2021)
186. Wallach, W.: From robots to techno sapiens: ethics, law and public policy in the development of robotics and neurotechnologies. Law Innov. Technol. **3**(2), 185–207 (2011)
187. Goering, S., Klein, E., Sullivan, L.S., Wexler, A., y Arcas, B.A., Bi, G., Carmena, J.M., Fins, J.J., Friesen, P., Gallant, J.: Recommendations for responsible development and application of neurotechnologies. Neuroethics 1–22 (2021)
188. Earp, B.D., Sandberg, A., Kahane, G., Savulescu, J.: When is diminishment a form of enhancement? Rethinking the enhancement debate in biomedical ethics. Front. Syst. Neurosci. **8**, 12 (2014)
189. Corcella, L., Manca, M., Nordvik, J.E., Paternò, F., Sanders, A.-M., Santoro, C.: Enabling personalisation of remote elderly assistance. Multimed. Tools Appl. **78**(15), 21557–21583 (2019)
190. Organization, W.H.: Classification of Digital Health Interventions v1. 0: A Shared Language to Describe the Uses of Digital Technology for Health. World Health Organization (2018)
191. Kostkova, P.: Grand challenges in digital health. Front. Public Health **3**, 134 (2015)
192. Recchia, G., Capuano, D.M., Mistri, N., Verna, R.: Digital therapeutics-what they are, what they will be. Acta. Sci. Med. Sci. **4**, 1–9 (2020)
193. Dang, A., Arora, D., Rane, P.: Role of digital therapeutics and the changing future of healthcare. J. Family Med. Prim. Care **9**(5), 2207 (2020)
194. Abbadessa, G., Brigo, F., Clerico, M., De Mercanti, S., Trojsi, F., Tedeschi, G., Bonavita, S., Lavorgna, L.: Digital therapeutics in neurology. J. Neurol. 1–16 (2021)
195. Kaufman, N.: Digital therapeutics: leading the way to improved outcomes for people with diabetes. Diab. Spectr. **32**(4), 301–303 (2019)
196. Kaldy, J.: Digital therapeutics: health care wired for the future. Senior Care Pharmacist **35**(8), 338–344 (2020)
197. Bevilacqua, R., Casaccia, S., Cortellessa, G., Astell, A., Lattanzio, F., Corsonello, A., D'ascoli, P., Paolini, S., Di Rosa, M., Rossi, L.: Coaching through technology: a systematic review into efficacy and effectiveness for the ageing population. Int. J. Environ. Res. Public Health **17**(16), 5930 (2020)
198. Khelassi, A., Estrela, V.V., Monteiro, A.C.B., França, R.P., Iano, Y., Razmjooy, N.: Health 4.0: applications, management, technologies and review. Med. Technol. J. (2019)
199. Chang, C.-J., Yang, T.-F., Yang, S.-W., Chern, J.-S.: Cortical modulation of motor control biofeedback among the elderly with high fall risk during a posture perturbation task with augmented reality. Front. Aging Neurosci. **8**, 80 (2016)
200. Wright, J.M., Regele, O.B., Kourtis, L.C., Pszenny, S.M., Sirkar, R., Kovalchick, C., Jones, G.B.: Evolution of the digital biomarker ecosystem. Digit. Med. **3**(4), 154 (2017)
201. Cavedoni, S., Chirico, A., Pedroli, E., Cipresso, P., Riva, G.: Digital biomarkers for the early detection of mild cognitive impairment: artificial intelligence meets virtual reality. Front. Human Neurosci. **14** (2020)
202. Rutkowski, T.M., Zhao, Q., Abe, M.S., Otake, M.: AI Neurotechnology for Aging Societies-- Task-load and Dementia EEG Digital Biomarker Development Using Information Geometry Machine Learning Methods (2018). arXiv:181112642
203. Ansado, J., Chasen, C., Bouchard, S., Northoff, G.: How brain imaging provides predictive biomarkers for therapeutic success in the context of virtual reality cognitive training. Neurosci. Biobehav. Rev. **120**, 583–594 (2021)
204. Sue, F.-M., Chang, Y.-S., Sheu, R.-K.: A platform for fusing psychological and physiological data from hybrid cloud. In: 2016 IEEE 13th International Conference on Networking, Sensing, and Control (ICNSC), pp. 1–6. IEEE (2016)
205. Tomassini C 5.5 National report: Ageing And Technologies, Italy, vol 165
206. Berger, R.P., Houle, J.-F., Hayes, R.L., Wang, K.K., Mondello, S., Bell, M.J.: Translating biomarkers research to clinical care: applications and issues for rehabilomics. PM&R **3**(6), S31–S38 (2011)

207. Dryden, E., Sahal, M., Feldman, S., Ayaz, H., Heiman-Patterson, T.: Amyotrophic lateral sclerosis disease progression presents difficulties in brain computer interface use. In: International Conference on Applied Human Factors and Ergonomics, pp. 70–77. Springer (2021)
208. Tun, S.Y.Y., Madanian, S., Mirza, F.: Internet of things (IoT) applications for elderly care: a reflective review. Aging Clin. Exp. Res. **33**(4), 855–867 (2021)
209. Pal, D., Funilkul, S., Charoenkitkarn, N., Kanthamanon, P.: Internet-of-things and smart homes for elderly healthcare: an end user perspective. IEEE Access **6**, 10483–10496 (2018)
210. Azimi, I., Rahmani, A.M., Liljeberg, P., Tenhunen, H.: Internet of things for remote elderly monitoring: a study from user-centered perspective. J. Ambient. Intell. Humaniz. Comput. **8**(2), 273–289 (2017)
211. Marques, G.: Ambient assisted living and internet of things. In: Harnessing the Internet of Everything (IoE) for Accelerated Innovation Opportunities, pp. 100–115 (2019)
212. Andrade, T., Bastos, D.: Extended reality in IoT scenarios: concepts, applications and future trends. In: 5th Experiment International Conference (exp. at'19), pp. 107–112. IEEE (2019)
213. Amorim, P., Santos, B.S., Dias, P., Silva, S., Martins, H.: Serious games for stroke telerehabilitation of upper limb-a review for future research. Int. J. Telerehabilitation **12**(2), 65–76 (2020)
214. Elayan, H., Aloqaily, M., Guizani, M.: Digital twin for intelligent context-aware IoT healthcare systems. IEEE Internet Things J. (2021)
215. Miraz, M.H., Ali, M., Excell, P.S., Picking, R.A.: Review on Internet of Things (IoT), Internet of everything (IoE) and Internet of nano things (IoNT). In: Internet Technologies and Applications (ITA), pp. 219–224. IEEE 2015
216. Javaid, M., Khan, I.H.: Internet of things (IoT) enabled healthcare helps to take the challenges of COVID-19 pandemic. J. Oral Biol. Craniofac. Res. **11**(2), 209–214 (2021)
217. DiGiovanni, G., Mousaw, K., Lloyd, T., Dukelow, N., Fitzgerald, B., D'Aurizio, H., Loh, K.P., Mohile, S., Ramsdale, E., Maggiore, R.: Development of a telehealth geriatric assessment model in response to the COVID-19 pandemic. J. Geriatr. Oncol. **11**(5), 761–763 (2020)
218. Vishnu, S., Ramson, S.J., Jegan, R.: Internet of medical things (IoMT)-an overview. In: 2020 5th International Conference on Devices, Circuits and Systems (ICDCS), pp. 101–104. IEEE 2020
219. Meng, W., Cai, Y., Yang, L.T., Chiu, W.-Y.: Hybrid emotion-aware monitoring system based on brainwaves for internet of medical things. IEEE Internet Things J. (2021)
220. Elmalaki, S., Demirel, B.U., Taherisadr, M., Stern-Nezer, S., Lin, J.J., Al Faruque, M.A.: Towards internet-of-things for wearable neurotechnology. In: 22nd International Symposium on Quality Electronic Design (ISQED), pp. 559–565. IEEE (2021)
221. Shirke, B., Wong, J., Libut, J.C., George, K., Oh, S.J.: Brain-IoT based emotion recognition system. In: 10th Annual Computing and Communication Workshop and Conference (CCWC), pp. 0991–0995. IEEE (2020)
222. Schiliro, F., Moustafa, N., Beheshti, A.: Cognitive privacy: AI-enabled privacy using EEG signals in the internet of things. In: 2020 IEEE 6th International Conference on Dependability in Sensor, Cloud and Big Data Systems and Application (DependSys), pp. 73–79. IEEE, (2020)
223. Maiti, M., Ghosh, U.: Next generation internet of things in fintech ecosystem. IEEE Internet Things J. (2021)
224. Yu, B., Hu, J., Funk, M., Feijs, L.: DeLight: biofeedback through ambient light for stress intervention and relaxation assistance. Pers. Ubiquit. Comput. **22**(4), 787–805 (2018)
225. Swan, M., Kido, T.: Ruckenstein M BRAINY–multi-modal brain training app for Google glass: cognitive enhancement, wearable computing, and the Internet-of-Things extend personal data analytics. In: Workshop on Personal Data Analytics in the Internet of Things 40th International Conference on Very Large Databases (2014)
226. Miralles, F., Vargiu, E., Rafael-Palou, X., Solà, M., Dauwalder, S., Guger, C., Hintermüller, C., Espinosa, A., Lowish, H., Martin, S.: Brain–computer interfaces on track to home: results of the evaluation at disabled end-users' homes and lessons learnt. Front. ICT **2**, 25 (2015)

Attention-Aware Recognition of Activities of Daily Living Based on Eye Gaze Tracking

B. G. D. A. Madhusanka, Sureswaran Ramadass, Premkumar Rajagopal, and H. M. K. K. M. B. Herath

Abstract Eye movements are essential in comprehending the environment. Users' attention may be directed via eye gazing, which can enhance Human–Computer Interaction (HCI). Gaze estimation can make HCI more natural in a non-intrusive way. For example, tiredness detection, biometric identification, illness diagnosis, activity recognition, an estimate of alertness level and gaze-contingent display are all possible uses of eye-tracking. It's been available for decades, but it's not been widely used in consumer applications. The high cost of eye-tracking technology and the lack of consumer-level applications are the main reasons behind this. When it comes to Activities of Daily Living (ADL), assistive robots may restore essential levels of independence for the elderly and others who are disabled. Although people can communicate their wishes in numerous ways, linguistic patterns and gaze-based implicit communication of intentions remain underdeveloped, such as bodily expressions or actions. In this study, based on the eye view, a new, implicit, nonverbal communication paradigm for HCI is introduced. Conventional gaze detection systems rely on infrared lights and cameras with high-resolution sensors to achieve outstanding performance and durability. But these systems need to be modified. Thus they are confined to laboratory research and challenging to apply in the real world. Here, we recommend that the gaze be followed using a webcam. Using a webcam to obtain 2D coordinates, we provide a practical visual monitoring framework based on models. This work on the platform is intended to ease HCI and thus increase useful technology and consumers' privacy in their daily lives. The test results of this experiment indicated that implicit human gaze patterns on visualized objects could efficiently be used for contact with people's intentions. Studies have also shown that it is simple to comprehend and use contact with the gaze. It is further suggested that the subject-dependent eye parameters are calculated using a specific reference system. Finally, an implicit

---

B. G. D. A. Madhusanka (✉) · S. Ramadass · P. Rajagopal
School of Science and Engineering, Malaysia University of Science and Technology (MUST), Petaling Jaya, Malaysia
e-mail: bgmad@ou.ac.lk

H. M. K. K. M. B. Herath
Department of Mechanical Engineering, Faculty of Engineering Technology, The Open University of Sri Lanka, Nugegoda, Sri Lanka

communication system for monitoring and interpreting purposes has been developed. After understanding the user's implicit intention to support the elderly with the action of the eye-gaze, the device can distinguish the activities/requirements required from the home environment. Finally, to direct caregivers to deliver the correct service, the implied purpose may then be used.

Keywords Activities of daily living (ADL) · Eye-gaze tracking · Gaze-based communication · Human–computer interaction (HCI) · Implicit intention inference · Webcam

1 Introduction

Nowadays, supplementary homes are employed regularly to provide the elderly who reside in these places' security, reassurance, and health assistance. The older people feel assured that they are doing their day-to-day work in such an atmosphere, as devoted employees provide 24/7 services during an emergency [1]. To enhance care services in supplementary care homes, nine distinct premises of the additional care home provider included in this study project have been provided with a monitoring system consisting of various kinds of non-intrusive sensors. This technique was not used to monitor seniors who have a specific sickness or problem with their health. However, data relating to daily life activities mainly were collected (ADLs). For example, volunteers facing a hearing, visual impairment, physical disability, diabetes, and other problems facing the project [2]. The distinction of the medical issues may change how anyone conducts ADLs as normal and abnormal conduct, which impact their detection, might be characterized differently in each scenario [3]. Identifying unwanted actions/conduct that can influence seniors' well-being considers various rooms of a particular care facility inspected. Thus, ADLs are monitored: (i) toilet and personal toilet, (ii) breakfasts, (iii) lunch breaks, (iv) evening meals preparation, (v) sleep preparation [4]. It should be noted that we evaluate these ADLs, which occur on a regular day in many or similar cases [5].

Human–computer interaction provides tailor-made help for various applications, including e-health and monitoring [5]. For several computer science companies, identifying human activity is an important study field. Human activity systems may now be defined by feature extraction as either a standard or a deep model. A conventional means of handling the problem of identifying the human activity is based on hand-made descriptors of functions divided into three types: local features, global characteristics and the two combinations [6–8]. The international aspects of the picture describe it as representing the whole spectrum of human body movements. Numerous commercial and non-commercial eye-tracking technologies are available to detect human activities in ADL. Several of them are costly or incorrect in real-world situations, and some need deliberate, time-consuming user calibration [9]. As a tip, current eye-tracking research focuses on constructing profound learning eye-tracking systems that do not require explicit human calibration [10].

Eye movement has been studied and recorded for over a century [11], with methodologies ranging from artificial observational methods to mechanical techniques, power techniques, and optical approaches [12]. In recent times, computing eye movement was adopted as a dominating method in many disciplines, such as cognitive science [13, 14], psychology [9, 15], medical diagnosis [16], identity authentication [17, 18] and eye-based interaction with the computer [17, 18]. Computer-based vision systems are less complicated, more intricate, and easier to operate. Eye-tracking and eye movement analysis have traditionally been applications that focused on eye movement. The gaze estimate and identification of important eye motion types are used for eye movement analysis [19].

According to Wong et al. [17], the current gaze estimation taxonomy includes feature and appearance-based techniques. The most often used gaze estimating approach is the feature-based technique, which removes gaze-related local elements. The approaches utilized based on components may be classified as corneal reflection or form-based procedures, depending on whether external light sources are employed. Tobii [20] and SMI [21] eye trackers have been successfully deployed using several cameras and IR LEDs. This technology is exact since the pupil centre and glint can be rapidly retrieved to calibrate the mistakes caused by head movement. However, their challenging calibration, expensive cost and poor health consequences mean that IR light is inevitable.

IR light systems are also unstable for outdoor applications [22]. Shape-based approaches with precisely reconstructed pupil, iris, and eyelid edges [23, 24] are imprecise [25–29] and required sufficient picture quality. On the other hand, the pupil and the shine are usually missing from webcam films. Camera calibration or geometry data, in general, is not needed for appearance-based approaches [30, 31]. Instead, the visual content is employed to assess the function underneath for the gaze points or direction of the gaze. Although this approach is more adaptive to head movements and has low accuracy, it is more vulnerable. Recently, deep learning has emerged as a viable answer to applications for computer vision which has significantly improved performance [32].

A typical deep learning technique, Convolutional Neural Networks (CNNs), have been widely studied and utilized in recent years in computer vision, natural language processing, and voice recognition [32]. Convolutional and subsampling layers of CNN's feature extractor extract implicit features from training data automatically, eliminating human feature selection requirements. To counteract this problem, CNN has adopted the empirical risk reduction concept, which is infamous for overfitting and requiring large training sets [33].

During a period in which profound learning is booming, gaze estimating models based on CNNs are becoming more popular and common. It gained popularity when Akinyelu et al. [32] successfully used it to classify handwritten numbers. Several domains, including computer vision [34–39], voices recognition [40], and language modelling [41], have been effectively applied in CNN models. They are ideal for large-scale data collections. CNN models can map picture properties like pupils and glint positions without hand-designed features to viewpoints directly [42]. Thus, CNN can obtain higher performance on gaze assessment to learn representations from enormous quantities of data. The multimodal, in-the-wild, CNN gaze dataset technique has been suggested by Lemley et al. [43]. A comprehensive moving eye-tracking system has been created by Liaqat et al. [44]. In the training of CNN models, a large dataset was used, which significantly decreased mistakes. These techniques may be used with any head position in an unconstrained ADL setting since the profound and multimodal networks and large-scale training datasets are used. The precise estimation of these methods is, however, insufficient for eye-based human–computer interaction [45].

Precise gaze estimation is an essential guarantee for eye movement analysis technology. Although strong convolutional nets in low-cost and real-world gaze assessments have progressed, the accuracy remains inadequate [46]. Many domains, like the diagnosis of nystagmus or dyslexia, eye-based detection, tiredness detection, and activity identification, do not need a gaze-point or direction to study eye movements [47]. Instead, a mapping function should be accessible between the length of the eye movement and a given activity or scenario. Time-varying eye movement data may be utilized to examine eye movement without considering the eye and its associated calibration. The advantages of moving away from a gaze-centred paradigm are listed below [48]. (1) The gaze mapping error can be corrected. (2) Other eye motion metrics (other than the iris centre, which is incorrect due to eyelid blockage) can be used to compensate for an iris centre identification error. For example, the broad width of the eye may be a helpful complement to pictures of low quality. (3) Relative movement information is more straightforward to discern in low-quality video interframes than estimated position, which may also be highlighted.

This research makes a significant addition by providing a learning methodology for ADL-based CNN and Support Vector Machine (SVM) to identify home activities [49]. As a result, numerous researchers have combined CNN and SVM, a method based on structural risk reduction, to address challenges in various fields, including handwriting recognition, human action recognition, and face detection. Compared to CNNs used primarily for pattern recognition, CNNs used for regression estimation are rarely documented, even less so for time-series signals. The proposed system is trained and evaluated using a publicly accessible dataset. This chapter also recommends a novel method for studying eye movement using a webcam. Feature points are used to acquire eye movement information rather than computing the mapping function, in contrast to the feature-based gaze tracking methodology. The specific improvements are as follows as compared to [50–52] and include:

(1) The extraction of eye feature points is done using CNN-SVM, making the detection results more precise and robust.
(2) CNN-SVM extracts eye movement features instead of using artificial extraction.
(3) Examining eye movement patterns now includes additional indicators such as relative iris and pupil centre displacement and change in open width.

Experiments show that the recommended technique yields good results. The benefits of the webcam-based methodology in terms of less intrusiveness, lower cost, and more straightforward operation are critical components for the widespread adoption of eye movement-based applications.

2 Approach to Truly Affective ADL for Human-Centred Design

In addition to ADL, ideas, goods, and services may be defined as combining modern technology with a social context to enhance the quality of life for persons at all phases of life [53]. The quality of life might be seen as well-being from an individual point of view. In a person's life, it has emotional, social, and physical characteristics. People are social entities. Therefore, one of ADL's fundamental duties is to make social interaction easier [54]. This is achieved by implementing the effects, detecting, and processing processes of a system (a general word used to include feelings, mood, emotions, etc.). Affective data improves the capacity of a strategy to make sound judgments and accomplish its aims by providing additional information to recognize the situation and mediate communication.

Integration in ADL systems involves expertise in multiple domains, including cognitive psychology, neurology, medicine, and computer science. In a subject such as affective computing, this expertise was of essential relevance. It focuses primarily on the research and development of recognizable systems and devices. In addition, they analyze, analyze, and mimic human activity [54], which leads to considerable research, algorithms, and processes in this field.

ADL apps aiming at helping older persons and young people live independently and comfortably in their living environment (since health issues may impact anybody at any age). However, living areas include user dwellings and diverse surrounding settings, such as city streets, schools, stores, restaurants, and other sites. Therefore, these individuals have mobility, social interactions, health care and knowledge, and abilities connected to issue areas (e.g., mathematics) and needed for daily living, such as eating and cleaning. Therefore, four ADL areas, including healthcare, education (teaching/learning), mobility (trends) and social interaction, are evaluated concerning the previously mentioned effective processes to satisfy increasing emotional, physical, and mental demands in extended ADL contexts [55].

Eye movement is one of the most significant ways of collecting environmental information to activate motor activity, allowing a person to function in ADL. They are excellent markers of an individual's interest and attentiveness. Eye-motion is a natural aspect of our worldwide contact. The orientation of the view may indicate the user's concentration directly. Eye movement implies a transfer of focus, and a lot may be revealed about his activities by following one's look. This might be essential to improve the connection between Humans-Computer Interaction (HCI), establishing intelligent interfaces where machines can more naturally recognize and communicate with people [56]. Seamless and customized interaction is achievable if the computer can identify the user's identity, interests, intentions, context, and actions. While it has been there for many decades eye-tracking technology, has not been widely used at the consumer level. To make eye tracking a ubiquitous technique, many problems must be resolved. One of the main constraints which limit its use is the high cost of commercially available eye-trackers. Another aspect that restricts applicability is the reduced precision in real-world circumstances. Another problem is the lack of consumer cases [57].

The goal of this chapter is to improve the visual monitoring of systems. To do this, we have created programs for indoor and desktop contexts. We have created cost-effective gauze tracking methods in realistic situations. Most eye-trackers already in use need specific cameras and lighting systems, making the device more expensive. However, using shelf cameras without extra hardware, low precision systems may be constructed. The exactness for each application is different. For example, a somewhat low-precision eye tracker would provide the ability to locate the general area of the game. However, computational processes and spatial resolution could need applications such as biometric identification based on eye movements. The cost of eye-tracking should thus be reduced so that technology is everywhere. For this purpose, we propose constructing a camera eye tracker that can be used with Python without extra ADL hardware.

3 Materials and Methods

3.1 CNN-SVM Classifier Training for Visual Attention Detection

Since the CNN approach is popular in various other domains, we've chosen to use it for activities in a frame-by-frame fashion. An additional benefit of CNNs is that they reduce the number of parameters and connections needed during the artificial neural network training phase. Visual attention detection remains an open research problem that necessitates exploring novel techniques and methodologies that improve recognition accuracy, processing time, and computational complexity. As a result, this study proposes a framework for visual attention detection using a hybrid CNN-SVM architecture. This paper uses CNN to extract features from different face images from the 300-W IMAVIS (image and vision computing) dataset [58]. These acquired characteristics are then sent into the proposed visual attention detection experiment's SVM classifier. Human actions are shown in each of the frames included in the video [59]. Extract from the raw RGB video frame the main characteristics. They have been used in a pre-trained deep CNN architecture with pretrained parameters in these trials. In the 300-W IMAVIS face dataset, a broad diversity of identities, emotions, light situations, location or occlusion were made utilizing 600-imagery pictures (300 indoor or 300 outdoor). Using a deep CNN network design, a probability vector for each input frame is created to reflect the likelihood of the different items in the frame [59].

A CNN model with pre-trained IMAVIS 300-W database parameters is used to extract light and precious video frame residual properties in each video sequence. The architecture consists of several CNN three-layered blocks, consisting of small, 64 × 64 kernels, 128 × 128, 256 × 256, 512 × 512, and finally 512 × 512. This network is supposed to receive an input of 292 × 292 pictures followed by a fully interconnected [60] layer. The display of the features gathered from a pretrained repeating model is the resulting vector from the final bundling layer. Although the data are relatively small, this technique lowers the time needed for training and prevents the data from being overpowered with the correct weight. However, the last layer of the selected CNN model is a classification layer in the proposed study. The output of the previous layer is a framework in the categorization process. The SVM classifier was used instead of the deleted layer to predict human detection of visual attention. Figure 1 shows the architecture of the suggested model for detecting visual attention.

It is a machine learning approach that excels other classifiers in terms of discriminating between various classifications. Since it's used to treat tiny datasets and significant areas, we choose it for our inquiry. The concept behind employing a supervised learning methodology with SVM is that the best hyperplane for dividing feature space may be used. While training, the SVM uses vectors generated in the high-dimensional area to identify the training dataset. The training data is moved to a new vector space when the collection of training data is not linearly separable. With sufficient training data, SVM delivers reliable and effective results.

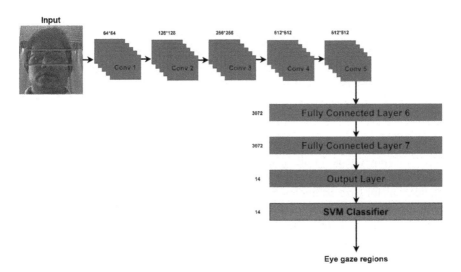

Fig. 1 The architecture of the proposed visual attention detection model

3.2 Implementation Details

Python was used for the profound CNN model. This technology is based on the NVIDIA GeForce 930 M (2 GB DDR3), 8 GB DDR3 RAM, an Intel Core i5-5200U CPU, and the 64-bit Windows Pro Edition. The proposed method is based on the CNN model with the modified dataset. Additionally, the model avoids the issue of overfitting datasets, which is a frequent occurrence. Each video frame in the dataset was divided into frames and added to the model using the previously trained CNN model. A 292 × 292 frame is altered from the chosen frame and shifted horizontally and vertically on a random basis throughout training. Increase the training dataset, and these operations are conducted at each cycle. The CNN model's final pooling layer was employed to create a 3072-sized vector during training and testing. The 300-W IMAVIS database offers more than "neutral" and "smiling" pictures and emotions such as "surprise" and "scared" partial oversight. The facial landmarks are accessible from the whole database, and 68 points for each facial landmark have been provided. The resultant vectors have been utilized for both the multi-class SVM classification training and testing data. The training procedure is finished with a training error of 0.02038 and a test error of 0.02045. A multi-class SVM classifier is used, which allows a linear and improved SVM performance to projects the original linear and nonlinear dataset into more dimensional space using the linear function kernel.

3.3 Gaze Estimation

Gaze estimates are an approach to detect users' intents and interests [61]. The method for gaze estimates [62] examines the link between visual information and the direction of the gaze. Eye properties retrieved from imagery data acquired from single and many cameras (pupil and corneal reflection) are utilized to estimate the gaze directions [63]. There are two types of approaches for gaze estimation in general: model and appearance [64]. Further detail on the two strategies is provided in the following subsections. In the handy field, the mobile gaze interaction [65], driver gaze monitoring [66], screen type keyboard [67] and virtual reality [68] are practical applications for gaze estimation.

In appearance-based approaches, the photometric appearance of the eye is utilized to determine the gaze [69]. They usually need just a single camera to collect pictures of the eye, which are used to construct gaze estimation models that can map the images in a specific direction of the gaze. These models need not be created; they may deduce picture attributes from data instead. Compared with model-based technologies, appearance-based systems need additional eye pictures for training, enabling them to acquire a discrepancy in appearance [70].

Based gaze estimate algorithms in real-world scenarios are likely to provide excellent results [71]. However, these coordinates can only be utilized for one setup and guidance [72] since their gaze position is computed directly inside the coordination system on the target screen [73] and means that screen coordinates may be utilized only for a single device and orientation. In various research [74], algorithms were developed to estimate the position of the gaze concerning the camera. These systems structure the gaze as a virtual plane in the camera coordination system [75].

The models for estimating the gaze and the eye's geometric model are integrated with the eye's characteristics, including the corneal and pupil centres [76]. The geometric portrayal of the eye is seen in Fig. 2. As depicted in Fig. 2, the optical axis is the line between the heart and the pupil centre. The visual axis between the centre of the cornea and the fovea determines the direction of the gaze. Thus, the gaze point is defined as the crossroads of the visual axis and the display surface [77]. Finally, kappa angles are the angles that are created by the intersecting optical and visual axes. The angle difference between the optical axis and the visual axis is a constant vector [78]. Personal calibration is usually used to estimate the value for each participant in model-based procedures. Corner precision at degrees [79], cm/mm distance precision [80], and gauze estimate precision at percentage [81] all provide instances of gazing metrics published in the literature for accurate monitoring.

Elderly people who are lonely or depressed may appreciate their attention when reading or eating a diary to help with daily living skills. Computationally efficient and high performing, our real-time estimation solution for the typical webcam footage is. According to educational psychology, it is expected that the methodology recommended will be used in the future to examine the behaviour.

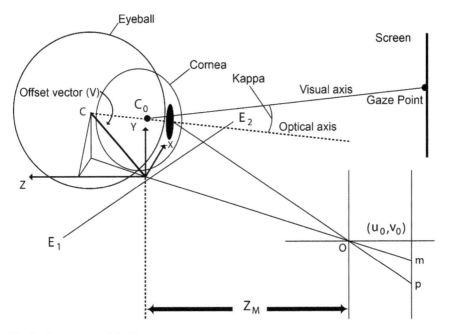

Fig. 2 Geometric model of the eye

Fig. 3 Environment setup

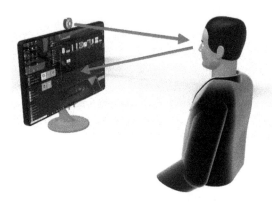

A high-resolution webcam with a broad-angle lens was usually placed on the top of the monitor screen in prior eye-tracking research. The camera was set below the subject, resulting in the original elevation angle. You may use this setup strategy to avoid the impact of eyelid movement. For most users, the camera is located on the top of the display. Thus, we broaden our scope and study the eye-tracking issue without employing a camera or costly eye-tracking equipment. [82] This illustration in Fig. 3 illustrates the primary light source of the ceiling light, which is a desktop computer with a camera hooked to the display. 50–70 cm from the camera to the user is required due to the common usage of low resolution and because the extracted eye block resolution is at least 20 × 20.

The eyes can be identified appropriately and monitored carelessly utilizing precise iris and pupil detection without changes in lighting. Measuring how effectively a model predicts a gaze and a discrepancy between the forecast and the actual gaze coordinates. The following section contains numerous computations on the accuracy of the gaze estimate.

3.4 Visual Gaze Estimation

This section builds on prior work in Fig. 3 by studying camera setups and gaze estimation algorithms to increase tracking resilience under real-world settings. User calibration, in addition to hardware setup calibration, is critical to user experience and convenience. For example, user calibration is required to represent the individual-specific features necessary for estimate bias correction. When the amount of calibration data rises, the calibration quality improves to some level. However, increasing the number of calibration sites to increase the data volume might be cumbersome and negatively impact the user experience.

Furthermore, the trade-off between the quality and simplicity of user calibration has been extensively researched in the literature [61]. Significant progress has been achieved, for example, more robust geometric eye models and more effective bias correction models have been constructed, and implicit calibration approaches have been implemented. This section also describes the proposed webcam-based eye gaze tracking approach in depth. Figure 4 depicts an overview of the process. It consists of a concurrently functioning webcam system with blink and gazes feature recognition, gaze estimation, and user calibration operations. The primary addition is that gaze outputs from both the eye and the camera are incorporated into the proposed gaze estimation mechanism, which produces an overall Point of Regard (PoR). The process begins with eye localization, which determines the presence of the eyes. Next, a robust non-rigid face tracker based on a well-supervised algorithm is used to locate and track the eyes. According to the decent supervised approach, the cascade of regression models may infer an appropriate final face shape using 68 markers. The method is based on 68 features. Marks around the eyes may be used to precisely remove the eye areas after matching the form of the face.

A. **Iris detection**

Once the preceding procedures have been used to remove the eye, the centre of the iris is located. To begin, we measure the width of the pupil's iris. A high-energy and fast-edge data combination will then find the iris's core. This method of smoothing the eye region using the L_0 gradient minimization technique is used to eliminate noisy pixels while keeping the eye's boundary shape to calculate the radius. For the intensity calculations, a proper iris centre estimate may be employed. After the eye-tracking locations, the Canny edge detector is applied. When dealing with short lengths and distance filters, several incorrect edges are used. The point of intersection between the pupil and the iris is too near

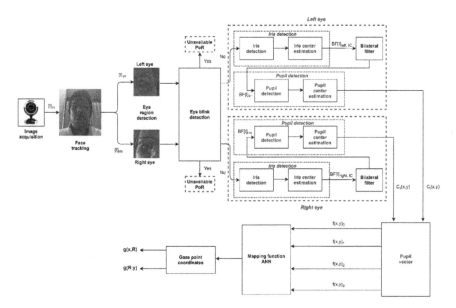

Fig. 4 Overview of a camera system, which comprises gaze tracking for both eye

or too far away. In the model of the iris circle, the parameters are calculated using the Random Sample Consensus (RANSAC) methodology [83, 84]. Once the RANSAC has been applied on the iris edges, the iris radius r may be computed. The last step is to set the iris's central location by combining extreme energy and edge strength. These two letters, E_1 and E_2, respectively reflect the intensity energy and edge strength.

$$E_1 = \sum (I \times S_r) \qquad (1)$$

$$E_2 = \sqrt{g_x^2 + g_y^2} \qquad (2)$$

where I is the eye region, and S_r is a circle window with the same radius as the iris. The g_x and g_y are the horizontal and vertical gradients of the pixel, respectively. To detect the iris centre, we should minimize the intensity energy in the circle window and maximize the edge strength of the iris edges. The trade-off is controlled by the parameter τ. That is,

$$\left(x_{BF[I]_{IC}}, y_{BF[I]_{IC}} \right)$$
$$= \min_{(x,y)} \left\{ E_1(x,y) - \tau \cdot \left(\int_{-\pi/5}^{+\pi/5} E_2(x,y) \cdot ds + \int_{4\pi/5}^{6\pi/5} E_2(x,y) \cdot ds \right) \right\} \qquad (3)$$

where $\left(x_{BF[I]_{IC}}, y_{BF[I]_{IC}} \right)$ is the estimation coordinate of the iris centre. The integral intervals are ranges of the iris edge that do not overlap with the eyelids.

Because of its enhanced resilience to light and eye type differences, a dark-pupil-based technique rather than a bright-pupil-based method is used for pupil centre identification. The equation of bilateral filtering is conducted on the input eye area with the dark pupil to smooth the pupil area while retaining the pupil to iris crisp (3). Bilateral filtering considers a Gaussian filter in space and another Gaussian filter, the pixel difference function [85]. The Gaussian function of space ensures that only pixels close to each other are evaluated for blurring. The Gaussian function of intensity difference, on the other hand, ensures that only pixels with similar intensities to the centre pixel are considered for blurring. As a result, it preserves the edges since pixels near the margins will have significant intensity variance. The critical element in bilateral filtering is that two pixels are close to one other if they occupy neighbouring spatial positions and have some photometric range similarity. Because bilateral filtering may preserve edges according to equations, it overcomes the disadvantages of different approaches such as Averaging Blur, Gaussian Blur, and Median Blur (4).

$$BF[I]_p = \frac{1}{W_p} \sum_{q \in s} G_{\sigma s}(p - q) G_{\sigma r}(I_p - I_q) I_q \qquad (4)$$

where W_p is a normalization factor,

$$W_p = \sum_{q \in s} G_{\sigma s}(p-q) G_{\sigma r}(I_p - I_q) I_q \qquad (5)$$

Equation (4) and (5) are used for the bilateral filter, where p is the target pixel, and q is one pixel around the target pixel, I_p is the colour of the target pixel, I_q is the colour of a pixel around the target pixel, s is the pixel group around the target pixel, $G_{\sigma s}$ is the weighted pixels according to the distance, and $G_{\sigma r}$ is the weighted pixels according to pixel colour difference.

B. Pupil detection

After calibrating parameters, we used bilateral filters to smoothen the image and preserve the edges of the image content of $BF[I]_{(x,y)}$. That was suitable for retaining the pupil's features. Following that, normalize the histogram to increase the contrast. Then, by injecting the average intensity into the surrounding areas, we may approximate the pupil's average intensity. The pupil blob is then highlighted by inverting the picture and using the average intensity inside the pupil as a threshold. However, the binary image contains a few other blobs that are as black as the pupil area, such as eyelashes, eyelids, and shades. Morphological methods are used to distinguish the actual pupil area from the distracting blobs. The final pupil is determined by the form, size, and position of the remaining candidate blobs. The object's centre of gravity is then utilized to calculate the pupil's centre.

A Canny Edge Detector and a Hough Circular Transform [86–89] compute the pupil iris frontier. A Combination of Profile and Mask The pupil detection iris borders are defined utilizing methods. The Hough circular transformation creates an edge map with vertically slanting gradients to the iris's outer rim. The difference between the pupils and iris centres and radii is identified using a threshold and accurate detection. For example: when the pupil divergences are T_1 in the X-direction and T_2 in the Y-direction, followed by T_3 and T_4 to show pupil and iris variations in the radius, as shown in Fig. 5.

Determine the centre of the pupil by X_c and Y_c, respectively,

$$x_c = x_{c-\text{iris}} - x_{c-\text{pupil}} \qquad (6)$$

$$y_c = y_{c-\text{iris}} - y_{c-\text{pupil}} \qquad (7)$$

where $(x_{c-\text{iris}}, y_{c-\text{iris}}) = BF[I]_{(x,y)}$ which describes iris centre estimation coordinates.

Also, $x_c < T_1$, the threshold for pupil and iris centre is different in x direction. Then, the system can detect the user's gaze move either left or right direction, respectively. Then, $y_c < T_2$, the threshold for pupil and iris centre is different in y direction.

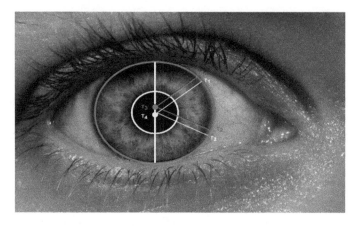

Fig. 5 Both iris and pupil centre determination

Then, the system can detect the user's gaze move either up or down direction, respectively. If $T_4 < R_d < T_3$ correct centre of the eye detected, where R_d is the radius difference between the iris and pupil centre.

Further, the masking technique will be implemented to determine the pupil's radius, as shown in Fig. 6.

By averaging of both R_1 and R_2, the radius of pupil labelled as R, can be computed where the radius R_1 is determined by computing the difference between $x_{\max}$ and $x_{\min}$ followed by division by two using Eq. (8):

$$R_1 = \frac{x_{\max} - x_{\min}}{2} \qquad (8)$$

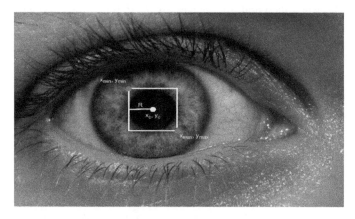

Fig. 6 Pupil detection based on masking

The same method is used to compute the value of radius R_2 as in the following equation as in (9):

$$R_2 = \frac{y_{max} - y_{min}}{2} \tag{9}$$

Finally, the pupil radius denoted by R is computed using Eq. (10) whilst pupil centre estimation coordinates represented by x_c and y_c are determined based on Eqs. (11) through (12), respectively.

$$R = \frac{R_1 + R_2}{2} \tag{10}$$

$$x_c = x_{min} + R \tag{11}$$

$$y_c = y_{min} + R \tag{12}$$

According to the respective pupil centre estimation coordinates derived from Eqs. (11) and (12) of both the left and right eye, a 2D gaze estimation method based on pupil vector is proposed in this research. An improved artificial neural network is developed to solve the mapping function between pupil vector and gaze point coordinates and then calculate the gaze direction of $g(x, R)$ and $g(R, y)$.

4 Calibration of Camera and Screen Parameters

Calibration approaches are intended to assist systems that wrongly calculate the Point of Gaze (PoG). The number of calibration points must be chosen carefully. A successful calibration method must contain as many calibration points as feasible to familiarize the user with the device. On the other hand, it should be basic enough not to pose problems for the user. For this system, a simple 4-point calibration method has been created. The purpose behind creating such a calibration method is that it might help calculate the eye area that will be utilized to scan the laptop screen. This basic technique enables the user to examine all corner locations to access mode. In this situation, accessible mode means the user may stay at a corner point for as long as they like. This notion supports the system in decreasing calibration errors caused by erroneous gaze detections. It starts by diverting the user's attention to the laptop's top left corner.

Meanwhile, the system begins its detection cycle, beginning with face detection and progressing through iris detection, pupil detection, gaze estimate points, and gaze locations until the user clicks again in the user interface. The system no longer saves gaze location results. The system saves the averaged findings to the top left corner location of the eye area scanning the laptop screen. This procedure is repeated for the remaining three corner locations. After calibration is complete, it enters the main eye gaze tracking loop, allowing the user to interact with their eyes. PoG is the critical stage since it incorporates computing PoG based on previously collected feature points. Errors detected during the detecting step must be corrected at this step.

PoG computations are impossible to conduct without a reference point. It can aid PoG computations by reducing the number of computations necessary to transform gaze motions into cursor movements on the laptop screen. The centre of the eye (CoE) is a good choice for a reference point. During the calibration step, the moveable area of the eyes was already calculated. CoE may be calculated by simply averaging the x and y coordinates. Equations (13) and (14), respectively, explain this notion.

$$CoE_x = \frac{CP2_x + CP1_x}{2} \qquad (13)$$

$$CoE_y = \frac{CP2_y + CP1_y}{2} \qquad (14)$$

where, CoE_x and CoE_y denote x and y coordinates of the centre point of the eye's movable region, respectively. $CP2$, $CP1$, $CP4$ and $CP3$ construct a rectangular region representing the eye's movable region, as shown in Fig. 7.

Furthermore, it was shown that cursor and gaze movements are connected; each cursor movement traverses many pixels to perform a single-pixel movement of the gaze. Determine the width and height of the eyes; the screen width and height were employed. The width and height are fixed for a laptop screen, whereas the eyeball's moveable zone will fluctuate based on the scenario. The width and height of the movable zone of the eye may be calculated using Eqs. (15) and (16).

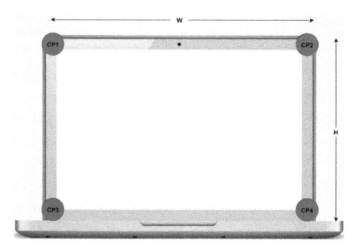

Fig. 7 4-point simple calibration

$$W_{eye} = CP1_y - CP2_y \tag{15}$$

$$H_{eye} = CP2_y - CP4_y \tag{16}$$

where, W_{eye} and H_{eye} represent width and height of the eye's movable region, respectively. Then, the scaling factor is computed for x and y coordinates using Eq. (17) and (18), respectively.

$$R_x = \frac{W_{screen}}{W_{eye}} \tag{17}$$

$$R_y = \frac{H_{screen}}{H_{eye}} \tag{18}$$

where, W_{screen} and H_{screen} denote width and height of laptop screen. Also, R_x and R_y represent scaling factor for x and y coordinates.

The PoG is computed to take into consideration the reference point's relevance. The gaze movements in the eyes are used to move the pointer on the laptop screen. Equations (19) and (20) may convert eye movements into cursor movements if the reference point in the eye coincides with the centre point on the laptop screen.

$$PoG_x = \frac{W_{screen}}{2} + R_x \times g(x, R) \tag{19}$$

$$PoG_y = \frac{H_{screen}}{2} + R_y \times g(R, y) \tag{20}$$

where, PoG_x and PoG_y represent x and y coordinates of PoG, respectively, and $g(x, R)$ denotes gaze point coordinate in x direction from the reference point, and $g(R, y)$ denotes gaze point coordinate in y direction from the reference point. They can be computed according to the output of the neural network. Also, the reference point R is calculated according to CoE described in Eqs. (13) and (14), respectively.

5 Results

After the calibration process is done, define the screen grid reference area according to Fig. 8. As per the user's attention area to the computer screen is defined the centre point of the screen as (x_R, y_R), an upper centre position as y_{min}, below centre position as y_{max}, left the centre position as x_{min} and right-centre position as x_{max} to initialize the system.

Figure 9a depicts the user eye gaze move to the 'centre' position of the screen. 'Center' coordinates are (587, 365), and the response time to detect the gaze point

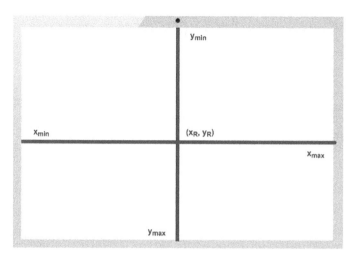

Fig. 8 Screen grid reference area

is 93.745 ms. Figure 9b depicts the user eye gaze move to the 'left' position of the screen. 'Left' position coordinates are (509, 429), and response time to detect the gaze point is 75.054 ms. Figure 9c depicts the user eye gaze move to the 'right' position of the screen. 'Right' position coordinates are (671, 396) and the response time to detect the gaze point is 124.998 ms. Figure 9d depicts the user eye gaze move to the 'top' position of the screen. 'Top' position coordinates are (605, 182) and response time to detect the gaze point is 93.768 ms. Figure 9e depicts the user eye gaze move to the 'bottom' position of the screen. 'Bottom' position coordinates are (542, 634), and response time to detect the gaze point is 78.140 ms.

We have recorded a series of films with 20 participants to assess their eye gaze performance. The right gaze direction was human-labelled for each frame of the images. Twenty images were shot in various lighting circumstances, with or without glasses, and in front of computer screens in multiple postures. They were told to begin recording the video by focusing on the centre of the screen and then moving their gaze to the left, right, top, and bottom of their eyes. We investigated the algorithm's performance in various picture circumstances to get a quantitative evaluation of the qualitative features of the photos.

In Fig. 10, a confusion matrix depicts one comprehensive inference performance of the mean of the intention to the "gaze direction." The horizontal axis represents predicted intention, whereas the vertical axis represents actual intention. The absolute mean accuracy and precision were calculated to be 0.92. Notably, the intention to eye gaze variance accounts for 0.08 of the mean absolute error. It is more challenging to characterize the purpose from the object aspect when there are less dominant eye gaze fluctuations. The CNN-SVM model is less forgiving of the attention detection classifier's errors.

The mean accuracy and precision for each type of intention are summarized in Fig. 11. The mean precision of the intention to "gaze direction to centre" was inferred

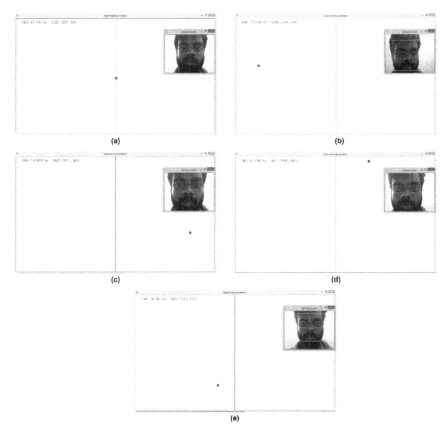

Fig. 9 User eye gaze moves to different locations. Figure 9a: User eye gaze move to the 'centre' position of the screen. Figure 9b: User eye gaze moves to the 'left' position of the screen. Figure 9c: User eye gaze move to the 'right' position of the screen. Figure 9d: User eye gaze moves to the 'top' position of the screen. Figure 9e: User eye gaze move to the 'bottom' position of the screen

		Predicted				
		Center	Left	Right	Top	Bottom
Actual	Center	1	0	0	0	0
	Left	0	0.9	0	0.05	0.05
	Right	0	0	0.9	0.05	0.05
	Top	0.05	0.05	0	0.9	0
	Bottom	0	0.05	0.05	0	0.9

Fig. 10 Confusion matrix for the gaze direction

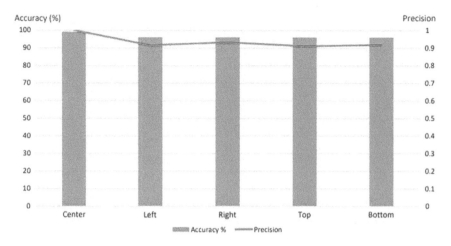

Fig. 11 Mean accuracy and precision for each intention

in 1 of the cases, and the mean precision of the intention to "gaze direction to left" was inferred in 0.9 of the cases. The mean precision of the intention to "gaze direction to the right" was inferred in 0.9 cases. The mean precision of the intention to "gaze direction to top" was inferred in 0.9 cases. Finally, the precision of the intention to "gaze direction to the bottom" was inferred in 0.9 of the cases.

Further, the mean accuracy of the intention to "gaze direction to centre" was inferred in 0.99 of the cases. The mean accuracy of the intention to "gaze direction to left" was inferred in 0.96 cases. The mean accuracy of the intention to "gaze direction to the right" was inferred in 0.97 of the cases. The mean accuracy of the intention to "gaze direction to top" was inferred in 0.96 cases. Finally, the accuracy of the intention to "gaze direction to the bottom" was inferred in 0.96 of the cases.

6 Conclusion

The eyes are a vital part of the human body that may be studied and extracted as necessary characteristics for various applications. Also, those with disabilities or older adults often use assistive gadgets that use eye control. Likewise, psychological studies have looked at eye fixation and saccade research, while identity and iris recognition is found in security systems. The two primary methods for collecting eye characteristics are eye detection and gaze estimation. Many previous articles have presented various ways for eye recognition and gaze estimation, but they were mainly concerned with problems at the high-resolution level. Without high-resolution cameras or other specialized/expensive equipment, users will be unable to use the site. It may be said that general webcam-based applications have become more popular and vital in recent years. Many consumers use consumer-grade PCs or laptops with ordinary webcams. However, there are presently just a few research dedicated to the issues with webcam-based applications. Many webcam-based applications need the user's attention to be acquired accidentally while using his ordinary personal computer and webcam without the need to purchase or wear any additional equipment. This chapter describes eye detection and gazes tracking methods that employ a typical webcam to accurately identify eyes and monitor gaze in real-time without the need for costly or specialist equipment. We proposed an eye-gaze detection method based on images captured by a single web camera set on the display's top. We were able to validate the system's accuracy by doing the research. Even though the proposed method seems simple, it has a high success rate in identifying eye gaze.

The program assessed the eye gaze performance of 20 participants in a series of films with varying lighting conditions. The findings indicated that the overall mean accuracy and precision for the five directions were 0.92 (92%). In addition, many alterations were applied to the image to test its resilience in terms of qualitative picture features. Among them are noise applications, brightness and contrast increase and reduction applications, axis rotation and blurring applications. The findings of the algorithm in these modifications revealed that the noise application had the greatest influence. Furthermore, the suggested method has significant limitations, and changes in light impact accuracy. Our future research will aim to increase the accuracy of the suggested eye-gaze detection method, making the system more resilient and faster at navigating the home environment.

References

1. Ahmad, A., Mozelius, P.: Critical factors for human computer interaction of ehealth for older adults. In: Proceedings of the 2019 the 5th International Conference on e-Society, e-Learning and e-Technologies, January, pp. 58–62. (2019)
2. Thakur, N., Han, C.Y.: A review of assistive technologies for activities of daily living of elderly (2021). arXiv preprint arXiv:2106.12183
3. Kaur, P., Sharma, M., Mittal, M.: Big data and machine learning based secure healthcare framework. Procedia Comput. Sci. **132**, 1049–1059 (2018)
4. Wang, Y.L., Hwang, M.Y.: Daily activities and psychological need satisfaction of elderly adults: the experience sampling method. Educ. Gerontol. **46**(9), 551–562 (2020)
5. Mishra, P., Biswas, S., Dash, S.: Deep learning based biomedical named entity recognition systems. In: Deep Learning Techniques for Biomedical and Health Informatics, pp. 23–40. Springer, Cham, (2020)
6. Zhang, R., Hummelgård, M., Örtegren, J., Yang, Y., Andersson, H., Balliu, E., Blomquist, N., Engholm, M., Olsen, M., Wang, Z.L., Olin, H.: Sensing body motions bd on charges generated on the body. Nano Energy **63**, 103842 (2019)
7. Goyal, L.M., Mittal, M., Kumar, M., Kaur, B., Sharma, M., Verma, A., Kaur, I.: An efficient method of multicolor detection using global optimum thresholding for image analysis. Multimedia Tools Appl. 1–23 (2021)
8. Mittal, M., Verma, A., Kaur, I., Kaur, B., Sharma, M., Goyal, L.M., Roy, S., Kim, T.H.: An efficient edge detection approach to provide better edge connectivity for image analysis. IEEE Access **7**, 33240–33255 (2019)
9. Joseph, A.W., Murugesh, R.: Potential eye tracking metrics and indicators to measure cognitive load in human-computer interaction research. J. Scientif. Res. **64**(1) (2020)

10. Zheng, C., Usagawa, T.: A rapid webcam-based eye tracking method for human computer interaction. In: 2018 International Conference on Control, Automation and Information Sciences (ICCAIS), October, pp. 133–136. IEEE (2018)
11. Bekteshi, S., Konings, M., Vanmechelen, I., Deklerck, J., Ortibus, E., Aerts, J.M., Hallez, H., Karlsson, P., Dan, B., Monbaliu, E.: Eye gaze gaming intervention in children with Dyskinetic cerebral palsy: a pilot study of task performance and its relation with dystonia and Choreoathetosis. Dev. Neurorehabil. **23**(8), 548–556 (2020)
12. Zuniga, R., Magee, J.: Camera Mouse: Dwell versus computer vision-based intentional click activation. In: International Conference on Universal Access in Human-Computer Interaction, July, pp. 455–464. Springer, Cham (2017)
13. Kabanda, G.: In: Review of Human Computer Interaction and Computer Vision. GRIN Verlag (2019)
14. Majaranta, P., Räihä, K.J., Hyrskykari, A., Špakov, O.: Eye movements and human-computer interaction. In: Eye Movement Research, pp. 971–1015. Springer, Cham (2019)
15. Kabir, A.U., Shahin, F.B., Islam, M.K.: Design and implementation of an EOG-based mouse cursor control for application in human-computer interaction. J. Phys.: Conf. Ser. **1487**(1), 012043 (2020). IOP Publishing
16. Lin, C.T., King, J.T., Bharadwaj, P., Chen, C.H., Gupta, A., Ding, W., Prasad, M.: EOG-based eye movement classification and application on HCI baseball game. IEEE Access **7**, 96166–96176 (2019)
17. Fahim, S.R., Sarker, Y., Rashiduzzaman, M., Islam, O.K., Sarker, S.K., Das, S.K.: A human-computer interaction system utilizing inertial measurement unit and convolutional neural network. In: 2019 5th International Conference on Advances in Electrical Engineering (ICAEE), September, pp. 880–885. IEEE (2019)
18. Karunachandra, R.T.H.S.K., Herath, H.M.K.K.M.B.: Binocular vision-based intelligent 3-D perception for robotics application. Int. J. Scientif. Res. Publicat. (IJSRP) **10**(9), 689–696 (2021). https://doi.org/10.29322/ijsrp.10.09.2020.p10582
19. Onyemauche, U.C., Osundu, U., Etumnu, R.C., Nwosu, Q.N.: The use of eye gaze gesture interaction artificial intelligence techniques for PIN entry (2020)
20. Hohn, M.J.: Use of Tobii Dynavox gaze viewer to track progress of child with physical and cortical visual impairments (CVI): a case study (2020)
21. Weiss, K.E., Hoermandinger, C., Mueller, M., Daners, M.S., Potapov, E.V., Falk, V., Meboldt, M., Lohmeyer, Q.: Eye tracking supported human factors testing improving patient training. J. Med. Syst. **45**(5), 1–7 (2021)
22. Ahmed, A.P.H.M., Abdullah, S.H.: A survey on human eye-gaze tracking (EGT) system "a comparative study." Iraqi J. Inform. Technol. V **9**(3), 2018 (2019)
23. Fan, C.P.: Design and implementation of a wearable gaze tracking device with near-infrared and visible-light image sensors (2014)
24. Liu, J., Chi, J., Lu, N., Yang, Z., Wang, Z.: Iris feature-based 3-D gaze estimation method using a one-camera-one-light-source system. IEEE Trans. Instrum. Meas. **69**(7), 4940–4954 (2019)
25. Ou, W.L., Kuo, T.L., Chang, C.C., Fan, C.P.: Deep-learning-based pupil center detection and tracking technology for visible-light wearable gaze tracking devices. Appl. Sci. **11**(2), 851 (2021)
26. Zhu, Y., Sun, W., Yuan, T.T., Li, J.: Gaze detection and prediction using data from infrared cameras. In: Proceedings of the 2nd Workshop on Multimedia for Accessible Human Computer Interfaces, October, pp. 41–46. (2019)
27. Sanjeewa, E.D.G., Herath, K.K.L., Madhusanka, B.G.D.A., Priyankara, H.D.N.S.: Visual attention model for mobile robot navigation in domestic environment. GSJ **8**(7) (2020)
28. Herath, K.K.L. et al.: Hand gesture command to understanding of human-robot interaction. GSJ 8.7 (2020)
29. Madhusanka, B.G.D.A., Jayasekara, A.G.B.P.: Design and development of adaptive vision attentive robot eye for service robot in domestic environment. In: 2016 IEEE International Conference on Information and Automation for Sustainability (ICIAfS), December, pp. 1–6. IEEE (2016)

30. Chi, J., Liu, J., Wang, F., Chi, Y., Hou, Z.G.: 3-D gaze-estimation method using a multi-camera-multi-light-source system. IEEE Trans. Instrum. Meas. **69**(12), 9695–9708 (2020)
31. Hochreiter, J., Daher, S., Bruder, G., Welch, G.: Cognitive and touch performance effects of mismatched 3D physical and visual perceptions. In: 2018 IEEE Conference on Virtual Reality and 3D User Interfaces (VR), March, pp. 1–386. IEEE (2018)
32. Ahmed, N.Y.: Real-time accurate eye center localization for low-resolution grayscale images. J. Real-Time Image Proc. **18**(1), 193–220 (2021)
33. Kattenborn, T., Leitloff, J., Schiefer, F., Hinz, S.: Review on convolutional neural networks (CNN) in vegetation remote sensing. ISPRS J. Photogramm. Remote. Sens. **173**, 24–49 (2021)
34. Yeamkuan, S., Chamnongthai, K.: 3D point-of-intention determination using a multimodal fusion of hand pointing and eye gaze for a 3D display. Sensors **21**(4), 1155 (2021)
35. Moladande, M.W.C.N., Madhusanka, B.G.D.A.: Implicit intention and activity recognition of a human using neural networks for a service robot eye. In: 2019 International Research Conference on Smart Computing and Systems Engineering (SCSE), March, pp. 38–43. IEEE (v) (2019)
36. Appuhamy, E.J.G.S., Madhusanka, B.G.D.A.: Development of a GPU-based human emotion recognition robot eye for service robot by using convolutional neural network. In: 2018 IEEE/ACIS 17th International Conference on Computer and Information Science (ICIS), June, pp. 433–438. IEEE (2018)
37. Milinda, H.G.T., Madhusanka, B.G.D.A.: Mud and dirt separation method for floor cleaning robot. In: 2017 Moratuwa Engineering Research Conference (MERCon), May, pp. 316–320. IEEE (2017)
38. Vithanawasam, T.M.W., Madhusanka, B.G.D.A.: Dynamic face and upper-body emotion recognition for service robots. In: 2018 IEEE/ACIS 17th International Conference on Computer and Information Science (ICIS), June, pp. 428–432. IEEE (2018)
39. Vithanawasam, T.M.W., Madhusanka, B.G.D.A.: Face and upper-body emotion recognition using service robot's eyes in a domestic environment. In: 2019 International Research Conference on Smart Computing and Systems Engineering (SCSE), March, pp. 44–50. IEEE (2019)
40. Palmero, C., Selva, J., Bagheri, M.A., Escalera, S.: Recurrent CNN for 3d gaze estimation using appearance and shape cues (2018). arXiv preprint arXiv:1805.03064.
41. Ahn, H.: Non-contact real time eye gaze mapping system based on deep convolutional neural network (2020). arXiv preprint arXiv:2009.04645
42. Chen, Z.: Enhancing human-computer interaction by inferring users' intent from eye gaze (Doctoral dissertation) (2020)
43. Lemley, J., Kar, A., Drimbarean, A., Corcoran, P.: Convolutional neural network implementation for eye-gaze estimation on low-quality consumer imaging systems. IEEE Trans. Consum. Electron. **65**(2), 179–187 (2019)
44. Liaqat, S., Wu, C., Duggirala, P.R., Cheung, S.C.S., Chuah, C.N., Ozonoff, S., Young, G.: Predicting ASD diagnosis in children with synthetic and image-based eye gaze data. Signal Process.: Image Commun. **94**, 116198 (2021)
45. Cha, X., Yang, X., Feng, Z., Xu, T., Fan, X., Tian, J.: Calibration-free gaze zone estimation using convolutional neural network. In: 2018 International Conference on Security, Pattern Analysis, and Cybernetics (SPAC), December, pp. 481–484. IEEE (2018)
46. Liu, H., Li, D., Wang, X., Liu, L., Zhang, Z., Subramanian, S.: Precise head pose estimation on HPD5A database for attention recognition based on convolutional neural network in human-computer interaction. Infrared Phys. Technol. **116**, 103740 (2021)
47. Chen, J., Wang, G., Kun, Z.: Personalized intelligent intervention and precise evaluation for children with autism spectrum disorder. In: Proceedings of DELFI Workshops 2020. Gesellschaft für Informatik eVz (2020)
48. Wöhle, L., Gebhard, M.: Towards robust robot control in cartesian space using an infrastructureless head-and eye-gaze interface. Sensors **21**(5), 1798 (2021)
49. Basly, H., Ouarda, W., Sayadi, F.E., Ouni, B., Alimi, A.M.: CNN-SVM learning approach based human activity recognition. In: International Conference on Image and Signal Processing, June, pp. 271–281. Springer, Cham (2020)

50. Madhusanka, B.G.D.A., Sureswaran, R.: Understanding activities of daily living of elder/disabled people using visual behavior in social interaction (2021)
51. Madhusanka, B.G.D.A., Ramadass, S.: Implicit intention communication for activities of daily living of elder/disabled people to improve well-being. In: IoT in Healthcare and Ambient Assisted Living, pp. 325–342. Springer, Singapore (2021)
52. Madhusanka, B.G.D.A., Sureswaran, R.: Recognition of daily living activities using convolutional neural network based support vector machine (2021)
53. Yatbaz, H.Y., Ever, E., Yazici, A.: Activity recognition and anomaly detection in E-health applications using color-coded representation and lightweight CNN architectures. IEEE Sensors J. (2021)
54. Carvalho, L.I., Sofia, R.C.: A review on scaling mobile sensing platforms for human activity recognition: challenges and recommendations for future research. IoT **1**(2), 451–473 (2020)
55. Javed, A.R., Faheem, R., Asim, M., Baker, T., Beg, M.O.: A smartphone sensors-based personalized human activity recognition system for sustainable smart cities. Sustain. Cities Soc. **71**, 102970 (2021)
56. Blobel, B.: A machine learning approach for human activity recognition. In: pHealth 2020: Proceedings of the 17th International Conference on Wearable Micro and Nano Technologies for Personalized Health, September, vol. 273, pp. 155. IOS Press (2020)
57. Chen, L., Fan, S., Kumar, V., Jia, Y.: A method of human activity recognition in transitional period. Information **11**(9), 416 (2020)
58. Bose, A.J., Aarabi, P.: Adversarial attacks on face detectors using neural net based constrained optimization. In: 2018 IEEE 20th International Workshop on Multimedia Signal Processing (MMSP), pp. 1–6. IEEE, (2018)
59. Chen, W.X., Cui, X.Y., Zheng, J., Zhang, J.M., Chen, S., Yao, Y.D.: Gaze gestures and their applications in human-computer interaction with a head-mounted display (2019). arXiv preprint arXiv:1910.07428
60. Moschoglou, S., Papaioannou, A., Sagonas, C., Deng, J., Kotsia, I., Zafeiriou, S.: Agedb: the first manually collected, in-the-wild age database. In: Proceedings of the IEEE Conference on Computer Vision and Pattern Recognition Workshops, pp. 51–59. (2017)
61. Modi, N., Singh, J.: A review of various state of art eye gaze estimation techniques. Adv. Computat. Intell. Commun. Technol. 501–510 (2021)
62. Kar, A., Corcoran, P.: A review and analysis of eye-gaze estimation systems, algorithms and performance evaluation methods in consumer platforms. IEEE Access **5**, 16495–16519 (2017)
63. Singh, J., Modi, N.: Use of information modelling techniques to understand research trends in eye gaze estimation methods: an automated review. Heliyon **5**(12), e03033 (2019)
64. Zheng, Y., Fu, H., Li, R., Hsung, T.C., Song, Z., Wen, D.: Deep neural network oriented evolutionary parametric eye modeling. Pattern Recogn. **113**, 107755 (2021)
65. Park, S., Mello, S.D., Molchanov, P., Iqbal, U., Hilliges, O., Kautz, J.: Few-shot adaptive gaze estimation. In: Proceedings of the IEEE/CVF International Conference on Computer Vision, pp. 9368–9377. (2019)
66. Adithya, B., Hanna, L. and Chai, Y., 2018. Calibration techniques and gaze accuracy estimation in pupil labs eye tracker. TECHART: Journal of Arts and Imaging Science, 5(1), pp.38–41.
67. Lemley, J., Kar, A., Drimbarean, A., Corcoran, P.: Efficient CNN implementation for eye-gaze estimation on low-power/low-quality consumer imaging systems (2018). arXiv preprint arXiv:1806.10890
68. Wang, K., Ji, Q.: 3D gaze estimation without explicit personal calibration. Pattern Recogn. **79**, 216–227 (2018)
69. Kanade, P., David, F., Kanade, S.: Convolutional neural networks (CNN) based eye-gaze tracking system using machine learning algorithm. Europ. J. Electri. Eng. Comput. Sci. **5**(2), 36–40 (2021)
70. Lin, S., Liu, Y., Wang, S., Li, C., Wang, H.: A novel unified stereo stimuli based binocular eye-tracking system for accurate 3D gaze estimation (2021). arXiv preprint arXiv:2104.12167
71. Heck, M., Edinger, J., Becker, C.: Conditioning gaze-contingent systems for the real world: insights from a field study in the fast food industry. In: Extended Abstracts of the 2021 CHI Conference on Human Factors in Computing Systems, pp. 1–7. (2021)

72. Han, S.Y., Cho, N.I.: User-independent gaze estimation by extracting pupil parameter and its mapping to the gaze angle. In: 2020 25th International Conference on Pattern Recognition (ICPR), pp. 1993–2000. IEEE (2021)
73. Gu, S., Wang, L., He, L., He, X., Wang, J.: Gaze estimation via a differential eyes' appearances network with a reference grid. Engineering (2021)
74. Chen, W., Xu, H., Zhu, C., Liu, X., Lu, Y., Zheng, C., Kong, J.: Gaze estimation via the joint modeling of multiple cues. IEEE Trans. Circuits Syst. Video Technol. (2021)
75. Nagamatsu, T., Hiroe, M., Arai, H.: Extending the measurement angle of a gaze estimation method using an eye model expressed by a revolution about the optical axis of the eye. IEICE Trans. Inf. Syst. **104**(5), 729–740 (2021)
76. Barbara, N., Camilleri, T.A., Camilleri, K.P. Modelling of blink-related eyelid-induced shunting on the electrooculogram. In: ACM Symposium on Eye Tracking Research and Applications, pp. 1–6. (2021)
77. Spiller, M., Liu, Y.H., Hossain, M.Z., Gedeon, T., Geissler, J., Nürnberger, A.: Predicting visual search task success from eye gaze data as a basis for user-adaptive information visualization systems. ACM Trans. Interact. Intell. Syst. (TiiS) **11**(2), 1–25 (2021)
78. Anitta, D.: Human head pose estimation based on HF method. Microprocess. Microsyst. **82**, 103802 (2021)
79. Huang, T., Fu, R., Chen, Y.: Deep driver behavior detection model based on human brain consolidated learning for shared autonomy systems. Measurement 109463 (2021)
80. Jiang, H., Jiao, R., Wang, Z., Zhang, T., Wu, L.: Construction and analysis of emotion computing model based on LSTM. Complexity (2021)
81. Pant, Y.V., Kumaravel, B.T., Shah, A., Kraemer, E., Vazquez-Chanlatte, M., Kulkarni, K., Hartmann, B., Seshia, S.A.: Model-based Formalization of the Autonomy-to-Human Perception Hand-off (2021)
82. Kim, K.B., Choi, H.H.: Resolution estimation technique in gaze tracking system for HCI. J. Convergence Inform. Technol. **11**(1), 20–27 (2021)
83. Wan, Z.H., Xiong, C.H., Chen, W.B., Zhang, H.Y.: Robust and accurate pupil detection for head-mounted eye tracking. Comput. Electri. Eng. **93**, 107193 (2021)
84. Mittal, M., Sharma, R.K., Singh, V.P.: Performance evaluation of threshold-based and k-means clustering algorithms using iris dataset. Recent Patents Eng. **13**(2), 131–135 (2019)
85. Vasudevan, B., Rajeshkannan, S., Kumar, J.S.: An adaptive chromosome based cost aggregation approach for developing a high quality stereo vision model. J. **21**(1), 11–11 (2021)
86. Qasmieh, I.A., Alquran, H., Alqudah, A.M.: Occluded iris classification and segmentation using self-customized artificial intelligence models and iterative randomized Hough transform. Int. J. Electri. Comput. Eng. (IJECE) **11**(5), 4037–4049 (2021)
87. Herath, H. M. K. K. M. B.: Internet of things (IoT) enable designs for identify and control the COVID-19 pandemic. In: Artificial Intelligence for COVID-19, pp. 423–436. Springer, Cham (2021)
88. Herath, H. M. K. K. M. B., Karunasena, G. M. K. B., Herath, H. M. W. T.: Development of an IoT based systems to mitigate the impact of COVID-19 pandemic in smart cities. In: Machine Intelligence and Data Analytics for Sustainable Future Smart Cities (pp. 287–309). Springer, Cham (2021)
89. Herath, H.M.K.K.M.B., Karunasena, G.M.K.B., Ariyathunge, S.V.A.S.H., Priyankara, H.D.N.S., Madhusanka, B.G.D.A., Herath, H.M.W.T., Nimanthi, U.D.C.: Deep learning approach to recognition of novel COVID-19 using CT scans and digital image processing. In: 4th SLAAI-International Conference on Artificial Intelligence, pp. 01–06. Sri Lanka (2021)
90. Lindsay, G.W.: Convolutional neural networks as a model of the visual system: past, present, and future. J. Cognit. Neurosci. 1–15 (2020)

Internet of Things and Cloud Activity Monitoring Systems for Elderly Healthcare

Joseph Bamidele Awotunde ⓘ, Oluwafisayo Babatope Ayoade, Gbemisola Janet Ajamu ⓘ, Muyideen AbdulRaheem ⓘ, and Idowu Dauda Oladipo ⓘ

Abstract According to the World Health Organization, people aged 60 years and above globally will be 2 billion in 2050 by increasing from its present 841 million populaces. With the recent advances in smart healthcare systems that make treatment available for all, it is expected that longevity becomes the norm for humans. Providing a convenient platform for elderly patients has therefore become the attraction of various researchers from different fields, and this makes the smart healthcare system become a point of desirability for many. The advancement in information technology especially in the area of Internet of Things (IoT), cloud computing, and wearable devices has helped bring healthcare nearer to the rural areas and improve elderly care globally. Ambient Assisted Living (AAL) makes it possible to incorporate emerging technology into our everyday activities. Therefore, this chapter explains the important role of IoT and Cloud activity monitoring systems for elderly healthcare in medicine to reduce caregivers' needs and help the aged live an active life. Also, proposes a framework of an intelligent IoT and cloud activity monitoring system for elderly healthcare using a wearable body sensor network. The suggested system educates and warns healthcare workers in real-time about changes in the health status of aged patients in order to recommend preventative steps that can save lives. The proposed system can accommodate any number of wearable sensors devices and a

---

J. B. Awotunde (✉) · O. B. Ayoade · M. AbdulRaheem · I. D. Oladipo
Department of Computer Science, University of Ilorin, Ilorin, Nigeria
e-mail: awotunde.jb@unilorin.edu.ng

O. B. Ayoade
e-mail: 15-68hg004.pg@students.unilorin.edu.ng

M. AbdulRaheem
e-mail: muyideen@unilorin.edu.ng

I. D. Oladipo
e-mail: odidowu@unilorin.edu.ng

G. J. Ajamu
Department of Agricultural Extension and Rural Development, Landmark University, Omu Aran, Nigeria
e-mail: ajamu.gbemisola@lmu.edu.ng

huge number of applications. The platform also enables remote health monitoring, and real-time monitoring, thus reduce the workload on the medical personnel. IoT and cloud activity monitoring system is a quick and rapid way of monitoring, and diagnosis of elderly patients by depriving them of diffusion of the infection to others.

Keywords Internet of Things · Elderly patient · Activity monitoring · Cloud computing · Smart healthcare system

1 Introduction

The constant aged of the world's population places greater strain on society and welfare systems, making it critical to develop better programs and inventions capable of treating medical problems associated with old age. E-Health provides initiatives to assist seniors in living longer in their homes, as well as innovative services to help pay for specific treatment or recuperation. Population aging is a visible phenomenon with significant social and economic implications. Over 70-year-olds will increase in number from 64 million in 2010 to 122 million in 2060 [1]. To address the problems that these phenomena has produced, the concept of Ambient Assisted Living (AAL) has been elevated as a target solution to healthcare, describing a network that is interconnected, context-aware, ubiquitous, customizable, responsive, and anticipative.

The ProActive Ageing initiative ("Prolonging ACTIVE life for an active and stable AGEING") offers web services for the successful (re) integration of older people into societal and operational life, for the enhancement of an elderly person's self-well-being and freedom through continuous learning and knowledge exchange, and for the delivery of structured training programs for structured workers [2]. According to the Internet of Things Technology Initiative (AIOTI), 110 European provinces have defined Active and Safe old age as a target for intelligent expertise [3, 4]. The AAL Joint solutions built health monitoring (HM) as a significant group of use cases established in European projects FP6 and FP7, with other thematic areas being behavior tracking, mobility associate, fitness instructor, grocery, and diet planner, socializing with Smart TV [5]. IoT has always been the crucial information technology for building such use cases because of its ability to upgrade real-world things and merge them into the Cloud [6]. Despite the limitations of IoT devices' storage and processing capabilities in comparison to continuously increasing criteria for the amount of device-generated data and their decision theory, cloud computing is emerging as a very appealing alternative solution with the potential to provide omnipresent, accessible, on-demand network access to a shared configuration database [7].

Apart from communicating and exchanging data between health professionals, cloud computing is widely used in many other areas of healthcare, including medical imaging (storage, exchanging, and processing), public health and patient self-management, hospital management and clinical information systems, and preparing, coordinating, or reviewing therapeutic interventions (Statistical analysis, text analysis, or medical trials) [8].

IoT devices, such as satellites, may have applications in the healthcare industry for Heart rate monitors, blood sugar supervises, and endoscopic capsules [9–11]. Sensors, actuators, and other mobile technologies are used devices in the therapeutic business will revolutionize it, especially during pandemic outbreaks [12, 13]. The Internet of Medical Things (IoMT) is a linked network of smart healthcare devices that accept data from internet communications networks and transmit it to healthcare information systems [14, 15]. Currently, 3.7 million therapeutic devices are in use that are linked to and monitored by various areas of the body in order to offer medical alerts [16, 17].

These IoMT networks communicate to public cloud such as Google Cloud Technology, Microsoft Azure Cloud, Amazon Web Services, and others bespoke network services in order to collect storage and analytics data. Patients with lingering or long-term illnesses can benefit from remote medical monitoring using IoT services. These systems can track and monitor patients who use embedded sensor equipment in medical centers.

They can transmit the fitness data across to their doctor. Medical gadgets that can be coupled or launched as IoT technology include infusion pumps that link to analytical monitors and hospital beds with sensors for monitoring patients' health status. Items like "Smart" objects with various sensors and actuators that are completely equipped to operate in their respective surroundings, as well as incorporated communication infrastructure to link with any imaginable alternative, assist the Internet of Things (IoT) in reaching its full potential. As shown in Fig. 1, the most common usage of IoT for old persons is activity monitoring.

The IoT is a large-scale machine deployment, such as machine type communication (MTC), that conducts sensing and actuation activities with little or no human participation. The number of Internet-connected items is predicted to outweigh the world's population. The number of linked health devices is fast expanding [18], as the IoT is concerned with the realism of connecting specific physical commodities to the internet. In addition, healthcare is the largest target market for IoT, with pulse rate tracking being the most advantageous use [19]. Simple devices like glucose meters and heart rate monitors, as well as IoT systems that feed data into more complicated technologies, might be used to create emergency alarm systems and remote medical monitoring systems.

This chapter presents (1) the integration of devices into an IoT- driven remote healthcare system and (2) the utilization of an IoT-based platform to track the health of older patients.

The rest of this chapter is organized as follows: Sect. 2 discusses deployment of IoT in elderly monitoring scheme. Section 3 has a detailed discussion of applications of IoT and Cloud computing in elderly monitoring systems. Section 4 presents the ICEAMS framework for activities monitoring of the elderly patient. Section 5 presents a practical case of ICEAMS for monitoring elderly people, and finally Sect. 6 concluded the chapter and presents future direction for the chapter.

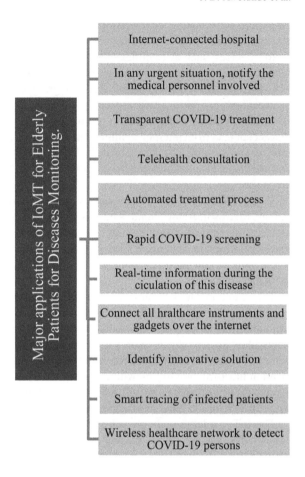

Fig. 1 Major application of IoT for elderly patients for diseases monitoring

2 Application of Internet of Things in Elderly Activity Monitoring Systems

2.1 IoT Operations

The latest breakthroughs in IoT, wearable sensors, and telecommunication technologies have made human living smarter in the age of universal computing, allowing smart healthcare services to be delivered [9, 10, 20]. The IoT has the ability to completely change the medical industry. Patients, medical staff, and carers, as well as monitoring devices are all connected by software and ICT technologies [9].

The healthcare sector in most emerging countries is facing severe economic issues, owing to the expanding number of reliable and high-quality services necessary for the aged. Elderly persons require extra care and attention because even a little illness or injury can result in irreversible damage [21].

According to the results of a poll performed by the United States of Elderly, 90% of elderly inhabitants want to be able to dwell in their own residences [22]. Many older persons choose to age in their own homes, according to recent studies [23], but they need caretakers or medical professionals to pay attention to them and keep an eye on or assist them. As a result, developing new tools and technology to assist elder individuals in aging in place is critical [24].

Increases technical advancements have resulted in an increase in lifespan breakthroughs the share of old individuals has grown in recent years. Age-related frailty, chronic diseases, and disabilities are all difficulties that these elderly persons must cope with on a daily basis. Recently, there has been a surge in interest in establishing aged care services based on cutting-edge technology with the goal of allowing seniors to live independently. The IoT has been established as a cutting-edge concept for linking real and virtual items in order to improve services, and it has the potential to significantly improve remote geriatric monitoring. Several recent initiatives have been made to address elderly care needs using IoT-based solutions [21].

There is a growing need for unique technology that can deliver effective remote geriatric monitoring services. To this goal, a variety of current disciplines should be used to serve the needs of the aged, taking into account their limits in everyday life. IoT, as a promising paradigm, has the capacity to provide such essential services to the elderly [25]. The IoT is a cutting-edge technology that combines sensor development, data gathering, network resources and services required, database administration, and information processing are all examples of data computing, and other disciplines to enable objects (e.g., entity, individuals) having distinct identities in order to communicate to a central server and build local connections [9]. IoT-enabled systems' connection allows entities to communicate and combine data to get a more thorough understanding of their functioning as well as the features of their surroundings, allowing them to provide more advanced services that are sophisticated and effective. One of the primary advantages of IoT application is that they enable continuous (i.e., 24/7) remote monitoring systems, which help to raise people's standard of living [26].

By linking items and people, the IoT has the capability to fundamentally influence numerous human characteristics existence. The system architecture may be partitioned into three levels depending on the characteristics and functionalists of IoT-enabled systems (data collecting, communication, and exploration), as stated by various academics. The architecture of an IoT-enabled system, on the other hand, may be redefined in terms of its use cases. As illustrated in Fig. 2, the system in our situation is defined as follows in order to meet the needs of elderly monitoring:

Perception layer: This is the first stratum and the one closest to the individual being tracked. The core objective of the insight level is to acquire necessary data from the client, as well as communication with upper levels. The perception layer, as shown in Fig. 2, may be classified into two parts: the body area network (BAN) and fixed/mobile sensors in the vicinity. The BAN may be seen as a web of vital signs peripherals (e.g., chest belts, infusion pumps, and blood stress monitors) or sensing gadgets (e.g., smartwatches, fitness trackers, and smart headwear) that gather user data. Medical data such as vital symbols (e.g., rate of heartbeat and rate of breathing),

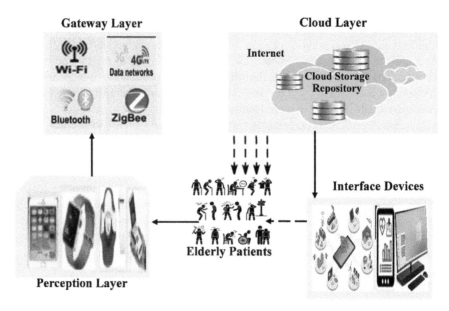

Fig. 2 A multi-layer IoT-based elderly monitoring system architecture

these devices record blood sugar levels, galvanic skin responses (GSR), and location information like position, exercise habits, and rest amount. The second type consists of fixed contexts sensors, which are commonly seen in residences and other public locations (e.g., surveillance camera, Smart TV, etc.). Environmental elements are also detected and responded to using mobile context sensors. This section includes a wide range of robotics.

Gateway Layer: The gateway layer accepts sensual information through mobile and wireless methods from the sensor node (such as Bluetooth, 6LoWPAN, and Zigbee) and transfers it to the Cloud layer for processing. In Fig. 2, the layer is separated into two clusters. The first is for fixed access points that transmit data indoors and are put in senior homes. The mobile access point is the second type, which is utilized for outside purposes. A smartphone is an excellent example of a data transmission and processing mobile access point.

The **Cloud layer**: In the data center, this is a distant layer. As seen in Fig. 2 the layer is divided into several divisions. Incoming data is stored in data centers before being analyzed using the Cloud's great computing capacity. Reasoning [27], machine learning algorithms [28], pattern recognition approaches [29], and other data analysis techniques are used. In order to successfully respond to the requirements of the elderly, decisions and reactions are made based on the results. These backend apps are capable of detecting lifestyle patterns in the elderly, like Mild Cognitive Impairment (MCI) [30], as well as anticipate chronic and acute disorders, such as blood glucose concentration prediction for a diabetic [10]. End-users, such as the monitored individual, their caregivers, and medical professionals, can be provided with a variety of apps and services, like a mobile user application, to communicate the outcomes.

2.2 IoT and Elderly Monitoring Systems

Meeting the needs of the elderly is one of the most important uses of IoT-based distant surveillance systems. On one side, senior fragility makes people more sensitive to a number of illnesses (severe and lingering), deficiencies (e.g., graphic, physical, and verbal), and limitations (e.g., poor memory) and, on either hand, raises the risk of being unaware on the other (e.g., computer illiteracy). As a result of disregarding the need of senior care, an increase in old dependency or the requirement for them to reside in a treatment facility may ensue. In this situation, IoT-based distant sensor observing can help resolve the aforementioned concerns, reduce the repercussions, and allow seniors to live freely. Given the projected high growth of the elderly population in the near future, major investments in innovative senior care concepts and technologies, such as the IoT are required. A number of methods have been offered to fulfill the standards of the aged by compensating for deficiencies or avoiding the unavoidable effects.

2.2.1 Health Monitoring

Due to aging's fragility and sensitivity to viral infections (e.g., acute and chronic ailments), monitoring system becomes the most significant aspect of aging remote monitoring. Remote health monitoring raises the standard of care to elderly's quality of life by identifying and alerting caretakers in the case of an emergency, as well as reducing nursing and hospital visits, and hence healthcare costs. In 2011, older people accounted for more than a one-third of all clinic charges and visits in the United States, according to a research conducted by the Agency for Healthcare Research and Quality (AHRQ) [31]. As a result, providing remote health monitoring services at home is critical to improving care services and lowering hospital expenditures and stays for the elderly. Besides, as the world's potential supporting ratio declines, a large number of older citizens may confront a future with a restricted quantity of care and supportive services.

The improvements are then applied based on sensor feedback, and a customized workout regimen is proposed without the requirement for direct human supervision. Acceptance of new technology is typically difficult, especially when the system's target users are the elderly. This reduced the use of traditional equipment (e.g., television) in various health monitoring techniques to provide more user-friendly services for old folks. In this context, Spin-sante and Gambi [32] propose a remote patient monitoring system related to digital television that incorporates a range of wire-free medical devices (e.g., oximeter, breathing tester, and glycaemia meter). Macis and colleagues worked on the HEREiAM programme [33], it explains how a

TV-based system may give greater aid and support to the elderly. The project uses a TV set at home to provide a variety of services to solve remote healthcare technology acceptability as well as other challenges such as security and social communication [34].

Another indicator that represents the health status of the elderly is daily activity. Physical activity, eating (meal frequency and length), sleeping, and other activities are only a few of them. Several efforts have been taken to this end, leveraging various techniques and sensory data to offer activity monitoring for the aged. Kasteren and colleagues [35] discuss a system (created as part of the CARE project) that tracks and recognizes older people's activity levels using wireless sensors and recognition mode.

2.2.2 Nutrition Monitoring

Malnutrition is a common aging problem that may be handled, whether it is caused by a deficit (undernutrition), excess (overnutrition), or a lack of appropriate nutrition. The elderly are more likely to suffer from malnutrition [36, 37]. Malnutrition has been linked to a number of health problems in the elderly, including cardiovascular and cerebrovascular disease, osteoporosis, and diabetes [10]. Nutrition monitoring, particularly weight and nutrition tracking, along with health tracking via IoT-based wearable sensors, are critical to enhancing people's health and well-being of senior citizens.

Various approaches and systems have previously been offered in this area. ChefMyself is a nutrition-related monitoring app that presents a methodology to help older people track their food intake [38]. It provides remote nutrition monitoring, including weight tracking (through cordless scales), diet tracking, a recipe repository, and grocery and cooking aid for the aged are all available via a Cloud-based connection. It also provides access to social networking sites to encourage the elderly to engage in more social activities.

Added method, DIET4Elders Sanchez et al. [39], shows a scheme (hardware and software) for monitoring, advising, and providing facilities for day-to-day events connected to senior people's dining habits in order to avoid malnutrition. The following are the three tiers of their suggested system: (1) Surveillance Module contains relevant data from everyday experiences, Evaluation and Appraisal Layer extracts information [40] and expertise about daily self-feeding, and Support Service Layer provides additional information (including interactions) from medical sources professionals and caretakers.

A wearable IoT-based gadget called eButton [41, 42] has been devised for those with specific requirements, such as the elderly, to accomplish multi-function remote monitoring. The eButton gadget uses a pictorial sensor on the patient chest to track his or her nutrition. Based on earlier models of food forms, the food volume is also approximated from the photos. The collected data, when combined with supplemental data (e.g., meal information), displays the user's daily nutrition and calories. In addition, the gadget provides services for tracking physical activity, such as sedentary occurrences and daily calorie consumption.

2.2.3 Safety Monitoring

One of the most pressing concerns in the lives of the elderly is security. As people age, they develop impairments, frailty, and forgetfulness, making it necessary to monitor their safety in order to live independently. An actual tracking system, on either hand, is capable of identifying risky circumstances can offer aged users with a sense of security as well as knowledge of their status for family who may not be there. In this field, several strategies and efforts to address remote safety monitoring of elderly people have been described. The most important ones are included in the following sections, which cover various phases of sensor watching in day-to-day undertakings. As an effect of illnesses or restrictions brought on by age, as well as visual and physical problems, elderly people are more likely than younger people to fall. Falls can cause serious injury or even death [43].

Dedicated fall detection approaches have been proposed to alleviate such problems. Fall detection technologies can be split into two groups, according to Igual et al. [44]: Remote monitoring devices and situationally systems. Wearable sensors are divided into two types on the sensory level: cellphones and small sensors put on a band or cloth. For some users, wearing sensors instead of being continually filmed by cameras in context-aware systems provides a more pleasant user experience. When a fall is detected, Technologies including a 3D accelerometer, gyroscope, and magnetometer are utilized to evaluate a patient's sudden positioning and orientation changes situations, evaluate the data, and execute additional operations (e.g., show warnings). Smartphone-based techniques are presented by Fang et al. [45], Sposaro and Tyson [46] and Habib et al. [47], while wearable sensor-based techniques are presented by Habib et al. [47], Cheng [48] and Odunmbaku [49].

Context-aware methods, on either hand, are being designed to measure collapses using optical sensors. Context-aware systems have limitations as compared to wearable sensors, such as geographic coverage of mounted cameras or disquiet for certain elder individuals who feel continually observed. Context-aware systems, on the other hand, provide a number of benefits for the examined individual, including eradicating the necessity to wear the device all of the time and lowering the risk of overlooking to convey the sensors. In this vein, [50, 51] have suggested two important fall detection projects, which employ a complexity camera and an automaton vision system, separately, to detect falls.

Moreover, as part of a comprehensive geriatric monitoring strategy employing ocular sensors, the FEARLESS scheme targets to monitor ageing individuals without the need of wearable sensors [52]. Elderly people are constantly monitored by a system that collects records from 3D depth sensors (such as Kinect), lenses as well as speakers and sends it to a computer [53]. In addition, a comprehensive fall detection system is suggested [54], which employs a number of approaches to identify persons and their activity. When an emergency happens (for example, a fall), the system sends the data to the server, which analyzes it and delivers necessary notices and outcomes via application procedures (for example, healthcare/medical professionals' cellphones) [55].

3 Application of Internet of Things and Cloud Computing in Elderly Activity Monitoring Systems

3.1 The Role of IoT and Cloud Computing in Elderly Activity Monitoring Systems

The nation's well-being and the livelihood of its citizens are inextricably links and solely depends on the healthcare services and the medical information technology of such nations. To move a step forward in healthcare services, the utilization of cloud computing (CC) and the IoT has really changed the modern medicine in developed nations. Due to the various merits of cloud computing like virtualization, efficiency, high reliability and scalability have helped smart healthcare to change the prospects of healthcare industries. The development of a high-efficiency medical monitoring and management systems, cost reduction, and the building of a public cloud in a hospital to promote resource sharing are some other importance of cloud computing in the healthcare sectors. Medical information transmission, tracking, and intelligent patient monitoring can be achieved using the RFID and other acoustic electromagnetic sensors in smart healthcare system [56–58]. The use of modern healthcare technology and Internet has really support the healthcare sectors to realize real-time patient monitoring system, safe and efficient medical management system. Internet integration with cloud computing has open up new potential for medical system for real-time patient monitoring and management even in social domains, thanks to the rapid growth of the Internet [59, 60].

The two worlds of cloud and IoT have evolved in their own ways. However, a number of common advantages have been identified in the literature, which can be used to forecast the future. On the one hand, the IoT can take advantage of cloud computing's nearly limitless capacity and resources to compensate for technical limitations. CC, in particular, can be an effective option for managing Internet services as well as the composition and use of things or data applications. CC, on the other hand, can benefit from the IoT by expanding its reach to deal with things in the real world in a more distributed and dynamic manner, as well as deliver new services in a wide range of real-world scenarios.

By definition, the IoT involves a huge number of data sources, generates huge amount of both unstructured and structured data with the following three primary characteristics: volume, velocity, and variety. As a result, huge amounts of data must be collected, processed, visualized, archived, shared, and searched. The data generated by IoT can be effectively managed by the cloud, thus created the most convenient and cost-effective ways of dealing with such data [61] because it provides practically unlimited and on-demand storage capacity at a cheap cost. Sharing of such huge data with third parties becomes easier with this integration and new potential for data aggregation, integration [62].

Because of platform flexibility, operational compatibility, and on-demand service delivery, cloud computing has the ability to realize data integration and interoperation for pervasive health monitoring [63, 64]. Cloud databases have been presented as a means of providing users with transparent and safe access to heterogeneous databases and platforms. CC platforms can help elderly activity monitoring systems improve system interoperability in a cost-effective manner. Developing a monitoring system combining these two technologies has been proved efficient in providing healthcare facilities in remote areas in helping caregivers and physicians to provide quality healthcare services to the elderly patients. The CC is used as a supportive technology in an IoT-based system in terms of computational capability, storage, resource utilization, and reduced energy consumption. Also, the cloud has been a favorite of IoT-based system by enhancing service deliveries globally and deliver unspeakable services in a distributed and dynamic manner. The IoT-based cloud framework can still be extended in the smart environment for the development and application of new service delivery.

3.2 IoT and Cloud Challenges in Elderly Activity Monitoring Systems

The IoT connects and communicates with billions of devices and sensors, allowing us to provide knowledge that helps us in our everyday lives. CC, on either hand, provides internet connectivity that is on-demand, easy, and expandable, letting users to share computer resources and, as a result, allowing for dynamic data integration from a variety of source. Various challenges that are associated with the implementation of IoT in healthcare systems can be overcome by the integration of CC with the IoT. This will address the concerns of IoT implementation in medical sectors. The various resources provided by the CC can be of merits to the IoT-based system, while the Cloud can acquire greater visibility in order to enhance its constraints in a more flexible and dispersed approach with physical objects.

The Cloud-based IoT approach has been successfully integrated in an aging activity monitoring system may face several challenges. Some of the issues are as follows:

Security and privacy: Data may be transported from the real world to the Cloud using cloud-based IoT. The major challenge in the implementation of cloud in IoT-based system is the authorization guidelines and regulations for clients to gain access to sensitive information on the platforms. This is very critical for protecting users' identity, especially when data quality is necessary, and sensitive medical information are on transit [65]. Furthermore, when key IoT applications migrate to the

Cloud, problems developed due to a lack of trust in the service provider, information about service level agreements (SLAs), and data placement [66, 67]. Multi-tenancy can potentially lead to the leakage of sensitive data. Furthermore, due to the processing power limits imposed by IoT items, digital signatures cannot be used for anything [65]. New concerns require extra care; for example, the distributed system is vulnerable to SQL injection, session hijacking, cross-site scripting, and side-channel attacks. Critical issues like session hijacking and virtual server exit are also possibilities for an issue [68].

Patient data is collected using portable devices and sensors. Medical facilities must be adequately protected so that patients can use their smartphones to receive health status updates. The implementation of a smart healthcare system opens up the possibility of expanding healthcare to the entire population. The implementation of an intelligent healthcare system can minimize the time it takes for patients to see doctors or the time it takes for diagnosis results to come back. This also allows for immediate access to medical care and services. The scalability of a smart healthcare system must be taken seriously in order to retain confidence between patients and medical experts, and this will save quality time. It is the primary issue, and obtaining information from end-users through illegal companies is not only inappropriate, but also poses a risk to the personal safety of medical data. The key issue with the smart healthcare system's introduction and adoption is security and privacy. Security is required in various layers of the IoT-based system like in cloud, fog, and system as a result of the integration of these layers [69].

Performance: High bandwidth is required to transfer the huge volumes of data sent to the internet by IoT devices. As an aftermath, acquiring appropriate network performance to transfer data to cloud infrastructures is a major concern; unfortunately, broadband development is not keeping up with storage and compute progress [70]. In a variety of contexts, great reactivity is required for service and data provision [68]. This is due to the fact that timeliness can be altered by unforeseen events, and real-time applications are highly dependent on performance efficiency [71].

Big data: With several specialists predicting that Data Mining would outnumber 50 billion connected devices by 2020, it's vital to focus on the transportation, accessing, retention, and analysis of the huge volumes of data. Indeed, it is clear that the IoT will be one of the key sources of big data due to the recent technological development in smart healthcare systems. The Cloud can permit long-term preservation of the data produced by IoT and allow complex analysis on such data [72]. Because the application's whole performance is strongly based on the features of this data management service, analysis of the huge data produced is a serious concern. Finding the ideal data management system that will enable the cloud to handle massive volumes of data remains a big difficulty [73]. Information security is extremely important, not only because of the influence it has on quality of service, but also because of security issues on the devices that are connected to cloud services [74].

Heterogeneity: One of the major challenges encounter in cloud-based IoT system is choosing the best from variety of devices, software products, and other resources that might be employed for new or advanced applications in healthcare system.

Cloud systems have heterogeneity difficulties; for example, most Cloud services have proprietary interfaces, permitting resource integration dependent on individual providers [75]. Likewise, when end-users adopt multi-Cloud solutions, the heterogeneity problem may intensify, as services would rely on many providers to improve application performance and robustness [72].

Because of the heterogeneity that exists within IoT-based systems during data processing, data formatting, and data clearing, it is challenging to process medical data. In a smart healthcare system for patient monitoring, enabling a network to link with numerous sensors is an example problem. When data is moved to another system for processing or analysis, heterogeneity must be present for this to happen. As you progress through the fog layer, you'll encounter many nodes, clusters, switches, and other devices that are required for data processing and communication [76]. In order to communicate with end-users using IoT-based devices and sensors, heterogeneity is a key element to consider when creating architecture that allows for numerous device monitoring [77].

Legal Issues: In recent research on specific applications, legal considerations have played a large role. Service providers, for example, must comply with a variety of international regulations. Users, on the other hand, should contribute to the data collecting effort [61]. There is no standard guide and regulations for computing the protocols and interfaces for various products and services in a smart healthcare system. A dedicated agency is needed to handle this problem, and standards should be put in place to standardize the healthcare system. This will help with data dissimilarity and achieving real-time reaction. Communication protocol, data aggregation interfaces, system interfaces, and gateway interfaces should all be seriously addressed for proper standardization [78].

3.3 IoT and Cloud for Improving Elderly Healthcare

The problems of security, low performance, privacy, and reliability issues associated with IoT are due to the limited processing power and storage capacity. These challenges must improve the performance of IoT-based system and the healthcare sectors will be able to enjoy the benefits of using this platform. The combinations of both IoT and cloud has brought effective solution to address these problems. The IoT also expands the boundaries in which the cloud works with real-world items in a more dispersed manner, as well as enabling innovative services for billions of devices in a variety of real-world situations [79]. Furthermore, the Cloud simplifies the use of apps and services for end-users while lowering the cost of doing so. The Cloud also streamlines IoT data collection and processing, allowing for rapid, low-cost setup and incorporation for sophisticated data processing and utilization [80]. The advantages of incorporating IoT into the cloud for elderly monitoring are as follows.

The Cloud-based IoT paradigm has two important features: application and data exchange. IoT can be used to transmit ubiquitous applications, and automation can be used to simplify low-cost data distribution and gathering. Using built-in apps and bespoke gateways, the Cloud is a practical and cost-efficient option for connecting, managing, and tracking anything [81]. The accessibilities of quick Interactive surveillance and remote object management, and also data actual accessibility, are made possible by systems. Though the Cloud can considerably enhance and facilitate IoT interconnectivity, it does have drawbacks in several areas. The move of huge data from IoT to the cloud can create practical restrictions of such data to be moved to the cloud storage device [82, 83].

The Internet of Everything (IoE) collects billions of devices and sensors that create new opportunities with various medical threats [10]. The world is fast advancing toward the IoE domain, with billions of people talking among each other, as well as a range of data being gathered. The Cloud-based IoT technique expands the Cloud through IoT devices, allowing the Cloud to operate with a variety of real-world situations and resulting in the production of new innovations in medical sectors [72]. The devices, protocols, and technologies that make up the IoT are diverse. As a result, achieving dependability, scalability, compatibility, safety, accessibility, and effectiveness can be difficult. The majority of these concerns are resolved when IoT is integrated into the cloud [84]. Other benefits include ease of use and access, as well as inexpensive deployment costs [85, 86].

The IoT comprises a vast number of data sources that create a vast volume of semi-structured or unstructured data [87] since it may be utilized on billions of devices. Big Data has three qualities [88]: diversity like the data type, velocity such as data generation frequency, and the data size which is the volume. The cloud is the most appropriate and cost-effective options of dealing with the huge amount of data generated by IoT-based system. It also opens up new possibilities for data integration, aggregation, and sharing with others [9, 10]. Acquired data is transported to nodes with high capabilities due to IoT devices that have limited processing capabilities that make the data processing to be more complicated and sometimes impossible to process this huge data. The IoT generated data will be transported to where aggregation and processing takes place. Yet, without a suitable underlying infrastructure, achieving scalability remains a difficulty. The Cloud provided a virtual computing capabilities and an on-demand usage paradigm [10]. In order to improve income and decrease hazards at a cheaper cost, predictive techniques and data-driven policy making can be included into the IoT [9].

4 Framework for IoT and Cloud in Elderly Activity Monitoring Systems

The architecture of the IoT-Cloud Elderly Activity Monitoring System (ICEAMS) is a difficult task, and several solutions were investigated. One of the key problems facing IoT's reality in developing smart personalized healthcare systems is data collecting and integration from different IoT devices. Because IoT devices collect complex and dynamic data on medical evaluation, monitoring, and therapy plans, and predictions in healthcare, appraising or incorporating a large amount of data is difficult. Data aggregation from individual device data sources is a critical issue that requires immediate attention. As a result, it'll be fascinating to discover which IoT sensors boost the performance of intelligent systems that gather a variety of disease indications. As a result, it would be critical to look into whether there was any other background data that could help the model perform better. Furthermore, more research is needed to determine the quality of the properties chosen from each biomarker.

Evaluation, treatment planning, and prediction are other important aspects of IoT implementation for elderly activity monitoring systems. These are needed to create a system capable of switching among web and local storage categorization algorithms with little processing time while actually providing and onward patient information care. This chapter lays out the framework for ICEAMS, a system that monitors the health of elderly people via a network of wearable sensors. Body temperature and pulse, for example, aid in the collection of physiological pointers. Because of the sensitive data acquired from these embedded devices, it will be uploaded straight to the public cloud sensor nodes' limited computing and storage capabilities, as well as to prevent utilizing a smartphone as a sensor module.

The ICEAMS employs cellphones and wearable sensors to watch seniors in real time, resulting in increased medical productivity by providing a more efficient and effective healthcare network with home-based supervision. The main goal of the ICEAMS is to track clinical data collected from the elderly's wearable device, create a data record in the cloud server, as well as then make this data available to registered healthcare practitioners and clinicians at any time. The process is made up of three layers that work together to achieve the system's goals. For example, in the older person's layers, each layer has its own standards and methods, but the most important components are that the devices, as well as the pathways, should be able to link to cloud services to store patient data. Figure 3 depicts the system's primary layers.

4.1 Elderly Patients' Layer (Wearable Devices)

The patient's body is equipped with a wearable monitor and smartphone sensors to collect clinical data. There are many different types of healthcare sensors accessible today. These sensors calculate vital indicators like intensity of oxygen in the blood, temperature, pulse rate, blood glucose, and SPo2 [89]. It's critical to keep track of these warning sign in the patient's body because any suspicious data could lead to an infection. A drop in the human body's oxygen supply, for example, causes sleep apnea, which can lead to death. Unusual blood pressure can lead to kidney illness or diabetes, and should be monitored in elderly patients. The sensitive information is transferred to the patient's mobile app through Bluetooth and then to a database server. In addition, sensors can calculate and deliver data on a daily basis without the need for patient intervention (IoT), boosting the efficiency of interface design and making it more convenient.

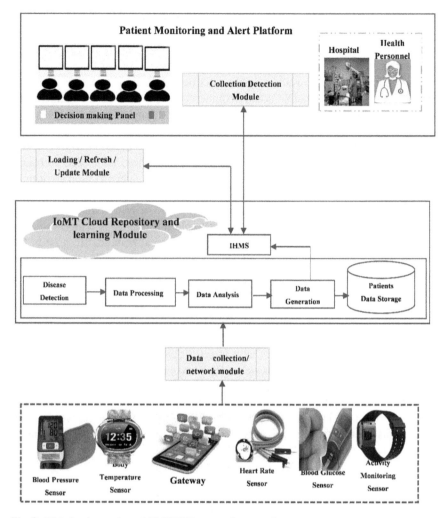

Fig. 3 High-level overview of CI-WBSN system framework

4.2 IoT-Cloud-Based (Data Layer)

The cloud is a network place where data is stored and processed. Patient data can be processed in the cloud and then made available for medical review through the network. As a consequence, all records will be gathered and disseminated in the cloud in order to identify any problem in medical data, and irregular disparities in patient records will be categorized based on the patient's condition and disease. All papers will be transmitted to the patient's and/or doctor's website, the emergency room, or both, depending on the patient's circumstance. Hence, the IoT web encourages collaboration and data transmission through its platform, which allows healthcare professionals to save client records, analyses, and diagnostics so that other specialists may immediately read information related to shared interests. It displays patient records in real-time updates and speedier medications.

4.3 Elderly Monitoring and Alert Platform (Hospital Layer)

The proposed system gives the medical doctor the opportunity of monitoring their patient in real-time using the information receive from the sensory data captured using various physiological devices. This can be done by study the data from cloud database which has been process by machine learning algorithm. The application gives the physicians update information about their patient conditions by replicates data and deleting all data in the IoMT server immediately it arrives to give real-time update on various signs. Therefore, making immediate decision in case of any emergency before the situation worsens.

The remaining components of a supported sensor network are mostly utilized for network pattern management and connections between device stages and their objects. In addition, domain-specific management within the computer system can be accessed and configured in the software program to access and configure similar device activities such active/inactive timestamps and sensing frequency. Domain-specific supervision, as a result, collaborates with both the public network and the component to install sensor network configuration and updates, as well as the component to inform/update the network's services about the new modifications. Similarly, the data analysis part of the cloud server exists, according to the services provided, to handle data processing tasks such as statistical analysis.

4.4 Elderly Monitoring and Alert Platform (Hospital Layer)

This framework allows the doctor to keep track of the information and sensory data of his or her patients. Physicians can study data from the program's cloud and take action based on it. This application replicates data in actual time by deleting all data from the IoMT server immediately it arrives, ensuring that physicians are up to date on the patient's condition and assisting paramedics in making an immediate decision in the event of an emergency before the situation worsens and hospital admission is avoided.

The remaining components of a supported sensor network are mostly utilized for network pattern management and connections between device stages and their objects. In addition, domain-specific management within the computer system can be accessed and configured in the software program to access and configure similar device activities such active/inactive timestamps and sensing frequency. Domain-specific supervision, as a result, collaborates with both the public network and the component to install sensor network configuration and updates, as well as the component to inform/update the network's services about the new modifications. Similarly, the data analysis part of the cloud server exists, according to the facilities provided, to handle data processing tasks such as statistical analysis.

4.5 The Gateway

This component is in charge of interfacing with patient devices that are used to diagnose patients' complaints and conduct initial data analysis. This component produces a description of the circumstances of patients who have been referred to healthcare. When an urgent condition is recognized, the Framework can also respond to indicators of irregularity by submitting a request for assistance (e.g., a demand for an assistant care provider) or an urgent request (e.g., a call for an ambulance).

5 The Practical Application of the Proposed Framework

5.1 Data Collection

IoT data should be acquired via IoT medical devices to observe the elderly's activities. The data obtained includes vital indicators like systolic and diastolic blood pressure, pulse rate, oxygen levels, sugar levels, and other physiological data detected by biomedical sensors distributed on the elderly's outfit or body using Body Area Network (BAN) and integrated devices in garments. A Personal Area Network (PAN) can also be used to monitor the elderly's behavioral changes and to respond to emergencies. The IoT devices continually detect and gather the data of health performance parameters in order to assess the operational technology for the aged. The extracted characteristics that keep track of your regular activities of human from MHEALTH dataset [20] were used for the proposed system, like old people's symptoms and body position connecting wireless body sensors. Devices on the chest, ankle, and wrist are utilized to track the different bodily parts moving.

The MHEALTH (Mobile HEALTH) dataset contains recordings of ten participants' body motion and vital signs while undertaking various physical activities. Sensors attached to the subject's chest, right wrist, and left ankle track the motion of various body components, including acceleration, rate of rotation, and magnetic field orientation. The sensor on the chest can also take 2-lead ECG readings, which can be utilized for basic cardiac monitoring, screening for various arrhythmias, or examining the effects of exercise on the ECG. The ECG data are recorded by sensors on the chest for heart rate monitoring [90, 91]. The dataset contains extracted features, with each subject being stored in its own log file: "MHEALTH subject SUBJECT

ID.log", which was then converted to "SUBJECT ID.CSV", with each record in the data file has the fields.

5.2 Data Preprocessing

For the data mining process, it is necessary to perform a data pretreatment step on the obtained IoT medical data to remove noise and inconsistencies. In addition, several feature selection strategies are used with the goal of reducing dimensions to make the classification portion of the senior monitoring system evaluation process easier. Since the dataset has performed feature selection on the IoMT-based data, the data preprocessing just concentrates on removing the noisy and inconsistencies in the data using rule-based method.

5.3 Prediction Algorithm for the Proposed Elderly Activity Monitoring System

The suggested system's goal is to label a recorded activity using the methods described in this chapter. Supervised machine learning algorithms were used, often known as classifiers, to achieve such labeling. The first stage is training, which involves using activities represented as features vectors and their labels to train the parameters of a given classifier. After that, the trained model is assessed by predicting the label of a specific assessment action in a way that is distinct from the training set.

For senior activity monitoring, a variety of classification methods have been investigated. However, there is no general classifier that surpasses all others when it comes to person identification [92]. KNN, NBNB, RFRF, Bayesian Networks, SVM, J48, Logistic Regression, Decision Tree, and ANN are among the most often used classifiers, hence, the proposed system used XGBooster classifier.

5.3.1 XGBoost Classifier

Chen and Guestrin [93] popularized XGBoost, a machine learning classifier that is both effective and scalable. The gradient enhancing decision tree first XGBoost ideal, which associations many decision trees in a boosting manner. Each new tree is created in order to lower the gradient boosting of the prior model's residual. Residual describes the differences between the real and expected values. The template has been trained until the quantity of decision trees defines the threshold. XGBoost follows the same notion of gradient boosting; to manage overfitting and enhance efficiency, it employs the quantity of spikes, training rate, subsampling ratio, and maximum tree depth are all variables to consider. Specifically, XGBoost optimizes the function goal, tree size, and scale of the weights, all of which are governed by typical variables for normalization. With many hyper-parameters, the XGBoost provides greater efficiency in a specific search space.

Gamma $\gamma \in (0, +\infty)$ denotes minimal loss reduction, which includes a split to render the partition on a tree's leaf node, according to the hyper-parameters. The minimum child weight $w_{mc} \in (0, +\infty)$ is defined as the minimum instance weight overall, implying that if the graph division stage yields a tree structure with the instance weight sum less than w_{mc}, the further partition will be discarded by the tree. The early stop algorithm works to find the optimum number of epochs that correspond to other hyper-parameters given. Finally, subsampling methods and $r_c \in (0, 1)$ column subsample ratio concepts were also provided by XGBoost in each tree. In the final step, to minimize the classification error, grid search is used to control the hyper-parameters.

Given $X \in \mathbb{R}^{n \times d}$ as training dataset with d features and n samples, XGBoost object function in tth is represented by

$$\text{Obj}^{(t)} \simeq \sum_{i-1}^{n} \left\{ \ell\left(y_i, \tilde{y}_i^{(t-1)}\right) + g_i f_t(x_i) + \frac{1}{2} h_i f_t^2(x_i) \right\} + \Omega(f_t), \quad (1)$$

$$g_i = \partial_{\tilde{y}(t-1)} \ell\left(y_i, \tilde{y}_i^{(t-1)}\right), h_i = \partial_{\tilde{y}(t-1)}^2 \ell\left(y_i, \tilde{y}_i^{(t-1)}\right), \quad (2)$$

where the loss function ℓ is represented by the first gradient g_i, and, h_i is the second gradient of ℓ. To measure the complexity of the model, the regularization $\Omega(f_t) = \gamma T + \frac{1}{2}\varphi\varphi^2$ was used, where the number of leaf nodes is represented by T.

As demonstrated in Eq. (3), the logistic loss ℓ of the training loss measures how well the model fits on the training data,

$$\ell\left(y_i, \tilde{y}_i^{(t-1)}\right) = y_i \ln\left(1 + e^{-\tilde{y}_i}\right) + (1 - y_i) \ln\left(1 + e^{\tilde{y}_i}\right) \quad (3)$$

given the tth training sample $x_i \in \mathbb{R}^d$, assume that a XGBoost model of XGB contains K trees, the corresponding prediction $\tilde{y}_i$ is computed as

$$\tilde{y}_i = \sum_{k=1}^{k} F_k(x_i) \quad (4)$$

$$\text{s.t. } F_k \in \text{XGB, where XGB} = \{F_1, F_2, F_3, \ldots, F_K\}. \quad (5)$$

R programming language was used to implement the proposed classifier and the evaluations were done using various performance metrics. The dataset with the relevant activity monitoring recognition was used with seamlessly incorporate all characteristics. The dataset contains 12 activities monitoring of elderly people.

Split the physical activities dataset vectors into two groups in a 70:30 ratio, randomly selecting 70% for training and 30% for testing. To train the classifier on the training set, use the XGBoost machine learning approach. For the 12 physical activities, the label index includes class labels like Climbing stairs, Cycling, Jogging, Frontal Elevation of Arms, Jump Front and Back, Lying down, Running, Sitting and Relaxing, Standing, waist bends Forward, Walking, Knees bending. All vectors that have the same values are added together and preserved. To determine the performance of the classifier, use the test dataset.

Table 1 displays the performance of the projected system using activity observing MHEALTH dataset using numerous metrics. The results obtained different metrics showed that the projected system is essential and relevant in elderly activity monitoring system for prediction and classification. The model has the highest predicted classification accuracy of 98.7%, which is excellent and may be used to forecast the elderly physical activities. For the sake of simplicity, the classification system generates results for the 12 physical activities designated as A1–A12.

To show how machine learning technique affects a classification on the activities monitoring on the dataset, Table 2 compares the proposed approach with several known approaches. Table 2 displays the cumulative performance measures for the proposed system and other models using the decreased MHEALTH dataset. The accuracy of the suggested approach is better than other approaches. The suggested elderly activities monitoring system, in general, has a 98.7% accuracy, which is 1.6% higher than the Multinomial Naïve Bayes with the second-highest accuracy. When equated to other techniques using the reduced MHEALTH dataset, the proposed approach performed better across all evaluation metrics. The proposed method's marginally higher accuracy is due to its robust feature selection and rule-based fitness calculation.

The proposed model differs from previous elderly activities monitoring classification models in that it uses a basic XGBoost estimate parameters that are appropriate for input to create its classification effectively and efficiently. Moreover, the model

Table 1 Proposed method evaluation

Activities	Accuracy (%)	Precision (%)	Recall (%)	F-measure (%)	ROC (%)
A1	95.4	96.2	96.8	95.7	95.3
A2	95.8	97.3	95.6	95.3	96.6
A3	97.3	97.6	97.3	98.4	98.1
A4	95.6	95.5	95.8	95.2	96.6
A5	98.2	97.8	98.4	98.8	99.3
A6	98.4	99.0	99.1	98.8	98.6
A7	96.7	97.3	97.1	96.9	96.6
A8	97.4	97.3	96.8	98.6	97.9
A9	98.3	98.8	98.7	98.5	98.8
A10	98.9	90.2	90.6	98.4	98.7
A11	96.4	96.5	96.8	96.2	96.7
A12	98.7	99.5	99.1	98.0	98.9

Table 2 Summary of performance comparison of accuracy of existing work

Technique	Dataset	Accuracy (%)
Random Forest [94]	UCI-HAR	60.0
CNN [95]	UCI-HAR	90.9
K-Means [94]	UCI-HAR	60.0
ANN [96]	UCI-HAR	91.4
CNN [97]	UCI-HAR	94.8
IBK [94]	UCI-HAR	90.0
SVM [98]	UCI-MHEALTH	65.4
Multinomial Naïve Bayes [20]	UCI-MHEALTH	97.1
CNN-pff [98]	UCI-MHEALTH	91.9
Naïve Bayes [94]	UCI-HAR	79.0
Proposed Model	UCI-MHEALTH	98.7

knows and examines high-level functionality, automatically decreases data dimensionality, and effectively portrays important features due to the reduced hidden layer. As a consequence, the proposed model is optimal for use in classification in healthcare industries with a vast amount of unlabeled and unstructured data, such as medical data.

6 Conclusions

Continuous population growth and corresponding increases in life expectancy, combined with worldwide infectious disease outbreaks in recent years, has prompted a quest for novel ways to make the most of limited resources. Automated illness monitoring, diagnosis, prediction, and treatment of patients provides not only quick data but also trustworthy service at a lower cost and correct outcomes from medical specialists. However, the healthcare system faces issues such as a lack of proper medical information, misdiagnosis, data treatment, and medical information transmission delays. To solve these identified problems this chapter proposed IoT-based cloud elderly monitoring system. The design integrates a deep learning mechanism to train the data using a XGBoost for classification of the capture data from the IoT devices. The data collected from different wearable sensors like body temperature, glucose sensors, heartbeat sensors, and chest were transmitted through IoT devices to the integrated cloud database. Deep learning was used to extract features from the patient capture data and the sensor signal is analyzed using XGBoost for the monitoring of the elderly activity. The proposed system can be widely used to monitor and diagnose patient physiological health situations globally using an internal network, hence, eliminating medical faults, reduce healthcare costs, minimize pressure on medical experts, enhancing patient satisfaction, and increase productivity in the healthcare system. The proposed model used XGBoost for the classification of the capture data using IoT-based devices and sensors from elderly activities, the result shown an improvement when compare with the recent state-of-the-art model.

References

1. European Commission: Directorate-general for economic and financial affairs. In: The 2012 Ageing Report: Economic and Budgetary Projections for the 27 EU Member States (2010–60). Publications Office of the European Union (2012)
2. Ianculescu, M., Stanciu, A., Bica, O., Florian, V., Neagu, G.: Shaping a person-centric eHealth system for an age-friendly community. A case study. Int. J. Comput. **1** (2016)
3. Weck, M., Tamminen, P., Ferreira, F.A.: Knowledge management in an open innovation ecosystem: building an age-friendly smart living environment. In: ISPIM Conference Proceedings, pp. 1–14. The International Society for Professional Innovation Management (ISPIM) (2020)
4. Davoodi, L., Merilä, S.: Smart Living Environment for Aging Well (2019)
5. Neagu, G., Preda, Ş., Stanciu, A., Florian, V.: A cloud-IoT based sensing service for health monitoring. In: 2017 E-Health and Bioengineering Conference (EHB), pp. 53–56. IEEE (2017)
6. Bates, J.: Thingalytics: Smart Big Data Analytics for the Internet of Things. Software AG (2015)
7. Mell, P., Grance, T.: The NIST Definition of Cloud Computing (2011)
8. Griebel, L., Prokosch, H.U., Köpcke, F., Toddenroth, D., Christoph, J., Leb, I., Sedlmayr, M.: A scoping review of cloud computing in healthcare. BMC Med. Inform. Decis. Mak. **15**(1), 1–16 (2015)
9. Awotunde, J.B., Adeniyi, A.E., Ogundokun, R.O., Ajamu, G.J., Adebayo, P.O.: MIoT-based big data analytics architecture, opportunities and challenges for enhanced telemedicine systems. Stud. Fuzziness Soft Comput. **2021**(410), 199–220 (2021)
10. Adeniyi, E.A., Ogundokun, R.O., Awotunde, J.B. IoMT-based wearable body sensors network healthcare monitoring system. In: IoT in Healthcare and Ambient Assisted Living, pp. 103–121. Springer, Singapore (2021)
11. Adly, A.S. Technology trade-offs for IIoT systems and applications from a developing country perspective: case of Egypt. In: The Internet of Things in the Industrial Sector, pp. 299–319. Springer, Cham (2019)
12. Kumar, S., Nilsen, W., Pavel, M., Srivastava, M.: Mobile health: revolutionizing healthcare through transdisciplinary research. Computer **46**(1), 28–35 (2012)
13. Darwish, A., Ismail Sayed, G., Ella Hassanien, A.: The impact of implantable sensors in biomedical technology on the future of healthcare systems. Intell. Pervasive Comput. Syst. Smart. Healthc. 67–89 (2019)
14. Awotunde, J.B., Jimoh, R.G., AbdulRaheem, M., Oladipo, I.D., Folorunso, S.O., Ajamu, G.J.: IoT-based wearable body sensor network for COVID-19 pandemic. Adv. Data Sci. Intell. Data Commun. Technol. COVID-19, 253–275 (2022)
15. Manogaran, G., Chilamkurti, N., Hsu, C.H.: Emerging trends, issues, and challenges on internet of medical things and wireless networks. Pers. Ubiquit. Comput. **22**(5–6), 879–882 (2018)
16. Varshney, U. Pervasive healthcare computing: EMR/EHR, wireless, and health monitoring. Springer Science & Business Media (2009)
17. Awotunde, J. B., Ajagbe, S. A., Oladipupo, M. A., Awokola, J. A., Afolabi, O. S., Mathew, T. O., Oguns, Y. J.: An Improved Machine Learnings Diagnosis Technique for COVID-19 Pandemic Using Chest X-ray Images. Communications in Computer and Information Science, 1455, pp. 319–330, (2021)

18. Awotunde, J.B., Folorunso, S.O., Bhoi, A.K., Adebayo, P.O., Ijaz, M.F.: Disease diagnosis system for IoT-based wearable body sensors with machine learning algorithm. Hybrid Artif. Intell. IoT Healthc. **201**
19. Kaw, J.A., Loan, N.A., Parah, S.A., Muhammad, K., Sheikh, J.A., Bhat, G.M.: A reversible and secure patient information hiding system for IoT driven e-health. Int. J. Inf. Manage. **45**, 262–275 (2019)
20. Syed, L., Jabeen, S., Manimala, S., Alsaeedi, A.: Smart healthcare framework for ambient assisted living using IoMT and big data analytics techniques. Futur. Gener. Comput. Syst. **101**, 136–151 (2019)
21. Azimi, I., Rahmani, A.M., Liljeberg, P., Tenhunen, H.: Internet of things for remote elderly monitoring: a study from user-centered perspective. J. Ambient. Intell. Humaniz. Comput. **8**(2), 273–289 (2017)
22. Downer, M.B., Wallack, E.M., Ploughman, M.: Octogenarians with multiple sclerosis: lessons for aging in place. Can. J. Aging/La Revue canadienne du vieillissement **39**(1), 107–116 (2020)
23. Jeannotte, L., Moore, M.J.: The state of aging and health in America 2007 (2007)
24. Rashidi, P., Mihailidis, A.: A survey on ambient-assisted living tools for older adults. IEEE J. Biomed. Health Inform. **17**(3), 579–590 (2012)
25. Awotunde, J.B., Folorunso, S.O., Jimoh, R.G., Adeniyi, E.A., Abiodun, K.M., Ajamu, G.J.: Application of artificial intelligence for COVID-19 epidemic: an exploratory study, opportunities, challenges, and future prospects. Stud. Syst. Decis. Control **2021**(358), 47–61 (2021)
26. Folorunso, S.O., Awotunde, J.B., Ayo, F.E., Abdullah, K.K.A.: RADIoT: the unifying framework for IoT, radiomics and deep learning modeling. Hybrid Artif. Intell. IoT Healthc. **109**
27. Maarala, A.I., Su, X., Riekki, J.: Semantic data provisioning and reasoning for the internet of things. In: 2014 International Conference on the Internet of Things (IOT), pp. 67–72. IEEE (2014)
28. da Costa, K.A., Papa, J.P., Lisboa, C.O., Munoz, R., de Albuquerque, V.H.C.: Internet of things: a survey on machine learning-based intrusion detection approaches. Comput. Netw. **151**, 147–157 (2019)
29. Wang, Y., Yan, J., Yang, Z., Zhao, Y., Liu, T.: Optimizing GIS partial discharge pattern recognition in the ubiquitous power internet of things context: A MixNet deep learning model. Int. J. Electric. Power Energy Syst. **125**, 106484 (2021)
30. Tan, H.X., Tan, H.P.: Early detection of mild cognitive impairment in elderly through IoT: Preliminary findings. In: 2018 IEEE 4th World Forum on Internet of Things (WF-IoT), pp. 207–212. IEEE (2018)
31. Pfuntner, A., Wier, L.M., Steiner, C.: Costs for hospital stays in the United States, 2011: statistical brief# **168** (2014)
32. Spinsante, S., Gambi, E.: Remote health monitoring for elderly through interactive television. Biomed. Eng. Online **11**(1), 1–18 (2012)
33. Macis, S., Loi, D., Angius, G., Pani, D., Raffo, L.: Towards an integrated tv-based system for active ageing and tele-care. In: Quarto Congresso Nazionale di Bioingegneria, GNB2014. Patron Editore (2014)
34. Macis, S., Loi, D., Pani, D., Raffo, L., La Manna, S., Cestone, V., Guerri, D.: Home telemonitoring of vital signs through a TV-based application for elderly patients. In: 2015 IEEE International Symposium on Medical Measurements and Applications (MeMeA) Proceedings, pp. 169–174. IEEE (2015)
35. Van Kasteren, T.L.M., Englebienne, G., Kröse, B.J.: An activity monitoring system for elderly care using generative and discriminative models. Pers. Ubiquit. Comput. **14**(6), 489–498 (2010)
36. Stratton, R.J., Green, C.J., Elia, M.: Disease-related malnutrition: an evidence-based approach to treatment. Cabi (2003)
37. Hickson, M.: Malnutrition and ageing. Postgrad. Med. J. **82**(963), 2–8 (2006)
38. Lattanzio, F., Abbatecola, A.M., Bevilacqua, R., Chiatti, C., Corsonello, A., Rossi, L., Bernabei, R.: Advanced technology care innovation for older people in Italy: necessity and opportunity to promote health and wellbeing. J. Am. Med. Dir. Assoc. **15**(7), 457–466 (2014)

39. Sanchez, J., Sanchez, V., Salomie, I., Taweel, A., Charvill, J., Araujo, M.: Dynamic nutrition behaviour awareness system for the elders. In: Proceedings of the 5th AAL Forum Norrkoping, Impacting Individuals, Society and Economic Growth (2013)
40. Chifu, V.R., Salomie, I., Chifu, E.Ş., Izabella, B., Pop, C.B., Antal, M.: Cuckoo search algorithm for clustering food offers. In: 2014 IEEE 10th International Conference on Intelligent Computer Communication and Processing (ICCP), pp. 17–22. IEEE (2014)
41. Awotunde, J.B., Jimoh, R.G., Oladipo, I.D., Abdulraheem, M., Jimoh, T.B., Ajamu, G.J.: Big data and data analytics for an enhanced COVID-19 epidemic management. Stud. Syst. Decis. Control **2021**(358), 11–29 (2021)
42. Bai, Y., Li, C., Yue, Y., Jia, W., Li, J., Mao, Z.H., Sun, M.: Designing a wearable computer for lifestyle evaluation. In: 2012 38th Annual Northeast Bioengineering Conference (NEBEC), pp. 93–94. IEEE (2012)
43. WHO: Falls. Retrieved on May 2021. http://www.who.int/mediacentre/factsheets/fs344/en/ (2016b)
44. Igual, R., Medrano, C., Plaza, I.: Challenges, issues and trends in fall detection systems. Biomed. Eng. Online **12**(1), 1–24 (2013)
45. Fang, S.H., Liang, Y.C., Chiu, K.M.: Developing a mobile phone-based fall detection system on android platform. In: 2012 Computing, Communications and Applications Conference, pp. 143–146. IEEE (2012)
46. Sposaro, F., Tyson, G.: iFall: an Android application for fall monitoring and response. In: 2009 Annual International Conference of the IEEE Engineering in Medicine and Biology Society, pp. 6119–6122. IEEE (2009)
47. Habib, M.A., Mohktar, M.S., Kamaruzzaman, S.B., Lim, K.S., Pin, T.M., Ibrahim, F.: Smartphone-based solutions for fall detection and prevention: challenges and open issues. Sensors **14**(4), 7181–7208 (2014)
48. Cheng, S.H.: An intelligent fall detection system using triaxial accelerometer integrated by active RFID. In: 2014 International Conference on Machine Learning and Cybernetics, vol 2, pp. 517–522. IEEE (2014)
49. Odunmbaku, A., Rahmani, A.M., Liljeberg, P., Tenhunen, H.: Elderly monitoring system with sleep and fall detector. In: International Internet of Things Summit, pp. 473–480. Springer, Cham (2015)
50. Bian, Z.P., Hou, J., Chau, L.P., Magnenat-Thalmann, N.: Fall detection based on body part tracking using a depth camera. IEEE J. Biomed. Health Inform. **19**(2), 430–439 (2014)
51. Juang, L.H., Wu, M.N.: Fall down detection under smart home system. J. Med. Syst. **39**(10), 1–12 (2015)
52. Planinc, R., Kampel, M.: Emergency system for elderly–a computer vision based approach. In International Workshop on Ambient Assisted Living, pp. 79–83. Springer, Berlin, Heidelberg (2011)
53. Planinc, R., Kampel, M.: Introducing the use of depth data for fall detection. Pers. Ubiquit. Comput. **17**(6), 1063–1072 (2013)
54. Planinc, R., Kampel, M.: Robust fall detection by combining 3D data and fuzzy logic. In: Asian Conference on Computer Vision, pp. 121–132. Springer, Berlin, Heidelberg (2012)
55. Berndt, R.D., Takenga, M.C., Kuehn, S., Preik, P., Berndt, S., Brandstoetter, M., Kampel, M., et al.: An assisted living system for the elderly FEARLESS concept. In: Proceedings of the IADIS Multi Conference on Computer Science and Information Systems, pp. 131–138 (2012)
56. Mao, Y., Bhuse, V., Zhou, Z., Pichappan, P., Abdel-Aty, M., Hayafuji, Y.: Applied Mathematics and Algorithms for Cloud Computing and Iot (2014)
57. Wang, Y., Wang, X.: The novel analysis model of cloud computing based on RFID internet of things. J. Chem. Pharm. Res. **6**(6), 661–668 (2014)
58. Bonomi, F., Milito, R., Natarajan, P., Zhu, J.: Fog computing: a platform for internet of things and analytics. In: Big Data and Internet of Things: A Roadmap for Smart Environments, pp. 169–186. Springer, Cham (2014)
59. Soldatos, J., Kefalakis, N., Serrano, M., Hauswirth, M.: Design principles for utility-driven services and cloud-based computing modelling for the Internet of Things. Int. J. Web Grid Serv. **6, 10**(2–3), 139–167 (2014)

60. Fang, S., Da Xu, L., Zhu, Y., Ahati, J., Pei, H., Yan, J., Liu, Z.: An integrated system for regional environmental monitoring and management based on internet of things. IEEE Trans. Ind. Inf. **10**(2), 1596–1605 (2014)
61. Atlam, H.F., Alenezi, A., Alharthi, A., Walters, R.J., Wills, G.B. Integration of cloud computing with internet of things: challenges and open issues. In: 2017 IEEE International Conference on Internet of Things (iThings) and IEEE Green Computing and Communications (GreenCom) and IEEE Cyber, Physical and Social Computing (CPSCom) and IEEE Smart Data (SmartData), pp. 670–675. IEEE (2017)
62. Gebremeskel, G.B., Chai, Y., Yang, Z. The paradigm of big data for augmenting internet of vehicle into the intelligent cloud computing systems. In International Conference on Internet of Vehicles, pp. 247–261. Springer, Cham (2014)
63. Choudhary, V., Vithayathil, J.: The impact of cloud computing: should the IT department be organized as a cost center or a profit center? J. Manag. Inf. Syst. **30**(2), 67–100 (2013)
64. Suciu, G., Vulpe, A., Halunga, S., Fratu, O., Todoran, G., Suciu, V.: Smart cities built on resilient cloud computing and secure internet of things. In: 2013 19th International Conference on Control Systems and Computer Science, pp. 513–518. IEEE (2013)
65. Mousavi, S.K., Ghaffari, A., Besharat, S., Afshari, H.: Security of internet of things based on cryptographic algorithms: a survey. Wireless Netw. **27**(2), 1515–1555 (2021)
66. Alenezi, A., Zulkipli, N.H.N., Atlam, H.F., Walters, R.J., Wills, G.B.: The impact of cloud forensic readiness on security. In: CLOSER, pp. 511–517 (2017)
67. Dar, K.S., Taherkordi, A., Eliassen, F.: Enhancing dependability of cloud-based iot services through virtualization. In: 2016 IEEE First International Conference on Internet-of-Things Design and Implementation (IoTDI), pp. 106–116. IEEE (2016)
68. Doukas, C., Maglogiannis, I. Bringing IoT and cloud computing towards pervasive healthcare. In: 2012 Sixth International Conference on Innovative Mobile and Internet Services in Ubiquitous Computing, pp. 922–926. IEEE (2012)
69. Puthal, D., Obaidat, M.S., Nanda, P., Prasad, M., Mohanty, S.P., Zomaya, A.Y.: Secure and sustainable load balancing of edge data centers in fog computing. IEEE Commun. Mag. **56**(5), 60–65 (2018)
70. Li, Q., Wang, C., Wu, J., Li, J., Wang, Z.Y.: Towards the business–information technology alignment in cloud computing environment: anapproach based on collaboration points and agents. Int. J. Comput. Integr. Manuf. **24**(11), 1038–1057 (2011)
71. Mocnej, J., Pekar, A., Seah, W.K., Papcun, P., Kajati, E., Cupkova, D., Zolotova, I.: Quality-enabled decentralized IoT architecture with efficient resources utilization. Robot. Comput. Integr. Manuf. **67**, 102001 (2021)
72. Aceto, G., Persico, V., Pescapé, A.: Industry 4.0 and health: internet of things, big data, and cloud computing for healthcare 4.0. J. Ind. Inf. Integr. **18**, 100129 (2020)
73. Diène, B., Rodrigues, J.J., Diallo, O., Ndoye, E.H.M., Korotaev, V.V.: Data management techniques for Internet of Things. Mech. Syst. Sig. Proc. **138**, 106564 (2020)
74. ALmarwani, R., Zhang, N., Garside, J.: An effective, secure and efficient tagging method for integrity protection of outsourced data in a public cloud storage. Plos one, **15**(11), e0241236 (2020)
75. Ramalingam, C., Mohan, P.: Addressing semantics standards for cloud portability and interoperability in multi cloud environment. Symmetry **13**(2), 317 (2021)
76. Yi, S., Li, C., Li, Q.: A survey of fog computing: concepts, applications, and issues. In: Proceedings of the 2015 Workshop on Mobile Big Data, pp. 37–42 (2015)
77. Mouradian, C., Naboulsi, D., Yangui, S., Glitho, R.H., Morrow, M.J., Polakos, P.A.: A comprehensive survey on fog computing: state-of-the-art and research challenges. IEEE Commun. Surv. Tutorials **20**(1), 416–464 (2017)
78. Kumari, A., Tanwar, S., Tyagi, S., Kumar, N.: Fog computing for healthcare 4.0 environment: opportunities and challenges. Comput. Electr. Eng. **72**, 1–13 (2018)
79. Teece, D.J.: Profiting from innovation in the digital economy: enabling technologies, standards, and licensing models in the wireless world. Res. Policy **47**(8), 1367–1387 (2018)

80. Kristiani, E., Yang, C.T., Huang, C.Y., Wang, Y.T., Ko, P.C. The implementation of a cloud-edge computing architecture using OpenStack and Kubernetes for air quality monitoring application. Mob. Networks Appl. 1–23 (2020)
81. Simić, M., Perić, M., Popadić, I., Perić, D., Pavlović, M., Vučetić, M., Stanković, M.S.: Big data and development of smart city: system architecture and practical public safety example. Serbian J. Electric. Eng. **17**(3), 337–355 (2020)
82. Folorunso, S.O., Awotunde, J.B., Adeboye, N.O., Matiluko, O.E.: Data classification model for COVID-19 pandemic. In: Advances in Data Science and Intelligent Data Communication Technologies for COVID-19: Innovative Solutions Against COVID-19, vol. 378, pp. 93 (2021)
83. Wu, Y.: Cloud-edge orchestration for the internet-of-things: architecture and ai-powered data processing. IEEE Internet of Things J. (2020)
84. Jiang, D.: The construction of smart city information system based on the Internet of Things and cloud computing. Comput. Commun. **150**, 158–166 (2020)
85. Usak, M., Kubiatko, M., Shabbir, M.S., Viktorovna Dudnik, O., Jermsittiparsert, K., Rajabion, L.: Health care service delivery based on the Internet of things: a systematic and comprehensive study. Int. J. Commun. Syst. **33**(2), e4179 (2020)
86. Darwish, A., Hassanien, A.E., Elhoseny, M., Sangaiah, A.K., Muhammad, K.: The impact of the hybrid platform of internet of things and cloud computing on healthcare systems: opportunities, challenges, and open problems. J. Ambient. Intell. Humaniz. Comput. **10**(10), 4151–4166 (2019)
87. Azad, P., Navimipour, N.J., Rahmani, A.M., Sharifi, A.: The role of structured and unstructured data managing mechanisms in the Internet of things. Cluster Comput. 1–14 (2019)
88. Mayer-Schönberger, V., Ingelsson, E.: Big Data and medicine: a big deal? (2018)
89. Nienhold, D., Dornberger, R., Korkut, S.: Sensor-based tracking and big data processing of patient activities in ambient assisted living. In: 2016 IEEE International Conference on Healthcare Informatics (ICHI), pp. 473–482. IEEE (2016)
90. Banos, O., Garcia, R., Holgado-Terriza, J.A., Damas, M., Pomares, H., Rojas, I., Villalonga, C.: mHealthDroid: a novel framework for agile development of mobile health applications. In: International Workshop on Ambient Assisted Living, pp. 91–98. Springer, Cham (2014)
91. Nguyen, L.T., Zeng, M., Tague, P., Zhang, J.: Recognizing new activities with limited training data. In: Proceedings of the 2015 ACM International Symposium on Wearable Computers, pp. 67–74 (2015)
92. Cao, L., Wang, Y., Zhang, B., Jin, Q., Vasilakos, A.V.: GCHAR: an efficient group-based context—aware human activity recognition on smartphone. J. Parallel Distrib. Comput. **118**, 67–80 (2018)
93. Chen, T., Guestrin, C.: Xgboost: A scalable tree boosting system. In: Proceedings of the 22nd ACM sigkdd International Conference on Knowledge Discovery and Data Mining, pp. 785–794 (2016)
94. Chetty, G., White, M., Akther, F.: Smart phone based data mining for human activity recognition. Procedia Comput. Sci. **46**, 1181–1187 (2015)
95. Ignatov, A.: Real-time human activity recognition from accelerometer data using convolutional neural networks. Appl. Soft Comput. **62**, 915–922 (2018)
96. Davis, K., Owusu, E., Bastani, V., Marcenaro, L., Hu, J., Regazzoni, C., Feijs, L.: Activity recognition based on inertial sensors for ambient assisted living. In: 2016 19th International Conference on Information Fusion (fusion), pp. 371–378. IEEE (2016)
97. Ronaoo, C.A., Cho, S.B.: Evaluation of deep convolutional neural network architectures for human activity recognition with smartphone sensors. 한국정보과학회 학술발표논문집, 858–860 (2015)
98. Ha, S., Choi, S.: Convolutional neural networks for human activity recognition using multiple accelerometer and gyroscope sensors. In: 2016 International Joint Conference on Neural Networks (IJCNN), pp. 381–388. IEEE (2016)

IoT Based Fall Detection System for Elderly Healthcare

Ahsen Tahir, William Taylor, Ahmad Taha, Muhammad Usman, Syed Aziz Shah, Muhammad Ali Imran, and Qammer H. Abbasi

Abstract Falls are a leading cause of immobility, morbidity, and mortality in older adults. Falls incur high cost to health services with millions of bed days. Half of the older adults over 65 years old, fall in a span of 5 years with 62% sustaining injuries and 28% protracting extensive injuries. Automatic fall detection system for elderly healthcare through Internet of Things (IoT) human-centered design can provide timely detection and communication of fall events for immediate medical aid in case of injury or unconsciousness. Fall detection systems have been reported to provide reduction in death rates of up to 80% due to timely medical support. In this chapter, we discuss elderly-centric IoT based fall detection system for smart homes and care centers with emphasis on edge, fog and cloud IoT layers. Sensing edge devices with wearable/environmental sensors, vision-based systems, and radio frequency sensing systems, such as WiFi-based sensing and RADAR are presented for an IoT-centered fall detection system. IoT gateways and communication protocols for the fog layer

---

A. Tahir (✉) · W. Taylor · A. Taha · M. Usman · M. A. Imran · Q. H. Abbasi
James Watt School of Engineering, University of Glasgow, Glasgow G12 8QQ, UK
e-mail: ahsen.tahir@glasgow.ac.uk; ahsan@uet.edu.pk

W. Taylor
e-mail: 2536400t@student.gla.ac.uk

A. Taha
e-mail: ahmad.taha@glasgow.ac.uk

M. Usman
e-mail: muhammad.usman@glasgow.ac.uk

M. A. Imran
e-mail: muhammad.imran@glasgow.ac.uk

Q. H. Abbasi
e-mail: qammer.abbasi@glasgow.ac.uk

A. Tahir
University of Engineering and Technology, Lahore 54890, Pakistan

S. A. Shah
Centre for Intelligent Healthcare, Coventry University, Coventry CV1 5RW, UK
e-mail: syed.shah@coventry.ac.uk

© The Author(s), under exclusive license to Springer Nature Singapore Pte Ltd. 2022
S. Scataglini et al. (eds.), *Internet of Things for Human-Centered Design*,
Studies in Computational Intelligence 1011,
https://doi.org/10.1007/978-981-16-8488-3_10

are discussed in the context of a fall detection system. Cloud processing of edge device data for fall activity detection and classification from activities of daily life is explained. Machine and deep learning algorithms for detection of fall events from 1 and 2D signals (image/video) are presented and various deployment scenarios are discussed in the context of edge or cloud IoT layers. This chapter is concluded with results and performance comparison of several IoT centered fall detection systems in terms of various sensing systems and state-of-the-art machine and deep learning models for effective detection of falls for elderly healthcare. Furthermore, future work and prospective improvements in IoT centered design for fall detection in elderly healthcare is discussed.

Keywords Internet-of-Things · Fall detection system · Wearable systems · WiFi/Radar sensing · Machine learning · Deep learning

1 Introduction

A fall is defined as an inadvertent descent to the ground or floor. Falls may result in fatal or non-fatal injuries. Falls in elderly may result in fractures and are costly in terms of health services. They are usually associated with multifactorial causes including age, patient history, muscle weakness, visual impairment, poor balance and environmental causes. Falls are the second highest cause of unintentional deaths worldwide after road accidents [1]. Worldwide 37.3 million falls require medical attention with 0.68 million deaths. Adults over 60 years old suffer the highest number of deaths due to falls worldwide [1]. In the UK alone, half of the older adults over 65 years old fall in a span of 5 years with 62% sustaining injuries. Among those who suffer from falls, 28% sustain extensive injuries, 21% lose confidence and 10% lose independence [2]. Falls cost 4 million bed days to UK National Health Service, along with 4 billion pounds in health-related costs [3]. The cost of falls in terms of high morbidity and immobility has resulted in a focus on fall detection systems for older adults. The system can detect occurrence of fall events and are imperative for older adults who live alone and may not be able to call for help due to unconsciousness or injury. Fall detection systems can provide timely intimation of fall events resulting in immediate medical help and are known to improve hospitalization by 26% and death rates reduction by 80% [4].

Internet-of-Things (IoT) consists of a large number of smart physical devices connected to the Internet through gateways without human–computer interaction and can communicate data in real-time. IoT based fall detection system can transfer real-time fall events to the cloud with smart sensing devices acting as "things".

Figure 1 illustrates an IoT based fall detection system with IoT edge, gateway and cloud. The system can utilize various communication technologies for access to the Internet, such as WiFi, GSM and 5G. The sensing devices in a fall detection system can be categorized into three broad categories (1) wearable sensors, (2) vision-based sensors and (3) WiFi/Radar sensing devices. The devices gather human activity data,

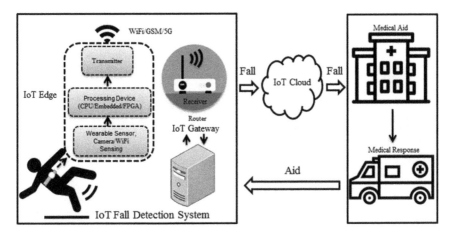

Fig. 1 Fall detection system overview

such as acceleration values from human body movements. The data can be processed at the transmitting embedded device for classification and detection of falls or at the receiver side on the IoT Gateway by the corresponding processing device. The processed data is transmitted to the IoT cloud from where it can be accessed through smartphones or desktop computers. The fall events can be communicated through cloud to a server in a medical emergency center in real-time, which is essential for dispatching timely medical aid. The level of processing done at the IoT edge device or gateway and the data to be sent to the server are flexible design decisions. Security and privacy issues that may not arise in traditional offline fall detection systems are important aspects for an IoT based fall detection system. Encryption and decryption process are part of the real-time processing tasks for IoT based sensing for fall detection.

Figure 2 illustrates the concept with three sensing devices, a wearable accelerometer, a camera and a WiFi sensing device. The accelerometer gives acceleration values of body movements in units of "g" (9.8 m/sec^2). The video frames and WiFi Channel State Information (CSI) are obtained from the camera and the WiFi sensing device. WiFi CSI values are variations in wireless channel estimation that vary over time due to changes in wireless channel caused by objects and human body movements in the vicinity. The signals from various sensing devices are processed with signal processing algorithms, such as time–frequency spectrograms for 1D signals or foreground–background segmentation for 2D/3D images or video frames to obtain moving objects. Machine Learning (ML) classification algorithms are applied to the processed data and features to detect falls at the IoT edge device.

Deep learning algorithms are also utilized for classification in fall detection systems [5, 6]. However, deep learning techniques are computationally intensive and may be deployed at the IoT gateway or cloud due to high processing requirements. In this scenario, the signals from sensing devices can be processed at the edge. Edge processing usually involves removal of outliers in sensor readings and use of

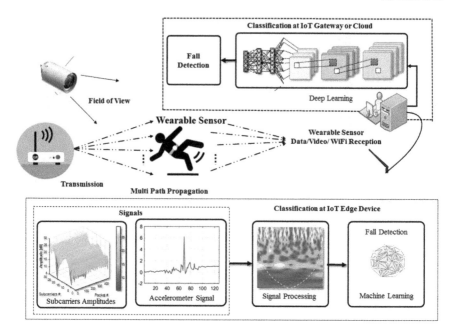

Fig. 2 IoT based fall detection system processing and classification

signal processing techniques, such as application of digital filters for de-noising or to obtain certain frequency ranges. The processing at edge device may also include compression along with encryption before transmission of signals. The transmitted signal can then be further processed at the IoT gateway. Deep learning techniques require higher throughput for training and can be applied at the processing device connected to the gateway, such as a desktop computer. Furthermore, the signal can be transmitted to the cloud where it can be visualized in real-time. The cloud offers more flexibility in computing resources and a large number of signals can be processed at the cloud with high throughput graphics processing units. More complex deep learning models can be utilized at the cloud for higher classification accuracy of fall events. Figure 2 illustrates both the scenarios with processing and classification performed at the edge device or at the gateway/cloud.

The next sections present different IoT layers. Section 2 discusses the edge IoT layer and its essential characteristics. Sections 3 and 4 present the fog IoT layer and the cloud layer, respectively. Section 5 presents the ML algorithms utilized for fall detection and Sect. 6 gives the performance results and metrics.

2 Edge IoT Layer

Edge IoT layer consists of edge devices which make up the sensing system end of the fall detection system and consists of sensors and embedded processors. Section 2.1 discusses the salient characteristics of edge devices and Sects. 2.2, 2.3 and 2.4 present the edge layer sensors and processing for wearable, vision-based and WiFi/Radar-based sensing systems.

2.1 Edge Devices

The edge devices are mostly made up of various embedded boards for processing and consist of embedded cores and Field Programmable Gate Array (FPGA) based reconfigurable System on Chip (SoC) devices. The smartphones are also part of the edge IoT layer. The IoT based fall detection systems have their own unique issues and demand stringent requirements compared to non-IoT based fall detection systems, such as privacy and security issues that may arise due to uniquely addressable devices and their global Internet connectivity.

The edge IoT layer embedded edge platforms should have most if not all the following characteristics with stringent requirements for security and privacy:

(1) **Uniquely Identifiable**: The edge devices used for fall detection should be uniquely identifiable. An IP address provides a globally unique address to identify a particular user with the wearable sensor or an environment where the sensor is installed.
(2) **Smart platform**: The device should provide a smart platform with sensor or wireless sensor connectivity with processing capabilities and an embedded core for running various tasks and algorithms.
(3) **Embedded ML cores**: Nowadays ML cores for learning and classification tasks are becoming a norm on edge devices. The custom application specific integrated circuits are an essential requirement for low-power and real-time edge Artificial Intelligence (AI).
(4) **Real-time processing**: Unlike the edge devices for measuring temperature and other environmental factors that can do with lower sampling rates of a sample per minute, the device for fall detection systems provide higher sampling rate in real-time to process or transmit data from sensors. The accelerometers can use a typical sampling rate of 50 samples per second, camera based systems should be able to provide higher rates from 30 to 60 frames per second and a wide range of resolutions. Typical WiFi sensing systems have sampling rates from 50 samples per second up to 400 samples per second for 5G software defined radios used for healthcare activity classification.
(5) **Energy efficiency**: The devices should provide higher energy efficiency. However, the requirements vary from system to system and depend upon the

type of sensors. Wearable sensors with Inertial Measurement Units (IMU) should typically work in a current range of micro Amperes.

(6) **Power management**: Power management is an important aspect and the devices should have support for sleep mode to save power, e.g., sensor readings may not be required, when the person with a wearable sensor is sleeping or resting.

(7) **Privacy and security**: Privacy and security are important aspects of sensing devices for IoT based fall detection systems. The unique IP addresses allow the sensors to be accessed globally and should provide encryption of data along with authentication mechanisms for the edge devices utilized for fall detection systems. The vision-based sensing platforms in this regard create a higher security risk and should have stringent access authentication to avoid hacking.

A large number of embedded platforms can be utilized for IoT based fall detection system. Embedded platforms such as Raspberry Pi Pico [7], Arduino [8] and NodeMCU [9] are ubiquitous in edge devices with IMU units. Low power and small form factor IoT capable boards are a good choice for fall detection systems. Embedded platforms, such as Adafruit FLORA [10] with 1.75 inch diameter are easily wearable and integrate Arduino compatible microcontroller with accelerometers and gyroscope sensors through Inter-Integrated Circuit (I^2C) bus. iNEMO [11] embedded platforms by STMicroelectronics integrate accelerometer, gyroscope and magnetometer with an embedded ML core in a small form factor. Similarly embedded vision platforms, such as iENSO vision board [12] combines edge based AI and image processing capabilities in a small form factor of 2.3 × 2.2 cm.

Reconfigurable SoC embedded platforms are a method of choice for edge IoT devices and have been utilized for fall detection system [13]. They provide a good trade-off between higher flexibility and low power for implementing signal processing techniques, feature extraction or ML classifiers on programmable logic. The signal processing can be implemented both in programmable logic and on hardware ARM cores on the SoC device depending upon the computational requirements. Xilinx Zynq SoC has been utilized for fall detection. The SoC provides ARM cores and programmable logic for implementing computationally intensive algorithms for fall detection. Figure 3 illustrates the Zynq SoC [14] architecture with ARM cores, programmable logic and Xilinx proprietary AXI bus for connecting the accelerator

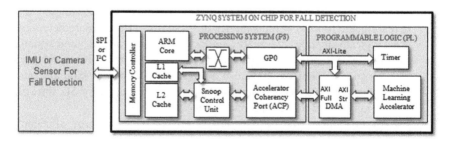

Fig. 3 Reconfigurable embedded platform for a fall detection system

IoT Based Fall Detection System for Elderly Healthcare 215

with the ARM cores. Fall detection sensors, such as an IMU with accelerometer and gyroscope sensors can be connected to the ARM core through the Serial Peripheral Interface or I^2C bus.

An example fall detection system presented by Tahir et al. [13] based on the Zynq platform is illustrated in Fig. 4. The system implements feature extraction in programmable logic and ML classification for fall detection in software on the ARM core. The sensor transmits accelerometer data from sensor to a Zynq edge device wirelessly. The signal is processed to compute mean and the zero meaned signal is wavelet transformed to obtain fractal features for fall detection on programmable logic. The features are passed to the ARM core for ML classification in software. The feature extraction process is implemented on programmable logic since it is more computationally intensive than the Linear Discriminant Analysis (LDA) algorithm. LDA is computationally less intensive than the feature extraction process [13]. Furthermore, apart from reconfigurable platforms, smartphone are ubiquitous edge devices with inbuilt sensors, such as accelerometer and gyroscope that can be utilized for fall detection. Smartphones can also be used with smart watches. Apple wearable

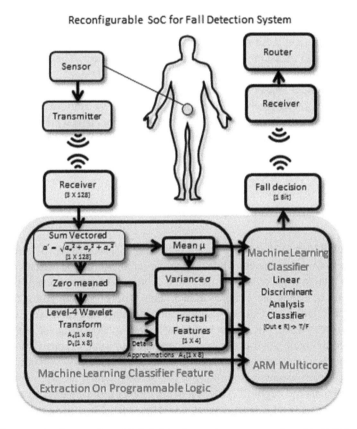

Fig. 4 An example of a reconfigurable fall detection system on a reconfigurable SoC device

watch can detect falls and send messages directly through the Apple smartphone to emergency contacts. The smartphone-based wearable's get Internet connectivity for fall event occurrence through the smartphone directly connected through GSM or WiFi router [15].

2.2 Wearable/Environmental Sensing System

Accelerometers and Gyroscopes can be used to track human motion via wearable devices or embedded in smartphones that users carry [16]. This can be advantageous if the user already owns a capable mobile device but is an expensive alternative otherwise. The wearable devices can be in the form of smart watches with embedded accelerometers. Accelerometers work together with gyroscopes to be able to determine the orientation of the user's body [17]. The data received from the accelerometers can be applied to ML algorithms to classify the human motion taking place [18]. Pressure sensors electrode arrays woven into fabric which can be worn by the user and allows for the detection of muscle movement and thus the detection of movement [19]. Pressure sensors can also be applied to furniture material to detect sit-to-stand and stand-to-sit motions [20]. Acoustic sensors are electrical devices that have the ability to measure sound waves in the environment. The sound waves can be used for fall detection systems by analyzing the acoustic signals [20]. The signals received from these sensors are then processed to remove noise from the signals. These noise removing filters can include high and/or low Butterworth filters [21]. These processed signals can then be used in AI to train models which can recognize the acoustic waves accompanying a fall [22]. Figure 5 shows the process followed for wearable fall detection systems.

2.3 Vision-Based Sensing Systems

Camera technology can be used to record individuals. This method will allow the user to not have to wear any devices while being monitored. ML can be used to remove the need for a human to be observing the video footage which can prevent the subject from feeling that they are being watched. This type of system can achieve high accuracy [23]. However, camera systems can sometimes be expensive. To decrease the costs of the systems, devices such as a low-cost Raspberry Pi device with a camera can be used to obtain good performance compared to more expensive devices [24, 25]. ML can be applied to the frames of the footage to establish if an individual has fallen [26]. Depth sensors work by using two sensors with a known range between them to calculate the depth [27]. As the depth changes, movement can be inferred. Kinect sensors are well known devices for Microsoft's Xbox gaming console. The device is allowed for gaming where people's movements would be sensed as input. An example of this is for games where the users are required to perform dancing

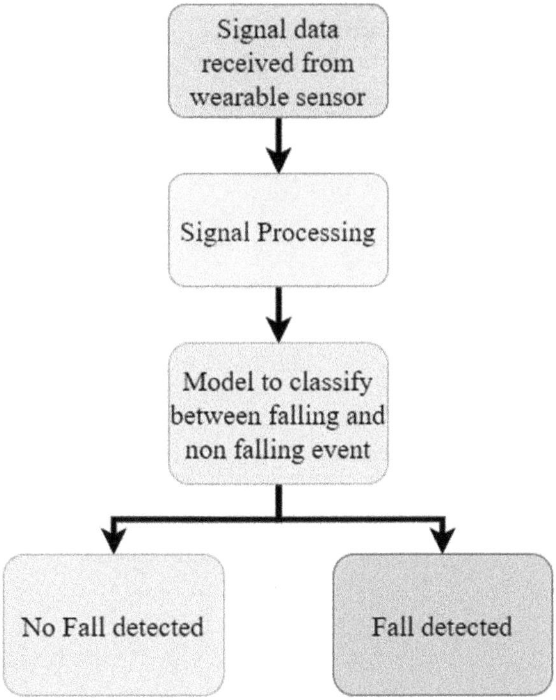

Fig. 5 Fall detection system using wearable sensors

[28]. These sensors can be applied with deep learning to be able to classify poses of humans within healthcare applications [29].

2.4 Contactless Non-interference Sensing

Radio Frequency (RF) and Radar are contactless methods that allow for detection of human movements without the need for the user to wear a device or have vision-based sensors raising privacy concerns. This removes the problem of users having to remember to wear devices and avoids any discomfort of either wearing devices or the intrusiveness of vision-based systems in the home. These methods are known as contactless non-intrusive methods of detection.

2.4.1 Radar Sensing

Radar technology provides sensing of the environment which can be used to monitor daily routine activities of elderly people [30]. Radar based sensing works by exploiting the Doppler signatures created on radar when movement occurs [31]. This can be used in healthcare applications for example if an elderly person experiences

Fig. 6 A Spectrogram displaying a falling action

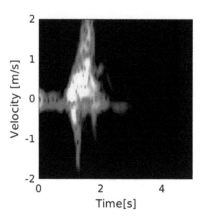

Fig. 7 Radar fall detection system processing

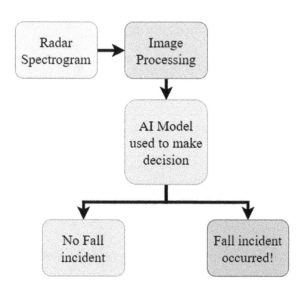

a fall. The Doppler signatures can be presented using spectrograms. Spectrograms are visual representations of the spectrum of frequencies of a signal. An example of a spectrogram containing a fall activity is shown in Fig. 6.

These spectrogram images can be used in AI for image classification of what activity takes place in that particular spectrogram [32–35]. Figure 7 displays the process used in a radar fall detection system.

2.4.2 Radio Frequency Sensing

Radio Frequency Sensing works by observing the state of a wireless communication link between devices such as the case with a WiFi network within the home. As the signals travel through the atmosphere, they will propagate differently depending on objects in the room. These objects can include humans and the signals will propagate differently depending on the positioning of the body. WiFi records the information of the signal propagation, and this is called the CSI. The CSI is used from WiFi to look at the amplitude of the RF signals while the human moves between the RF signals [36, 37]. Figures 8 and 9 show CSI amplitude samples of a falling motion and a non-falling action. The CSI describes how the wireless signal propagates between

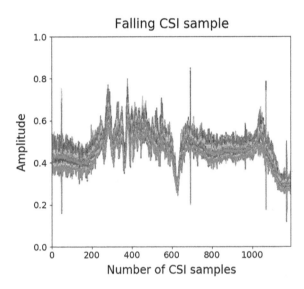

Fig. 8 Sample of a fall event captured using CSI amplitude

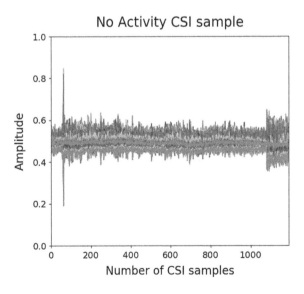

Fig. 9 Sample of a no fall event captured using CSI amplitude

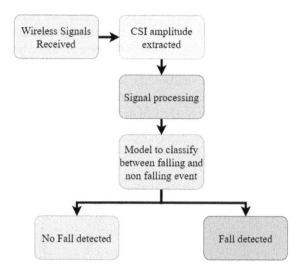

Fig. 10 RF fall detection system processing

the transmitting node and receiving node [38]. This data can be exploited to detect changes during a specific human motion such as the example of a fall occurring.

WiFi is considered superior due to its low cost and the extensive coverage already present in homes [39]. Another advantage of using WiFi is that it eliminates the need for excessive equipment which can feel invasive, and the additional equipment can be expensive and requires maintenance [38]. Systems that utilize minimal equipment for fall detection are economically viable. A system using RF signals will monitor the CSI of incoming signals. Signal processing is applied for noise reduction and to make changes within the signal more prominent. The signals are then input into a ML model, which can learn the CSI patterns and is trained to recognize a fall signature in the CSI values. Then a trigger can be sent to indicate a fall has been detected in the system. Figure 10 shows the process used in a RF fall detection system.

3 Fog IoT Layer

In fall detection systems, a fog IoT layer is composed of various components (mainly IoT gateways) and communication technologies that connect the components with the computing platforms. Particularly, the communication technologies in this context include, but are not limited to, cellular networks (such as 5G, 4G, and GSM), Zigbee, Bluetooth, NFC, WiFi, LoraWAN, and so on. IoT gateways have emerged as a key component of a robust IoT platform that can help enable an effective fall detection system. The gateway acts as a communication and computing hub wherein different sensors are connected to it via one of the communication technologies [40]. Furthermore, gateways connect those sensors to different users, applications, and the

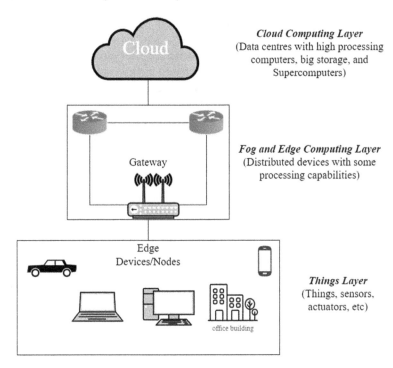

Fig. 11 The IoT communication architecture

Internet. In most cases, IoT gateways act as a bridge between sensors/actuators and the Internet. The communication architecture of IoT is given in Fig. 11.

In terms of features set, gateways generally host one or more of the following features:

(1) Gateways facilitate communication to/from sensors and Internet/non-Internet devices.
(2) Data caching, streaming, data aggregation, pre-processing, cleansing, filtering and optimization.
(3) System diagnostic and configuration management.
(4) Security-device and network security.

3.1 Communication Technologies

The communication architecture of IoT gateway depends on the underlying technology being used. The communication technologies can be divided into four categories, (i) Peer-to-Peer (P2P) technologies, (ii) Low-power and short-range mesh technologies, (iii) Local Area Network (LAN) technologies, and (iv) low-power and long distance technologies [41].

3.1.1 Peer-To-Peer (P2P) Technologies

P2P means that only two devices are connected together directly. In the context of IoT networks, a sensor node can be connected to the gateway in P2P fashion. P2P technologies include legacy Bluetooth, WiFi Direct, and near field communication (NFC). Bluetooth is the best known P2P technology, which is present in almost every smartphone and tablet. Due to low range communication, it is much more power efficient than WiFi and cellular technologies. WiFi Direct is an alternative to Bluetooth, which is native to almost every modern-day smartphone. WiFi Direct is P2P technology, which works without the need of an access point (AP). The working principle is similar to infrastructure mode WiFi wherein one of the participating devices takes roles of an AP while others act as clients. Generally, WiFi Direct is faster than Bluetooth. Near field communication is another P2P technology which uses electromagnetic field between coils to enable communication between two nodes. NFC works on the principle of electromagnetic coupling, the communication range is generally within an inch or two. This makes NFC a very secure technology with a very little chance of eavesdropping.

3.1.2 Low Power and Short-Range Mesh Technologies

There are two main technologies that create a low-power and short-range mesh network, which are Bluetooth low energy (BLE) and Zigbee. These technologies are very important when someone is dealing with an application which has battery-powered devices, sending a low amount of data to a shorter range. BLE is a highly power-efficient communication protocol, which works with different devices, transmitting data at different rates. BLE is highly scalable supporting up to 32, 767 devices connected in a mesh network. BLE is among the most adopted technologies in IoT networks, especially in the Internet of medical things settings. BLE uses the 2.4 GHz band. Zigbee is a competitor of BLE that uses the same 2.4 GHz band, operates in a mesh network topology and has the same range as of BLE. In terms of scalability, Zigbee supports twice as many devices as supported by BLE, that is, around 65,000 devices. Home automation and industrial automation are a few applications of Zigbee.

3.1.3 Local Area Network (LAN) Technologies

WiFi is a good option in the scenarios wherein sensors support wireless LAN and need direct access to the Internet. The coverage area provided by the WiFi is better than Zigbee and BLE. In addition, WiFi is a readily available technology and its coverage is ubiquitous. Another advantage of WiFi is the supported data rate, which is far better than Zigbee and BLE. However, these advantages come at the expense of power consumption. The power consumption of WiFi is a way more than Zigbee and BLE.

3.1.4 Long-Distance Low-Power Technologies

There can be scenarios where IoT devices are deployed at remote locations and they send a low amount of data to the Internet. For instance, weather monitoring sensors mostly have very low data to send. The cellular technologies, such as GSM and LTE are not suitable in this scenario as they generally do not support very low data rates. These kinds of scenarios are generally known as low-power wide area networks (LPWAN). The most popular technologies in LPWAN are LoRa/LoRaWAN, narrow-band IoT (NB-IoT), and LTE-M. LoRa is a long-range P2P technology having a range of more than 6 miles in some areas. The frequency range of LoRa varies in different regions. For instance, in North America, the operating frequency of LoRa is 915 MHz while in Europe it is around 868 MHz. In some areas it is also licensed at 169 MHz and 433 MHz. LoRa is the underlying technology while LoRaWAN is a network layer protocol. The only way to provide Internet access to LoRa devices is through a LoRa gateway. On the other hand, NB-IoT is a cellular based technology, which provides coverage to remote sensors. Being a cellular technology, it is complex and more expensive in terms of budget and power consumption. However, it provides a direct access to the Internet. NB-IoT supports low data rates but it is not yet deployed in many areas of the world. LTE-M is best suitable for long distance and high data rate scenarios. LTEM provides sensors a direct access to the Internet using 4G cellular network. LTE-M is fundamentally different from standard LTE technology as it is optimized for the low-power consumption suitable for battery powered devices.

The most common data communication protocols are Message Queuing Telemetry Transport (MQTT), Constrained Application Protocol (CoAP), Advanced Message Queuing Protocol (AMQP), Data-Distribution Service for Real-Time Systems (DDS), and Hypertext Transfer Protocol (HTTP). The details of these protocols can be found at [42].

4 Cloud IoT Layer

The cloud layer in an IoT network supports caching and processing capabilities that can be accessed by different IoT devices and applications. The resources at the cloud (caching, processing, etc.) can be accessed by different IoT applications anytime and anywhere. To this aim, different API are used which are generally made available to any HTTP client. For instance, Google cloud IoT Core API mainly comprises two sets of REST resources: cloud IoT and cloud IoT device. In order to get the information about different subscribers virtualization technology is used, which is also helpful in getting the segregation of IoT applications. With the help of APIs and virtualization, IoT applications can provide different quality of service (QoS) to different users over the same physical network.

5 Machine and Deep Learning Algorithms

Random forest algorithm works by using a collection of decision trees. These trees make predictions based on features found in the training data. Each trees prediction is considered a vote. The majority of predictions decide the final Random Forest prediction [43]. The K-Nearest Neighbors algorithm is well known for its simplicity. KNN makes direct comparisons between the testing data and training data [44]. The features of the training data are assigned a K sample then the testing data is assigned to the K sample with the nearest match [45]. During the training phase Support Vector Machine attempts to create boundaries known as hyper planes between classes. The hyperplane is positioned as far as possible from the closest data points of the classes present in the data. These points are known as the support vectors [46]. The hyper planes are used to divide the support vectors into the different categories. The features of new data are used to place the new data between the hyper planes and provide classification [47].

The Long short-term memory (LSTM) deep learning algorithm is an extension of a recurring neural network (RNN). A recurring neural network is a type of neural network which models the dynamic behavior of sequences of data between nodes of the neural network. LSTM expands on RNN with the use of three different gates on each node. The first gate decides if the current state should be erased. The second gate is used to control if input should be considered, and the final gate decides if the state should be included in the node output. These gates allow for LSTM to decide if the sequence of data is relevant to the output of the node [48]. Bi-directional long short-term memory (BiLSTM) is a further extension of LSTM. Where LSTM only considers past behaviors of data sequences, the BiLSTM considers data in both previous and upcoming data in the sequence. This is possible with the use of two LSTM networks. One LSTM network, the forward LSTM network, can review past data sequences and the backward LSTM network can review future data sequences [49]. The CNN algorithm is an emerging technology which is a powerful solution for image classification problems which were initially thought to require human intelligence [50–52]. The CNN algorithm is made up of densely connected layers that take the activations of all the previous layers as input. The layers produce feature maps from this input which are known as growth rates [53]. CNN algorithms come in the form of 1 Dimension (1D), 2 Dimensions (2D) and 3 Dimensions (3D) with 3D resulting in highest computational power requirements [38]. 1D, 2D and 3D CNN refers to the number of directions the kernel moves in. 1D CNN makes use of 2 dimensional inputs and outputs for example time-series data. 2D CNN uses inputs and outputs of 3 dimensions and is mostly used for image data. 3D CNN is 4 dimensional for input and output and is mostly used on 3d image data such as MRI and CT scans.

6 Performance Metrics and Results

The severe consequences of falls in the older population have called for the innovative use of technology to develop systems that are capable of detecting and reporting the fall events, if and when they happen. However, without the right metrics to evaluate such systems, the wider community and healthcare systems across the world, will not be able to confidently trust the technology and rely on it. This section therefore identifies and presents evaluation metrics for different fall detection systems.

6.1 Evaluation Metrics

To evaluate the performance of an FDS, it is important to consider the main building blocks of the system, from the technology used, to the hardware and software, to installation, and others. Accordingly, the following metrics have been identified to evaluate any fall detection system, for research or commercialization purposes:

(1) System accuracy in real-time detection—Essential to all fall detection systems.
(2) Alert generation feature—Essential to all fall detection systems.
(3) System portability and ease of deployment—Optional to some fall detection systems.

6.1.1 System Accuracy Metrics

An important aspect of fall detection systems is the real-time feature, meaning the system's ability to accurately report the activities of the monitored person, as they happen, to a user friendly web-interface or dashboard, in a near-instant timing. From this, three Key Performance Indicators (KPIs) need to be considered, to ensure a perfect score in this metric:

(1) Event detection accuracy
(2) Event logging in real-time
(3) User friendliness of the web-interface

The accuracy of detection has two folds. The first is the method implemented to capture the event, whether using contactless technology, wearable sensors, and/or vision-based sensing devices. The second is the accuracy of the AI-based algorithm implemented to intelligently classify or infer the event being a normal activity or a fall. This therefore needs to be considered in the system design phase where large datasets with inter and intra-class variations are collected, and extensive testing scenarios are considered. A typical framework to evaluate the accuracy of fall detection systems can be found in [54] where four binary classifications are considered: • True Positive (TP)—A fall event was correctly detected • True Negative (TN)—A non-fall event was correctly detected • False Positive (FP)—A non-fall event incorrectly detected as fall • False Negative (FN)—A fall event incorrectly detected as non-fall. The four binary classifications, TP, TN, FP and FN, are used to generate four algorithm performance metrics, that is, Accuracy, Precision, Recall, and $F1$-Score. The Accuracy displays the total number of correct classifications versus the total classifications made (see Eq. 1).

$$\text{Accuracy} = \frac{TP + TN}{TP + TN + FP + FN} \quad (1)$$

The Precision metric is used to measure one of the classifications against how precise it is in comparison to all classifications.

$$\text{Prescision} = \frac{TP}{TP + FP} \quad (2)$$

The Recall is used to show the ratio of the correct classification to all classifications for a particular class. This is usually run for all classes in the model and presented as an average.

$$\text{Recall} = \frac{TP}{TP + FN} \quad (3)$$

The $F1$-score is used to provide an average between the Precision and Recall metrics.

$$F1 - \text{Score} = 2 \times \frac{\text{Precision} \times \text{Recall}}{\text{Precision} + \text{Recall}} \quad (4)$$

A typical representation of the four values TP, TN, FP and FN, is in the form of a confusion matrix, see Fig. 12. A confusion matrix is one that is usually used to represent the performance of a classification model to tell how much of the test

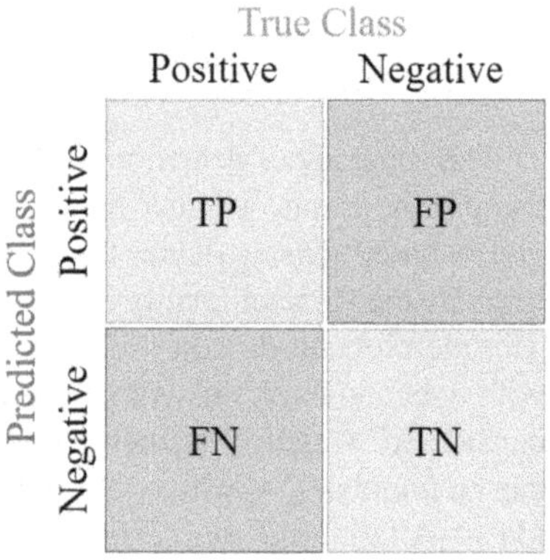

Fig. 12 Confusion matrix showing the true and false classifications

data has been correctly predicted. In other words, how many data samples have been confused to be a different classification as compared to the true class?

Although all four values are important and need to be scored and calculated with as much data as possible, the most serious one is the FN as it is the one that could mean patients or individuals can be in a serious condition, without the system reporting the status. The FP value, while it doesn't have a life-threatening impact, can result in resource waste and damage to the environment if the system was linked to emergency response and constant false alarms were generated. Event logging in real-time: It is crucial to ensure the system reports the event, regardless of what it is, in a timely manner. The severity of delayed reporting is usually associated with the "fall" only, however it is important to ensure a fully functional system. The time between incident and notification/reporting can differ and therefore it needs to be measured and evaluated during the early testing stages of such systems. This can be performed by comparing the reported times to the actual event. Nevertheless, the challenge in conducting this test is coming up with a non-invasive/intrusive method to record the actual event performed and exact timing. User-friendliness of the web-interface: This metric is rather a qualitative one, yet crucial to the success of such systems. To the end user, especially care takers or emergency services, the interface is "the system" as they will interact with it and not the sensing technology, majority of the time. Accordingly, design ideas could be shared with the target users, in focus groups, prior to implementing them or ideas collected through questionnaires and/or interviews. To develop a dashboard, the following can be considered:

(1) Dashboard accessibility
(2) Dashboard design—Color coded events reporting, animation for alerts etc.
(3) Security of the reported data and the personal information.

6.1.2 Alert Generation

A crucial design objective for remote healthcare monitoring in general and for fall detection systems in particular, is the generation of accurate alerts. The alert generation feature can be useful to indicate potential threats to the patients and/or monitored individuals, based on the recorded activity levels. This metric can also be used to reflect the accuracy of the system, as it is crucial to ensure alerts are generated only when and if necessary, as well as its real-time feature, previously discussed.

The alert generation metric therefore encompasses two things, the alert type and alert generation time. The type of alert means what the system would output to inform the target beneficiaries of the reported event. While it might seem trivial, it is crucial to design the system such that the alert is as informative as it can be while ensuring it is concise to enable the notified personnel to act upon it in a timely manner. Alerts can be generated based on recorded activities and can therefore be scored to reflect falls, sleep-time disturbance, sleeping time, room transition, wandering and general activity. Each category has a different severity level and therefore the corresponding alert/notification should be different. Secondly, comes the alert generation time, which is closely tied to the real-time feature of the system, previously explained, to ensure the serious events are reported as soon as they happen, as it may mean a person's life is saved.

6.1.3 System Portability and Ease of Deployment

This metric will not apply to all fall detection systems and the use case would decide on its application. The purpose of the metric is to evaluate the portability of the system, in cases where it won't be fixed in one place. Depending on the use, such systems can be used for temporary monitoring of patients that are recovering from accidents or surgeries, and so on. Thereby, it is important to have, in the market, systems that can be installed and cleared out in a timely manner. This evaluation metric will therefore be based on the number of hardware nodes/units associated with the implementation of the system and would involve measuring the following:

(1) Portability—Is the system mobile or fixed
(2) Setup time—Is it a "Plug & Play" system or requires pre-planned setup
(3) Maintenance—What level of intervention is needed to maintain the system? Can it be done remotely?

A score can be therefore given for every fall detection systems, based on the above-mentioned.

Metrics, to evaluate its portability and ease of deployment.

6.1.4 Comparison of Results and Systems

Table 1 illustrates some of the fall detection systems presented in literature and gives a comparison of four systems, each using a different technology to implement the fall detection. The table is used to highlight the main aspects of any fall detection system, i.e., the technology used, the applied algorithm (where applicable), and the performance of the system in terms of its accuracy.

Table 1 Comparison between fall detection systems that utilize various technologies

Source	Technology	Algorithm	System accuracy (%)
Aziz et al. [55]	Accelerometer	Support Vector Machine (SVM)	80
Bloch et al. [56]	Accelerometer and an infrared sensor	Data fusion	Sensitivity—62.5 Specificity—99.5
Debard et al. [57]	Camera	SVM	Sensitivity: 88 Specificity: 95.6
Wang et al. [58]	Radio Frequency	SVM and Random Forest	SVM: 90 Random Forest: 90

As can be seen in Table 1, the performance of every system is reported and from the figures, one can pick a favorite. However, as a whole system, the previously highlighted metrics in Sect. 6.1 need to be considered to arrive at an accurate evaluation of every system.

Nevertheless, the highlighted metrics can, to some extent, be quantified or scored for every system; the question remains. There are several other factors that research studies have highlighted and are used to favor one system over the other. For instance, some of the drawbacks of using camera-based systems include invasion of privacy, the need for ambient light, and line-of-sight requirement for detection. As for the wearable technology, concerns are usually around the inconvenience of having to mount the device on the body, whether through direct or indirect skin contact, and the severe consequences that can result from forgetting to wear them. The contactless sensing technology has the advantage over the vision-based and wearable technologies as they do not pose any privacy concerns and are completely non-invasive, however the accuracy is in occasions questioned, compared to sensor-based systems. Therefore, it is crucial to consider several factors when designing a fall detection system for research.

Edge IoT layer should be able to run computationally intensive deep learning algorithms. Future research in this domain includes implementation of deep learning algorithms on constrained edge devices for various classification tasks. The edge IoT devices for an elderly fall detection system should be energy efficient and able to perform power management for sustained real-time operation. Security and privacy guarantees are an essential part of an IoT system in general and edge devices in particular to ensure legal access to the sensing devices. Energy management and security issues are active research topics in the IoT based fall detection systems. Furthermore, use of RF systems allow contactless sensing through WiFi and radars. Contactless sensing is the future of smart homes and healthcare centers because of its non-invasive and non-intrusive nature. Future IoT cloud systems will also incorporate federated learning where edge devices can utilize locally available data to train local models and the parameters are sent to a centralized model for averaging. Federated learning in edge and cloud layers is an open area of research for IoT based fall detection systems.

7 Conclusions

This chapter explained IoT based fall detection system for older adults. Fall detection systems are essential tools for elderly healthcare and imperative for their health and wellbeing. The IoT edge layer with different sensing systems and embedded platforms was described. Essential elements of an IoT fall detection system system were discussed. Different fall detection systems including wearable sensor, vision based and radio frequency, such as WiFi and Radar were presented, and their processing steps were discussed. An overview of fall detection systems in terms of their focus on machine and deep learning techniques was given. The Fog and Cloud IoT layers were discussed and important communication technologies for Internet connectivity were presented. Finally, their performance metrics and evaluation criteria were explained.

References

1. World Health Organization: Falls. https://www.who.int/news-room/fact-sheets/detail/falls (2021). Accessed 1 July 2021
2. PCP market research: falls, measuring the impact on older people (2012)
3. Tian Y., Thompson J., Buck D., Sonola L.: Exploring the system-wide costs of falls in older people in Torbay. King's Fund (2013)
4. Noury N., Rumeau P., Bourke A.K., ÓLaighin G., Lundy J.E.: A proposal for the classification and evaluation of fall detectors. Innovation Res. Biomed. Eng. **29**(6), 340–349 (2008)
5. Tahir, A., Ahmad, J., Morison, G., Larijani, H., Gibson, R., Skelton, D.: HRNN4f: Hybrid deep random neural network for multi-channel fall activity detection. Probab. Eng. Informational Sci. 1–14 (2019)
6. Tahir, A., Morison, G., Gibson, R., Skelton, D.: A novel functional link network stacking ensemble with fractal features for multichannel fall detection. Cogn. Comput. **12**(5), 1024–1042 (2020)
7. RasberryPi Inc.: RP2040 A microcontroller chip designed by Raspberry Pi. https://www.raspberrypi.org/documentation/rp2040/getting-started/. Accessed 2 June 2021
8. Arduino Inc.: Arduino Nano. https://www.arduino.cc/en/pmwiki.php?n=Main/ArduinoBoard Nano. Accessed 2 June 2021
9. NodeMCU. https://www.nodemcu.com/index_en.html. Accessed 2 June 2021
10. Adafruit Inc.: Adafruit FLORA. https://learn.adafruit.com/category/flora. Accessed 2 June 2021
11. STMicroelectronics Ins.: iNEMO-Inertial Modules. https://www.st.com/en/mems-and-sensors/inemo-inertial-modules.html. Accessed 2 June 2021
12. iENSO Inc.: iVS-AWV3-AR0521. https://www.ienso.com/product/ivs-awv3-ar0521/. Accessed 2 June 2021
13. Tahir, A., Morison, G., Skelton, D.A. Gibson, R.M.: Hardware/software co-design of fractal features based fall detection system. Sensors **20**(8), 2322 (2020)
14. Xilinx: Zynq-7000 SoC data sheet: overview. July 2, 2018. https://www.xilinx.com/support/documentation/data_sheets/ds190-Zynq-7000-Overview.pdf. Accessed 2 June 2021
15. Apple Inc. https://support.apple.com/en-us/HT208944. Accessed 1 June 2021
16. DIrican, A.C., Aksoy, S: Step counting using smartphone accelerometer and fast Fourier transform. Sigma J. Eng. Nat. Sci **8**, 175–182 (2017)
17. Nez, A., et al.: Comparison of calibration methods for accelerometers used in human motion analysis. Med. Eng. Phys. **38**(11), 1289–1299 (2016)
18. Ignatov, A.D., Strijov, V.V.: Human activity recognition using quasiperiodic time series collected from a single tri-axial accelerometer. Multimedia Tools Appl. **75**(12), 7257–7270 (2016)
19. Meyer, J., Lukowicz, P., Troster, G.: Textile pressure sensor for muscle activity and motion detection. In: 2006 10th IEEE International Symposium on Wearable Computers, IEEE, pp. 69–72 (2006)
20. Uddin, M., Khaksar, W., Torresen, J.: Ambient sensors for elderly care and independent living: a survey. Sensors **18**(7), 2027 (2018)
21. Sigcha, L., et al.: Deep learning approaches for detecting freezing of gait in Parkinson's disease patients through on-body acceleration sensors. Sensors **20**(7), 1895 (2020)
22. Adnan, S.M., et al.: Fall detection through acoustic local ternary patterns. Appl. Acoust. **140**, 296–300 (2018)

23. Dorgham, O., Rass, S.A., Alkhraisat, H.: Improved elderly fall detection by surveillance video using real-time human motion analysis. Int. J. Soft Comput. **12**(4), 253–262 (2017)
24. De Miguel, K., et al.: Home camera-based fall detection system for the elderly. Sensors **17**(12), 2864 (2017)
25. Antony, A., Gidveer, G.R.: Live streaming motion detection camera security system with email notification using Raspberry Pi. IOSR J. Electron. Commun. Eng. (IOSRJECE), Special Issue-AETM'16, pp. 142–147 (2016)
26. Wang, S., et al.: Human fall detection in surveillance video based on PCANet. Multimedia Tools Appl. **75**(19), 11603–11613 (2016)
27. Bhattacharya, A., Vaughan, R.: Deep learning radar design for breathing and fall detection. IEEE Sensors J. **20**(9), 5072–5085 (2020)
28. Zhang, Z.: Microsoft kinect sensor and its effect. IEEE Multimedia **19**(2), 4–10 (2012)
29. Tripathi, U., et al.: Advancing remote healthcare using humanoid and affective systems. IEEE Sensors J. (2021)
30. Sehairi, K., Chouireb, F., Meunier, J.: Elderly fall detection system based on multiple shape features and motion analysis. In: 2018 International Conference on Intelligent Systems and Computer Vision (ISCV), IEEE, pp. 1–8 (2018)
31. Erol, B., Amin, M.G., Boashash, B.: Range-Doppler radar sensor fusion for fall detection. In: 2017 IEEE Radar Conference (RadarConf), IEEE, pp. 0819–0824 (2017)
32. Jokanovic, B., Amin, M., Ahmad, F.: Radar fall motion detection using deep learning. In: 2016 IEEE Radar Conference (RadarConf), IEEE, pp. 1–6 (2016)
33. Erol, B., et al.: Wideband radar based fall motion detection for a generic elderly. In: 2016 50th Asilomar Conference on Signals, Systems and Computers, IEEE, pp. 1768–1772 (2016)
34. Wang, M., Zhang, Y.D., Cui, G.: Human motion recognition exploiting radar with stacked recurrent neural network. Digit. Signal Process. **87**, 125–131 (2019)
35. Erol, B., Amin, M.: Generalized pca fusion for improved radar human motion recognition. In: 2019 IEEE Radar Conference (RadarConf), IEEE, 1–5 (2019)
36. Zhao, J., et al.: R-DEHM: CSI-based robust duration estimation of human motion with WiFi. Sensors **19**(6), 1421 (2019)
37. Chopra, N., et al.: THz time-domain spectroscopy of human skin tissue for in-body nanonetworks. In: IEEE Trans. Terahertz Sci. Technol. **6**(6), 803–809 (2016)
38. Lolla, S., Zhao, A.: WiFi motion detection: a study into efficacy and classification. In: 2019 IEEE Integrated STEM Education Conference (ISEC), IEEE, pp. 375–378 (2019)
39. Wang, T., et al.: Wi-Alarm: low-cost passive intrusion detection using WiFi. Sensors **19**(10), 2335 (2019)
40. Din, I.U., et al.: The Internet of Things: a review of enabled technologies and future challenges. IEEE Access **7**, 7606–7640 (2019)
41. Teel, J.: Comparison of wireless technologies: bluetooth, WiFi, BLE, Zigbee, Z-Wave, 6LoWPAN, NFC, WiFi Direct, GSM, LTE, LoRa, NBIoT, and LTE-M. url: https://predictabledesigns.com/wireless_technologies_bluetooth_wifi_zigbee_gsm_lte_lora_nb-iot_ltem/. Visited 24 June 2021
42. IoT Standards & Protocols. url: https://www.postscapes.com/internet-of-things-protocols/ (2020). Visited on 24 June 2021
43. Shaikhina, T., et al.: Decision tree and random forest models for outcome prediction in antibody incompatible kidney transplantation. Biomed. Signal Process. Control **52**, 456–462 (2019)
44. Saçlı, B., et al.: Microwave dielectric property based classification of renal calculi: application of a kNN algorithm. Comput. Biol. Med. **112**, 103366 (2019)
45. Li, K., et al.: Research on KNN algorithm in malicious PDF files classification under adversarial environment. In: Proceedings of the 2019 4th International Conference on Big Data and Computing, pp. 156–159 (2019)
46. Huang, S., et al.: Applications of support vector machine (SVM) learning in cancer genomics. Cancer Genomics-Proteomics **15**(1), 41–51 (2018)
47. Jain, M., et al.: Speech emotion recognition using support vector machine. arXiv preprint (2020). arXiv:2002.07590

48. Wang, J., et al.: Cnn-rnn: A unified framework for multi-label image classification. In: Proceedings of the IEEE Conference on Computer Vision and Pattern Recognition, pp. 2285–2294 (2016)
49. Wang, S., et al.: Bi-directional long short-term memory method based on attention mechanism and rolling update for short-term load forecasting. Int. J. Electr. Power Energy Syst. **109**, 470–479 (2019)
50. Chang, P.D., et al.: Hybrid 3D/2D convolutional neural network for hemorrhage evaluation on head CT. Am. J. Neuroradiol. **39**(9), 1609–1616 (2018)
51. Ren, A., et al.: Machine learning driven approach towards the quality assessment of fresh fruits using non-invasive sensing. IEEE Sensors J. **20**(4), 2075–2083 (2019)
52. Elbayad, M., Besacier, L., Verbeek, J.: Pervasive attention: 2d convolutional neural networks for sequence-to-sequence prediction. arXiv preprint (2018). arXiv:1808.03867
53. Yu, J., et al.: 2D CNN versus 3D CNN for false-positive reduction in lung cancer screening. J. Med. Imaging **7**(5), 051202 (2020)
54. Broadley, R.W., et al.: Methods for the real-world evaluation of fall detection technology: a scoping review. Sensors **18**(7) (2018). ISSN 1424-8220. https://doi.org/10.3390/s18072060. url: https://www.mdpi.com/1424-8220/18/7/2060
55. Aziz, O., et al.: Validation of accuracy of SVM-based fall detection system using real-world fall and non-fall datasets. PLOS ONE **12**(7), 1–11 (July 2017)
56. Bloch, F., et al.: Evaluation under real-life conditions of a stand-alone fall detector for the elderly subjects. Ann. Phys. Rehabil. Med. **54**(6), 391–398 (2011). ISSN 1877-0657
57. Debard, G., et al.: Camera-based fall detection using real-world versus simulated data: How far are we from the solution?. J. Ambient Intell. Smart Environ. **8**(2), 149–168 (Mar 2016). ISSN 18761364
58. Wang, Y., Wu, K., Ni, L.M.: WiFall: device-free fall detection by wireless networks. IEEE Trans. Mobile Comput. **16**(2), 581–594 (2017)

mHealth Apps for Older Adults and Persons with Parkinson's Disease

Mattia Corzani

Abstract Recent years observed massive growth in wearable technology, everything can be smart: phones, watches, glasses, shirts, crutches, etc. These technologies are prevalent in various fields: from wellness, sports, and fitness to the healthcare domain. The spread of this phenomenon led the World Health Organization to define the term "mHealth" as "medical and public health practice supported by mobile devices, such as mobile phones, patient monitoring devices, personal digital assistants, and other wireless devices". Furthermore, mHealth solutions are suitable to perform real-time wearable biofeedback systems: sensors in the body area network connected to a processing unit (smartphone) and a feedback device (loudspeaker) to measure human functions and return them to the user as (bio)feedback signal. Considering the COVID-19 pandemic emergency, never as today, we can say that the integration of mHealth systems in our society may contribute to a new era of clinical practice. After reporting a brief description of mHealth system architecture, this chapter explores several opportunities where innovative mHealth solutions could improve assessment and rehabilitation strategies for aging people and persons with Parkinson's disease. This chapter presents solutions that need medical support in a clinical context and others that can be self-administered and require only a smartphone as a stand-alone system. Finally, the Discussion highlights the challenges for future research and development of innovative mHealth systems.

Keywords Mobile Health applications (mHealth apps) · Wearable inertial sensors · Assessment · Rehabilitation · IoT · Gait · Biofeedback

1 Introduction

The evolution of mobile phones and electronic technology leads to continuous miniaturization, making the mobile phone a really wearable device. The use of mobile and

M. Corzani (✉)
Department of Electrical, Electronic, and Information Engineering, University of Bologna, Viale del Risorgimento, 4, 40136 Bologna (BO), Italy
e-mail: mattia.corzani@unibo.it

© The Author(s), under exclusive license to Springer Nature Singapore Pte Ltd. 2022
S. Scataglini et al. (eds.), *Internet of Things for Human-Centered Design*,
Studies in Computational Intelligence 1011,
https://doi.org/10.1007/978-981-16-8488-3_11

wireless technologies to support health objectives can transform the face of health service delivery across the globe [1]. In 2011, the spread of this phenomenon had led the Global Observatory for eHealth of the World Health Organization to define the term "mHealth" as "medical and public health practice supported by mobile devices, such as mobile phones, patient monitoring devices, personal digital assistants, and other wireless devices" [2]. In 2021, the number of smartphone users world-wide will grow to 3.8 billion, and today 45% of people in the world have smartphones [3]. This figure is up considerably from 2016 when there were 2.5 billion users, 34% of that year's global population [4].

mHealth apps appeared later, and they address a broad array of mHealth applications and the use of mobile phones, e.g., to monitor biological signals or support healthy lifestyles. Thus, mHealth apps allow mobile devices as healthcare systems: for prevention, assessment, therapeutic support, and rehabilitation of motor and non-motor functions [5–7]. Importantly, the deployment of mHealth can be achieved using the various sensors available inside smartphones (as a stand-alone system) or in conjunction with external wearable sensors (as an integrated system).

Nowadays, mHealth reality is considered the biggest technological breakthrough, and its potential is increasing together with the utility of mHealth apps [8]. In the context of the ongoing COVID-19 pandemic, these technologies have become more relevant than ever, thanks to the advantages they provide [9]. In fact, mHealth platforms, with appropriate information technology (IT) and health literacy, can empower patients to manage their condition better themselves [9]. For example, patients with diabetes can monitor their blood glucose through mobile apps improving both the quality of medical services and their safety [10].

In the following section of this chapter, Sect. 2. *"mHealth System Architecture connected with apps"*, a generic system architecture to understand mHealth components and workflow better is described. Section 3. *"mHealth apps—Requirements in the Healthcare field"* reports the main requirements related to mHealth systems. Section 4. *"mHealth apps for Clinical Assessment"* and Sect. 5. *"mHealth apps for Neuromotor Rehabilitation"* present an overview of mHealth solutions for the clinical assessment and rehabilitation of the principal neuromotor dysfunctions experienced by older adults (OA) and persons with Parkinson's disease (PD). Finally, the *Discussion* highlights the challenges for future research and development of innovative mHealth systems.

2 mHealth System Architecture Connected with Apps

As a result of the growing demand for mHealth system, important research and development efforts have been carried out during the last years both by academia and industry in this area, driving great breakthroughs on enabler technologies, such as wireless communications, micro- and even nano-electronics, or sensing techniques, and materials [11, 12]. Advances in microelectronics and wireless communications have made Body Area Networks (BAN), which represent the key functional component in a mHealth systems [5, 13]. BAN are composed of tiny smart sensors deployed in, on, or around a human body. These sensors are distributed on the human body consequently with the different physiological parameters or/and body function to measure. Thus, their location is an important aspect. It is possible to detect brain activity (Electroencephalography—EEG) using a sensor near the scalp. Then, with surface Electromyography (sEMG), it is possible to acquire the myoelectric activity of the specific muscles involved in the execution of selected motor tasks [14]. Besides, wearing on the shoes Inertial Measurement Units (IMUs), which contains triaxial accelerometer, gyroscope, and (optionally) magnetometer, it is possible to characterize the motor behavior during gait [15]. Lastly, in the management of type 1 diabetes, patients use sensors able to detect blood glucose (BG) in real-time without finger-pricks required [16].

Similarly for other main biosignals, as reported by Dias et al. [5]: Hearth Rate (HR), Skin Perspiration (SP), Respiration Rate (RR), Oxygen Saturation (OS). Importantly, locating the same sensors described above in inappropriate places would not correctly detect the physiological parameters and features reported.

In common, these sensors are connected with a portable processing unit, like a smartphone in mHealth systems connected with apps, to exchange information with clinicians and/or send it as feedback to the patient. A schematic mHealth architecture is designed based on literature review, where the BAN are composed of various sensors properly located in the human body, Fig. 1.

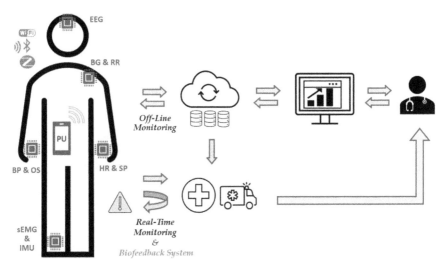

Fig. 1 Schematic mHealth system architecture connected with apps, adapted from [5, 13, 17, 18]. PU (red), Portable Unit (for example a Smartphone). List of sensors node or physiological parameters detected (blue): EEG, Electroencephalography; BG, Blood Glucose; RR, Respiration Rate; HR, Hearth Rate; SP, Skin Perspiration; BP, Blood Pressure; OS, Oxygen Saturation; IMU, Inertial Measurement Unit; sEMG, surface Electromyography

2.1 Sensor Node

At first, the sensor architecture or, better, the sensor node is described: a sensor network that is capable of performing some processing, gathering sensory information, and communicating with the data-logger present in the network [19], Fig. 2.

The main components of a sensor node are a microcontroller, transceiver, external memory, power source, one or more sensors, consisting of a transducer, and A/D converter:

- **Transducer**: varies its electrical properties to varying environmental conditions. Usually Micro Electro Mechanical Systems (MEMS) technology ensures higher efficiency, lower production costs, and less power consumption than other types of sensors such as piezoelectric. However, depending on the application, a piezoelectric transducer can be more accurate: to analyze human movement in high dynamic tasks, it is common to prefer piezoelectric accelerometers [20, 21].
- **A/D Converter—Analog to Digital Converter**: converts the transducer's voltage value to a digital value. The A/D converter's resolution implies a quantization of the input: this necessarily introduces a small amount of error/noise. Furthermore, an ADC converts the input periodically, sampling the data: this limits the input signal's allowable bandwidth.
- **Micro-controller**: it manages and controls the hardware of the sensor node, can perform local online signal processing (filtering/amplify the signal, data fusion, feature extraction).
- **Transceiver**: it connects the sensor node to the network. It can be an optical or radio-frequency device.
- **External memory**: it is needed to store the program's binary code running on the sensor node.
- **Power supply**: source of power for communication (usually most affecting factor), sensing, and data processing.

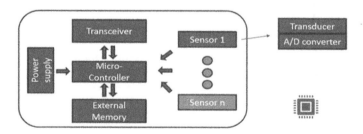

Fig. 2 Schematic overview of a sensor node

2.2 Portable Processing Unit (PU)

The portable processing unit (PU), also denominated as data-logger, is where all the information is gathered, containing the outputs and inputs of the mHealth system [5]. The communication between a node sensor and the data-logger is normally made through wireless protocols, avoiding loose wires around the body leading to a higher comfort and movement liberty. As Fig. 1 shows, PU can be a common smartphone with a custom application installed on it. PU can receive data from online monitoring devices and store it in a local memory. This two-way communication allows other devices to establish a wirelessly connection to a main device, which stores the data of several sensors. This system can also be helpful to label the timing of important events using external devices [13, 17, 22]. The wireless protocols most popular in mHealth systems are Radio Frequency Identification (RFID), ANT/ANT+, Bluetooth, Wi-Fi, ZigBee, and LoRa (Long Range radio).

RFID is widely used primarily for tracking and identification purposes: a reader or interrogator sends a signal to a tag or label attached to an object to be identified [23]. ANT/ANT+ is a proprietary protocol stack designed for ultra-low power, short-range wireless communications in sensor networks, especially for health and fitness monitoring systems [23]. It ensures low power consumption by using a low data rate and can operate for more extended periods. Bluetooth is a short-range radio-frequency-based connectivity between portables and fixed devices requiring low power consumption and with a low-cost. It is widely implemented in commercial devices like smartphones and laptops. The new Bluetooth technology named Bluetooth Low Energy (BLE) has even a lower power consumption with a smaller form factor. Interestingly, in Android devices, the data rate is highly dependent on the model used, with a maximum of around 10 Mbps. Using Bluetooth connectivity, one master device can communicate at a maximum with seven slave nodes, forming a star-type network structure. Wi-Fi protocol lower layers were adopted, allowing higher data throughput for low power requirements applications, not as low as the Bluetooth technology but can also be a good connection protocol to use, mainly when a higher distance of communication is needed [5]. ZigBee is another technology used for low power and low data rate communication protected using the Advanced Encryption Standard. This feature makes ZigBee ideal for medical applications because it can consume less energy than Bluetooth versions earlier than 4.0, but with a lower data transferring rate [5]. LoRa technology is a long distance coverage, low-cost and low power consumption wireless protocol. LoRa network architecture is deployed in a star-of-stars topology where gateways relay messages between end-devices and a central network server. The maximum number of nodes that can communicate with a gateway module depends on its specifications, usually defined by the number of packets it can support [24]. It has the disadvantage of low data rate but a huge advantage of scalability and customization of several parameters such as frequency channel, transmission power, and data rate. In the construction of a wearable device, the communication protocol is crucial to identify the number

Table 1 Wireless protocols main features. Adapted from Dias et al. [5], Majumder et al. [23]

Wireless protocol	Max nodes supported	Range	Max data rate	Power consumption
RFID	1	1–3 m	640 Kbps	200 mW
ANT/ANT+	65 533	30 m	60 Kbps	1 mW
Bluetooth	1 master + 7 slaves	1–100 m	3 Mbps	2.5–100 mW
BLE	1 master + 7 slaves	1–100 m	10 Mbps	10 mW
Wi-Fi	255	200 m	54 Mbps	1 W
ZigBee	65 533	100 m	250 Kbps	35 mW
LoRa	HIGH (depends on gateway and single packet)	50 km	700 bps	LOW (customizable)

and the distances of the devices involved. Besides, there is also the need to minimize energy consumption [25] and consider the wireless technologies available in commercial devices (such as smartphones).

Table 1 summarizes some of the main features of these wireless protocols. Mobile telecommunications technologies can also be used to transmit real-time data. However, it is essential to implement strong encryption and authentication technology to ensure a secure transmission channel over the long-range communication medium for the safeguarding of personal medical information [23]. Alternatively, it is also possible to handle sensors node inside the PU: for example, using only a smartphone as a stand-alone system, thus exploiting their built-in sensors [6].

2.3 Offline Monitoring

All data from vital signs can be stored in a portable unit (micro-SD memory card for example), for future use in medical analysis or just as a personal record. The data can be stored while a real-time monitoring is occurring. The main aim of such monitoring is to record vital data for clinic diagnosis and prediction by clinicians [5]. For example, sleep issues such as apnea, can be analyzed through saved data from the patient: a home sleep monitoring allows to monitor sleep in a familiar environment resulting in reliable data acquisition [22, 26]. Offline monitoring allows a high level of data processing to give much more information that is valuable to the end-users and clinicians, for example, using data mining techniques to have more in-depth knowledge representation [26].

2.4 Real-time Monitoring and Biofeedback System

With mHealth systems it is possible to perform clinical monitoring outside a medical environment, alert the patient in case of any physiological problem or monitor himself, and be updated on his vital signs during daily activities [17]. On the other hand, in a medical environment mHealth systems allows the patients monitoring inside the boundaries of a specific area, normally a hospital, where the patients can move while their vital information is being wirelessly transmitted to a remote monitoring center and thus made available to clinicians [5]. These live systems can also be configured with a set of alarms for each patient helping in the detection of some required anomaly. The vital signs can also be recorded in Medical Information Systems to be later analyzed by clinicians [5, 13, 27]. However, the biggest advantage of mHealth systems in real-time monitoring is the possibility of patient's monitoring at home and outdoors, using Internet communications. This feature allows the patient to has a normal life while being monitored, with his vital signs continuously or intermittently transmitted to a remote monitoring center, with health support and, if needed, inform the patient of his medical status [5].

Furthermore, vital signs and physiological parameters can also be transmitted to portable devices, such as smartphones and smartwatches, to visualize and analyze persons' health status, allowing the so-called Biofeedback (BF) process. BF is defined as a process in which a system or agent accurately measures and feeds back, to persons and their therapists, information with educational and reinforcing properties about their physiological processes in the form of analog or binary, auditory, and/or visual feedback signals. The objectives are to help persons develop greater awareness of, confidence in, and an increase in voluntary control over their physiological processes that are otherwise outside awareness and/or under less voluntary control [28]. With BF the information fed back to the patients adds or reinforces their physiological sensory channels: thus, BF was also defined as augmented feedback [29]. With such self-monitoring systems [5], clinicians must carefully teach patients how to use them at home, in particular, how to understand and react to BF alerts [28]. For example, this is what already happens in the treatment of type 1 diabetics' subjects. Several artificial pancreases have been developed to help manage type 1 diabetes [30, 31]. To obtain satisfactory results, the clinician's contribution to patient education is crucial [10, 32]. In the last decades, self-monitoring and BF systems were used in many areas such as instrumental conditioning of autonomic nervous system responses, psychophysiology, behavior therapy, and medicine, stress research and stress management strategies, electromyography, consciousness, electroencephalography, cybernetics, and sports [28]. Nowadays, thanks to mHealth and technological progress, BF systems will become more achievable.

3 mHealth Apps—Requirements in the Healthcare Field

Healthcare systems have recognized the advantages of using Information and Communication Technologies (ICT), including mHealth app systems, to improve the quality of care, and they are now working, although at a different pace worldwide, to turn traditional into smart healthcare [33]. To meet the increasing demands of an aging population with chronic diseases and comorbidities, technology appears to be to shift from clinic-centric to patient-centric healthcare [34]. Nevertheless, to accelerate the shift toward the brave new world of mHealth, technology must be appropriately designed with the aid of end-users. Many mHealth technologies have failed to innovate the current clinical practice because they ignored the interaction between technology, human characteristics, and socio-economic environment [35]. As an alternative to the technical industrial mindset, User-Centered Design has proven to be an effective tool to realize products and services for the Healthcare sector. User-Centered approach has to be included in the design process since the starting phases to develop a product or system that is effective due to the close relationship with the users' requirements and the high capacity of satisfaction of their needs [36–38].

In general, many important factors should be considered when developing a mHealth app [39, 40]. First, the main characteristics related to functionality and adoption of mHealth app are: wearability, monitoring duration, connectivity configuration, and maintainability of the system developed [40–42]. Last but not least the user's willingness and motivation: in this aspect, clinicians have a crucial role [42, 43].

Besides, there is the need to identify the key stakeholders. In evaluating a mHealth system, they are clinicians, developers, patients whose management may be affected, and people responsible for purchasing and maintaining the system [44]. Each may have different needs and requests to be satisfied, Fig. 3.

For example, from the developer's point of view, the algorithms used in the system must be validated, robust and well-written. In general, nobody should use a system or device that elaborated inaccurate measurements: the features implemented should be validated and tested within the proposed usage context [42].

Moreover, as already mentioned, the usability and user-friendliness of the apps are a fundamental determinant for technology adoption, in particular, among older adults [36–38, 45, 46]. In particular, usability is defined in the official International Organization for Standardization (ISO) guidelines as "the extent to which a system, product or service can be used by specified users to achieve specified goals with effectiveness, efficiency and satisfaction in a specified context of use" [47]. In addition, perceived usefulness and ease of use causes people to accept or reject information technology [45]. The first is defined as the "degree to which a person believes that using a particular system would enhance his or her functions". The latter, in contrast, refers to "the degree to which a person believes that using a particular system would be free of effort" [45].

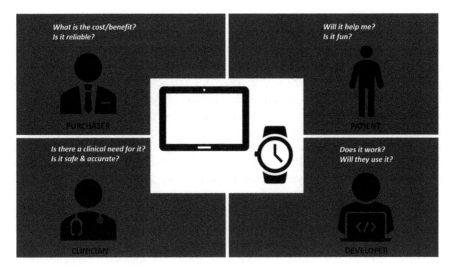

Fig. 3 Different stakeholders may have different needs and requests to be satisfied in the evaluation of a mHealth system. Adapted from Friedman et al. [44]

Furthermore, when measuring aspects of one's health, the accuracy of the results relies on the correct administration of the test. Thus, any usability problem associated with using a mobile app should be identified and addressed before it is made available to end-users. This is usually done through several iterations of testing with target user groups, ideally until no major usability problems exist with regards to using the apps and administering the test. Usability studies are most often carried out in a laboratory setting, convenient, and offer a high degree of control instead of field-based usability testing [44]. However, field-based testing, which, in this context, would be a home setting, provides insight into how the system is used under more realistic situations [44]. Depending on the system being tested and the development phase, usability should ideally be tested in both laboratory and home settings [48].

The use of smartphone apps as stand-alone systems provides a feasible solution in a fully wearable system. They have the significant advantages of pervasiveness, ubiquity, and exploitation of common apps usage experience. Moreover, the choice of off-the-shelf smartphones would also keep the mHealth system costs low, also increasing its compatibility with external commercial devices. On the other hand, there are several challenges associated with the development of mHealth apps:

- Design for all model and system available with the same performance (different smartphones have different capabilities);
- Built-in sensors do not have priority in the mobile operating system, OS (smartphones were born to handle calls and/or messages);
- Safety measures in order to ensure the patients' safety and privacy, developing strategies to ensure data are only accessible to those authorized to access [40].

In particular, to date, there is a lack of standardized regulation methods to evaluate the content and quality of mHealth apps [49–51]. The quality assessment of mHealth apps is challenging as it is difficult to identify the core components of quality and appropriate measures to assess them [52]. Besides, the different smartphone models available in the market make this assessment more complicated. For example, smartphone built-in inertial sensors do not have a fixed sample frequency: frequency changes dynamically around a fixed value depending on the OS requests, and it varies across the different smartphone models [53]. Moreover, some features are only available in certain smartphones and not in others (or in other cases, the feature could be limited): BLE connection could be absent in some smartphones or limited to only few megabytes in others, not allowing data exchange with external sensors [54].

On a more general ground and from a healthcare system perspective, introducing guidelines for app development and use may be highly effective in improving the quality standards. In the US, the FDA regulates mHealth within the existing framework for medical devices [55]. Only a limited number of apps meet the definition of medical device and are, as such, subject to the US FDA regulation [55]. In Europe, the new regulations on medical devices (MDR [EU] 2017/745) describe whether mHealth products must be medical devices [56]. As a result, apps that support a medical diagnosis and have medical use must be CE marked as medical devices [57]. While the implementation of the new, more stringent MDR might lead to the development of more high-quality apps and improved patient safety, it might also limit the development and release of new apps and software on the market. Classifying a device as class IIa or higher requires evaluation by a notified body, which can be very costly and, therefore, a barrier to entry for app developers [57].

4 mHealth Apps for Clinical Assessment

The health state's measurement is essential in both clinical practice and research to assess and monitoring the severity and progression of a patient's health status, the effect of treatment, and alterations in other relevant factors. The miniaturization of sensing, feedback, and computational devices has opened a new frontier for movement assessment and rehabilitation [58]. Wearable systems are portable and can enable individuals with various movement disorders to benefit from analysis and intervention techniques that have previously been confined to research laboratories and medical clinics [58].

4.1 Older Adults

The clinical assessment of frail older adults (OA) is challenging, as they often have multiple comorbidities and diminished functional and physiological reserves

[59]. Besides, the physical illness or adverse effects of drugs are more pronounced resulting in atypical presentation, cognitive decline, delirium or inability to manage routine activities of daily living (ADLs) [60]. ADLs include the fundamental skills typically needed to manage basic physical needs, comprised the following areas: grooming/personal hygiene, dressing, toileting/continence, transferring/ambulating, and eating [61]. Successful ADLs' performance is a significant health indicator that can predict mild cognitive impairments, dementia, and mortality in older adults [62, 63]. Hence, it is crucial to measure ADLs in older adults effectively. Several types of approaches have been used to quantify the level of independence in ADLs. ADLs may be measured by self-report, proxy/caregiver/informant report, and/or direct observation filling ad hoc scale/questionnaire [64–66]. These tools obtain a general sense of the level of assistance needed and the most appropriate setting for the patient [61]. Self-report measures are convenient to administer and are frequently used when direct observation is not possible or when individuals are relatively cognitively intact. However, they may be less valid when individuals have poor insight into their functional impairments [67, 68]. Informant-based ratings are commonly completed by caregivers who know the patient well, but how also may be biased by their own burden in caring for the individual or by over or underestimating the patient's true functioning [61]. The use of performance-based measures can provide objective data about ADL functioning and they may be able to detect change over time [69], but generally require more training to administer as compared with self or informant reports [61]. The need to improve these measurements and to objectively quantify how subjects engaged in physical activity (PA) led to the recent spread of wearable-accelerometer devices (or activity trackers) [70]. These devices allow daily monitoring of the behavior of the OA, also enhancing their aptitude for PA [71]. Historically, these accelerometry-based solutions employ summary threshold metrics to assess PA. To date, novel measures, such as fragmentation, allow for a deeper understanding of the quantities and patterns of daily PA, which are most informative for health outcomes [72].

Besides, falls are a major threat to the health and independence of OA. Quantitative methods for assessing fall risk factors are necessary to effectively implement preventative measures and reduce falls' incidence and severity [73]. In the last years, research groups developed different mHealth apps to monitor fall risk factors [73]. In general, mHealth app systems, due to their ubiquitous nature, offer the potential to provide fall risk screening in community settings [73] as an alternative to a qualitative approach.

Moreover, to objectively evaluate specific items of ADLs related to fall risk, in particular gait and balance [73], different instrumented tests can be performed, Table 2.

To date, thanks to the great advances in wearable technologies these instrumented tests are feasible not only in clinical, but also continuously at home in a self-administrable way [80]. This is crucial for the prevention of movement dysfunctions in OA. For example, a solution that permits objective evaluation of body posture and gait in OA is the mHealth systems proposed by Bergquist et al. [48]. They developed three smartphone apps for self-administering an instrumented version of the "Timed

Table 2 Gait and balance assessment tools. Adapted from Singh et al. [59]

	Description
Turn 180° test [74]	A measure of dynamic postural stability, asking a patient to take few steps and then turn around by 180° to face the opposite direction. Count the number of steps taken to complete a 180° turn
Timed-Up-and-Go test (TUG) [75]	A measurement of mobility. A person is asked to stand up from a seated position, walk for 3 m, turn and walk back to a chair and sit down. Measure the time taken in seconds
Tandem stand test [76]	A measure of balance and ankle strength. A person is asked to stand in a near tandem position with their bare feet separated laterally by 2.5 cm with the heel of the front foot 2.5 cm anterior to the great toe of the back with their eyes closed. A person can hold arms out or move the body to help keep the balance but do not move the feet
Alternate Step test [77]	A measure of strength, balance, coordination, and stair climbing. It provides a measure of mediolateral stability. A person should be asked to place alternate whole left and right barefoot onto a 19 cm high stepper for a total of eight times
10 m Walk test (10MWT) [78]	A measure of walking speed over a short duration. It requires a 20 m path that includes 5 m for acceleration and deceleration. Practically, a full 20 m walkway is not always available, thus there are several shorter distances commonly used to assess walking speed including 3, 4, and 6 m assessments
Sit-to-Standtest (StS) [79]	A measurement of functional mobility, balance, and lower limb strength. A person should be able to stand up and sit down five times with crossed arms from a 45 cm straight-backed chair

Up and Go" test (Self-TUG, Fig. 4), the "Standing tandem" test (Self-Tandem), and the "Five times sit-to-stand" test (Self-STS). The app uses the inertial sensors of the smartphone and real-time verbal instructions to guide the user during the test (Fig. 4c). The usability test of the apps was performed with target elderly groups [48].

Thus, mHealth solutions also allow pervasive and self-administered systems, feasible in daily life situations [48]. Nevertheless, the usability of the solutions proposed might be critical: it is essential to follow a User-Centered-Design (UCD) approach [37, 38], also considering that fine motor skills issues (such as tremor) in older people may hinder their interaction with these wearable systems [81]. In this perspective, Gabyzon et al. [82] developed and examined the feasibility of a tablet app to assess touchscreen ability in OA. This aspect is crucial for the correct interaction with modern devices. In general, a combination of self-report and performance-based measures of ADL performance may be the best way to fully capture the picture of disability for a given OA [83].

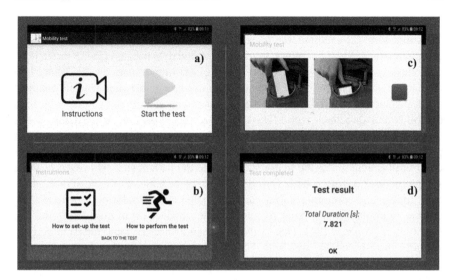

Fig. 4 The Self-TUG app. **a** Home screen. **b** Instructions tab to report how to correctly set-up and perform the test. **c** The inertial sensors of the smartphone and real-time verbal instructions guide the user during the test. **d** The total duration of the test automatically detect by the app. Adapted from Bergquist et al. [48]

4.2 Persons with Parkinson's Disease

Parkinson's disease (PD) is a complex disorder expressed through many motor and non-motor manifestations, which cause disabilities that can vary both gradually over time or come on suddenly. In addition, there is a wide interpatient variability making the appraisal of the many facets of this disease difficult [84]. Two kinds of measures are used for the evaluation of PD. The first is subjective, inferential, based on rater-based interview and examination or patient self-assessment, and consist of rating scales and questionnaires. These evaluations provide estimations of conceptual, nonobservable factors (e.g., symptoms), usually scored on an ordinal scale [84]. The new second type of measure is objective, factual, based on technology-based devices capturing physical characteristics of the pathological phenomena (e.g., sensors to measure the frequency and amplitude of tremor) [84].

Recently, there has been a growing interest in developing an objective assessment of the symptoms in PD, and its health-related outcomes, using new technology-based tools, worn or operated by patients either in a healthcare or domestic environment [84]. The most important new technologies to aid in the treatment monitoring of PD patients are based on the use of inertial measurement units (IMU). Most commercially available IMUs have a triaxial accelerometer and a triaxial gyroscope, although a magnetometer is also commonly included. Over time, sensors have become more sophisticated, and they can be worn unobtrusively and can be attached to almost any body part to measure movement. These wearable devices can record not only the orientation, amplitude, and frequency of movements [85]. These data allow clinicians to assess, for example, the presence and severity of the cardinal features and complications of PD (i.e., tremor, bradykinesia, and dyskinesias) [86]. Kinesia [87], a wireless system for automated assessment of PD tremor, uses an IMU placed on the patient's index finger or the heel and can differentiate between a healthy subject and a patient with bradykinesia. Kinesia system can also record tremor with high reliability and agreement with MDS-UPDRS rest and postural tremor items (one of the most common clinical scale used to provide an overall idea of the motor status of persons with PD) [87, 88]. Objective gait and balance quantification are important for the overall evaluation of the motor status of the PD patient [85]. However, as these symptoms in PD can be both episodic (Freezing of Gait—FOG, hesitation, difficult turning) and continuous (slow gait) associated with variability in performance, clinical examination at a point of time is often inadequate in elucidating the full spectrum of problems [84]. Thanks to the great advances in wearable technologies, various sensor-based and wearable technologies are now being used for the assessment and monitoring of movement patterns during clinical visits and the daily lives of PD patients [84, 85]. In addition, wearable sensors, frequently worn in the lower body segment, have emerged as a novel tool to quantitatively assess FOG during real life with more reliability than clinical measures alone [89, 90]. For example, a solution that permits objective evaluation of body posture and gait in PD subjects is the mTUG/mSWAY system [91, 92]. To date, numerous smartphone applications have been designed specifically for patients with PD. Existing applications include those devised for assessment of motor, cognitive, and psychological symptoms, as well as those intended to adjust and control treatment [93]. For example, Lopane et al. [94] implemented a system that allows optimizing the levodopa therapy in PD subjects according to disease progression to establish the minimum dose required over time, Fig. 5. Thanks to its integrated technology-based platform composed of a tablet app, a smartphone app, and a digital blood pressure monitor, the protocol can be performed under a physician's supervision, but also self-administer at home [94]. This mHealth system includes the following assessment tests that can be tailored and scheduled into a single assessment protocol:

- alternate finger tapping test (tablet app);
- reaction time test (tablet app);
- actual intake of the levodopa test dose (tablet app);
- measurement of the blood pressure (digital blood pressure monitor);
- measurement of the Timed Up and Go (TUG) test (smartphone app);
- identification of dyskinesia and the measurement of the tremor at rest (smartphone app).

Those two devices automatically connect to the tablet when the assessment protocol starts [94].

Thus, mobile devices seem to be a useful tool for the detection, assessment, and potential care of patients with PD [95–97]. However, high-quality studies are lacking, although they are certainly feasible, due to smartphones' accessibility and ease of use [85]. In conclusion, clinical scales are the most widely employed standards for

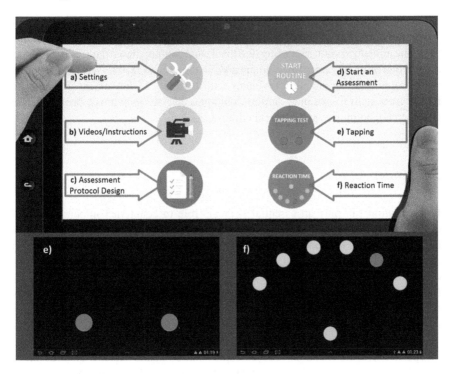

Fig. 5 Menu of the tablet app. **a** Settings. **b** Audio/video instructions. **c** Design the assessment protocol. **d** Start an assessment protocol. **e** Demo of the alternate finger tapping test. **f** Demo of the reaction time test. Adapted from Lopane et al. [94]

the evaluation of patients with PD [85]. Their limitations include subjectivity and the inability to monitor the disease continuously [85]. New sensors and wearable devices provide objective, accurate, and reproducible measurements that can overcome these barriers and complement the use of traditional methods. However, the use of these new technologies is still limited in practice because most of the studies performed to date were heterogeneous and non-standardized [85].

5 mHealth Apps for Neuromotor Rehabilitation

Neurorehabilitation aims to cement patients' existing skills, retrieve any lost skills, and promote the learning of new abilities, allowing people to function at their highest possible level despite their physical impairment. A variety of factors may have a significant effect on neurorehabilitation and influence motor learning processes. These factors include verbal instructions, characteristics, and variability of training sessions, the individual's active participation and motivation, positive and negative learning transfer, posture control, memory, and feedback. All of these factors are clinically applicable, and they provide the basis for emerging or established lines of research having to do with retraining sensorimotor function in neurological patients [98]. The miniaturization of sensing, feedback, and computational devices has opened a new frontier for movement assessment and rehabilitation [58, 99]. Wearable systems are portable and can enable individuals with a variety of movement disorders to benefit from analysis and intervention techniques that have previously been confined to research laboratories and medical clinics [58].

5.1 Older Adults

Rehabilitation can play an essential strategic role to counteract impairments and disability which characterize the aging process. Correct rehabilitative programs must be approached on the functional limitation and residual abilities of OA. Leading a more active lifestyle and regular physical activity including aerobic and resistance exercises have been demonstrated to improve cardiovascular, respiratory, musculoskeletal, and cognitive well-being in OA [100]. Physical activity interventions for people with an intact cognition are well documented and shown to be effective in improving balance and reducing falls [73]. A comprehensive physical activity guideline for all adults, including OA, was published by the American College of Sports Medicine (ACSM) [101]. People with dementia are two to three times more likely to fall and multimodal interventions that combine cognitive, as well as motor therapy, should be performed [102]. Physical activity is beneficial for reducing overall morbidity and mortality in OA [103]. The physical activity recommendations intended for all older adults may need to be modified for particular health conditions and disorders, using specific types of exercise to correct or ameliorate identified impairments and functional limitations [103]. Physical therapists, exercise physiologists, and physicians specializing in rehabilitation can help to tailor the exercise prescription to meet patient needs. In addition, healthcare providers are perceived as respected sources of health information and should take an active role in promoting physical activity. Primary care clinicians should emphasize the importance of physical activity for health maintenance, ask patients if they are physically active, and advise them to become physically active [103]. Innovatively, a recent European project (www.preventit.eu) developed and tested a personalized mHealth solution aimed at behavioral change in OA, to decrease the risk for age-related functional decline.

The project consists of a smartphone and smartwatch app to motivate older persons to exercise, and that shows how to integrate mobility exercises in daily living activities, Fig. 6. This app, created by a multidisciplinary team, was already developed in its final version [104] and a feasibility study was performed [105]. Results indicated that the developed interventions were feasible and safe. Participants liked the concept of lifestyle-integrated activities, managed to change their daily routines toward increased activity, and were positive about the app [105].

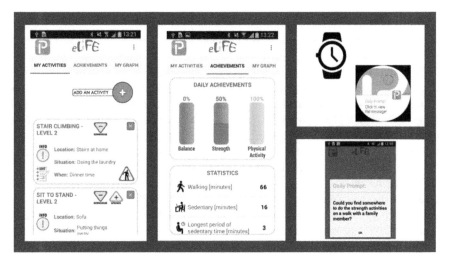

Fig. 6 A beta version of the PreventIT app

5.2 Persons with Parkinson's Disease

Despite optimal medical management, most patients with Parkinson's disease (PD) continue to experience a wide range of motor and non-motor symptoms [106, 107]. All of these influence activities of daily living and affect the patient's quality of life [108, 109]. Examples of motor symptoms that respond insufficiently to medication or surgery include impairments in speech, postural stability, and freezing of gait. Additional disability arises from the presence of non-motor symptoms (e.g., cognitive impairment, depression, or psychosis), that are sub-optimally controlled with current medical management [106, 110]. This situation creates treatment challenges, not only in advanced disease stages, but even early on in the course of PD [111]. Moreover, although it is recommended to early start rehabilitation, it should be considered that PD is a chronic progressive disorder and the intervention must be adjusted to changing clinical conditions and tailored to the individual patients' needs [112, 113]. A widely held belief holds that nonpharmacological management might offer symptomatic relief of motor or non-motor symptoms that are otherwise difficult to treat. Hence, a multidisciplinary approach involving non-pharmacological and pharmacological treatment is the standard nowadays [114].

The use of external sensory cues (e.g., auditory, visual) to reinforce attention toward the task [115] is an effective gait rehabilitation strategy for persons with PD; the cues stimulate the executive voluntary component of action [116–118] by activating the attentional-executive motor control system and bypassing the dysfunctional, habitual, sensorimotor BG network [116, 117, 119–122]. This strategy helps people with PD improve gait consistency and rhythmicity.

One of the most innovative developments in the quantitative assessment and management of PD symptoms is the use of wearable technologies during gait [123], which are able to overcome traditional open-loop cue, providing customized cueing: stimuli are triggered when gait deviates from normal, thus providing patients with immediate feedback on their performance. These closed-loop stimuli (audio [124–126], visual [127, 128], audio-visual [129] or proprioceptive [130]) are known as intelligent inputs [124]. Closed-loop systems are based on the Knowledge of Performance [29], which is indicated as one of the optimal techniques for motor rehabilitation in PD subjects [131]. In contrast to open-loop systems, in closed-loop systems the external information does not necessarily become part of the participants' movement representation (as explained by the "guidance hypothesis"), thus possibly decreasing the development of cue-dependency [132]. The possibility of real-time biofeedback represents an important step toward the maximum benefit and clinical impact of wearable sensors. Wearable systems also permit data collection in a more naturalistic environment [124, 129]. Casamassima et al. [133] developed a unique mHealth system (CuPiD-system) made of wearable sensors and a smartphone that provides real-time verbal feedback to improve the dynamic balance and gait performance of people with PD [124, 134].

Thanks to advances in technologies, visual feedback is possible through Smart Glasses (SG) [135]. SG represents an ideal modality to provide personalized feedback and assistance to people with PD in daily living situations. Indeed, McNaney et al. [136] reported that participants with PD were generally positive about SG as an everyday assistive device; however, usability issues and social stigma still hinder its general acceptance.

Innovatively, Imbesi et al. [137] proposed a wearable gait rehabilitation solution by integrating the Vuzix Blade SG [138] into the smartphone-based CuPiD-system [133], Fig. 7.

Although, the potential of real-time biofeedback in gait rehabilitation through wearable devices is underexploited [85], these new real-time systems seem to increase

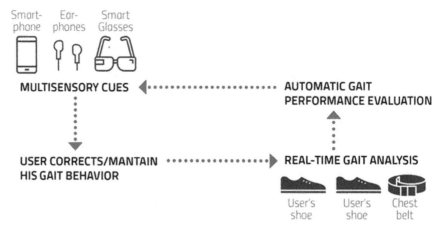

Fig. 7 Schematic representation of the mHealth system. Adapted from Casamassima et al. [133]

adherence to treatment, self-management, and quality of life [139], allowing also personalized and tailored rehabilitation on the individual patients' need [124].

6 Discussion and Future Scenario

Considering the pandemic emergency, never as of today, we can say that the integration of mHealth apps in our society may contribute to a new era of clinical practice. After reporting a brief description of mHealth system architecture, this chapter explored several different opportunities where innovative mHealth solutions could improve assessment and rehabilitation strategies for aging people and persons with Parkinson's disease. This chapter reported solutions that need medical support in a clinical context and others that can be self-administered and require only a smartphone as a stand-alone system.

However, the primary aim of a mHealth system is to improve the person's quality of life and increase his autonomy and independence. The huge development of technology in recent years leads to the manufacturing and use of miniature, low-cost sensors and powerful devices that open the way to non-invasive, non-intrusive, and continuous monitoring of an individual's health condition.

There are many challenges for future research and development to improve the performance and acceptance of the mHealth system.

First, to achieve widespread acceptance among the people, the systems need to be affordable, easy-to-use, unobtrusive. Nevertheless, many patients continue to depend on the clinician's support. They would request direct contact with them, and they would reject solutions that might create any distance between them and their clinician. Inclusive design principles might be helpful for designers to collect and elaborate on patients' requirements, next to the technical and technological ones, to improve these aspects.

Second, the new regulations on medical devices in Europe (MDR [EU] 2017/745) might lead to more high-quality mHealth systems, improving patient safety. On the other hand, it might limit the development and release of new solutions and software on the market [49].

Besides, the privacy and security of the sensitive medical information of the user must be guaranteed. More efforts are needed to develop algorithms to ensure highly secured communication.

Third, as we witness a digital transformation of the healthcare system, mHealth technologies are expected to become better integrated into the clinical workflow, especially to provide telemedicine. Thus, thanks to the Internet connection, mHealth systems can increase healthcare access and improve cost-effectiveness. During the COVID-19 pandemic, this transformation of the healthcare system has been dramatically accelerated by new clinical demands, including the need to assure continuity of clinical care services. For example, healthcare professionals could use mHealth systems to monitor patients' conditions remotely and continuously mitigate or prevent hospital surges.

In man's continuous aspiration to improve his well-being, we have to face the exponential growth of technology. Thus, we must deal with unknown challenges, unexpected situations and generate new uncertain solutions. In general, we are used to taking a predictable path, the so-called comfort zone. That is why we are used to choosing the options we already know. The challenge of future research, including the development of mHealth systems, requires a mental shift from linear and predictable to bold and spontaneous, handling the incoming technologies to the best of our abilities.

References

1. Park, S., Chung, K., Jayaraman, S.: Chapter 1.1—Wearables: fundamentals, advancements, and a roadmap for the future. In: Sazonov, Neuman, M.R. (eds.) Wearable Sensors, pp. 1–23. Academic Press, Oxford (2014). https://doi.org/10.1016/B978-0-12-418662-0.00001-5.
2. WHO Global Observatory for eHealth and World Health Organization: mHealth: New Horizons for Health Through Mobile Technologies. World Health Organization, Geneva (2011). Accessed: Sep. 28, 2020. [Online]. Available http://www.who.int/goe/publications/goe_mhealth_web.pdf
3. 'Smartphone users worldwide 2020', Statista. https://www.statista.com/statistics/330695/number-of-smartphone-users-worldwide/. Accessed Sep. 28, 2020
4. 'How Many People Have Smartphones Worldwide (Sept 2020)'. https://www.bankmycell.com/blog/how-many-phones-are-in-the-world. Accessed Sep. 28, 2020
5. Dias, D., Paulo Silva Cunha, J.: Wearable health devices—vital sign monitoring, systems and technologies. Sensors (Basel) **18**(8) (2018). https://doi.org/10.3390/s18082414
6. Majumder, S., Deen, M.J.: Smartphone sensors for health monitoring and diagnosis. Sensors (Basel) **19**(9) (2019). https://doi.org/10.3390/s19092164
7. Haghi, M., Thurow, K., Stoll, R.: Wearable devices in medical Internet of Things: scientific research and commercially available devices. Healthcare Inform. Res. **23**(1), 4 (2017). https://doi.org/10.4258/hir.2017.23.1.4
8. 'Emerging New Era of Mobile Health Technologies'. https://e-hir.org/journal/view.php?id=10.4258/hir.2016.22.4.253. Accessed Sep. 28, 2020
9. Adans-Dester, C.P., et al.: Can mHealth technology help mitigate the effects of the COVID-19 pandemic? IEEE Open J. Eng. Med. Biol. **1**, 243–248 (2020). https://doi.org/10.1109/OJEMB.2020.3015141
10. American Diabetes Association: 7. Diabetes technology: standards of medical care in diabetes-2020. Diabetes Care **43**(Suppl 1), S77–88 (2020). https://doi.org/10.2337/dc20-S007
11. Teng, X.-F., Zhang, Y.-T., Poon, C.C.Y., Bonato, P.: Wearable medical systems for p-Health. IEEE Rev. Biomed. Eng. **1**, 62–74 (2008). https://doi.org/10.1109/RBME.2008.2008248
12. Agoulmine, N., Ray, P., Wu, T.-H.: Communications in ubiquitous healthcare [Guest Editorial]. IEEE Commun. Mag. **50**(1), 16–18 (2012). https://doi.org/10.1109/MCOM.2012.6122527
13. Custodio, V., Herrera, F.J., López, G., Moreno, J.I.: A review on architectures and communications technologies for wearable health-monitoring systems. Sensors (Basel) **12**(10), 13907–13946 (2012). https://doi.org/10.3390/s121013907
14. Maranesi, E., et al.: The surface electromyographic evaluation of the functional reach in elderly subjects. J. Electromyogr. Kinesiol. **26**, 102–110 (2016). https://doi.org/10.1016/j.jelekin.2015.12.002
15. Corzani, M., Ferrari, A., Ginis, P., Nieuwboer, A., Chiari, L.: Motor adaptation in Parkinson's disease during prolonged walking in response to corrective acoustic messages. Front Aging Neurosci. **11** (2019). https://doi.org/10.3389/fnagi.2019.00265

16. 'How it Works', Dexcom, 30 July 2019. https://www.dexcom.com/g6/how-it-works. Accessed 24 June 2021
17. Pantelopoulos, A., Bourbakis, N.G.: A survey on wearable sensor-based systems for health monitoring and prognosis. IEEE Trans. Syst. Man Cybern. Part C (Applications and Reviews) **40**(1), 1–12 (2010). https://doi.org/10.1109/TSMCC.2009.2032660
18. Tennina, S., et al.: WSN4QoL: a WSN-oriented healthcare system architecture. Int. J. Distrib. Sens. Netw. **10**(5), 503417 (2014). https://doi.org/10.1155/2014/503417
19. Zanjireh, M.M., Larijani, H.: A survey on centralised and distributed clustering routing algorithms for WSNs. In: 2015 IEEE 81st Vehicular Technology Conference (VTC Spring), May 2015, pp. 1–6. https://doi.org/10.1109/VTCSpring.2015.7145650
20. Chen, K.Y., Bassett, D.R.: The technology of accelerometry-based activity monitors: current and future. Med. Sci. Sports Exerc. **37**(11 Suppl), S490-500 (2005). https://doi.org/10.1249/01.mss.0000185571.49104.82
21. Yang, C.-C., Hsu, Y.-L.: A review of accelerometry-based wearable motion detectors for physical activity monitoring. Sensors (Basel) **10**(8), 7772–7788 (2010). https://doi.org/10.3390/s100807772
22. Cunha, J.P.S., Cunha, B., Pereira, A.S., Xavier, W., Ferreira, N., Meireles, L.: Vital-Jacket®: a wearable wireless vital signs monitor for patients' mobility in cardiology and sports. In: 2010 4th International Conference on Pervasive Computing Technologies for Healthcare, March 2010, pp. 1–2. https://doi.org/10.4108/ICST.PERVASIVEHEALTH2010.8991
23. Majumder, S., Mondal, T., Deen, M.J.: Wearable sensors for remote health monitoring. Sensors (Basel) **17**(1) (2017). https://doi.org/10.3390/s17010130
24. Mikhaylov, K., Petaejaejaervi, J., Haenninen, T.: Analysis of capacity and scalability of the LoRa low power wide area network technology. In: European Wireless 2016; 22th European Wireless Conference, May 2016, pp. 1–6
25. Asensio, Á., Marco, Á., Blasco, R., Casas, R.: Protocol and architecture to bring things into Internet of Things. Int. J. Distrib. Sens. Netw. **10**(4), 158252 (2014). https://doi.org/10.1155/2014/158252
26. Banaee, H., Ahmed, M.U., Loutfi, A.: Data mining for wearable sensors in health monitoring systems: a review of recent trends and challenges. Sensors (Basel) **13**(12), 17472–17500 (2013). https://doi.org/10.3390/s131217472
27. Shahriyar, R., Bari, Md.F., Kundu, G., Ahamed, S.I., Akbar, Md.M.: Intelligent mobile health monitoring system (IMHMS). In: Electronic Healthcare. Berlin, Heidelberg, pp. 5–12 (2010). https://doi.org/10.1007/978-3-642-11745-9_2
28. Biofeedback: A Practitioner's Guide, 3rd ed., pp. xiv, 930. Guilford Press, New York, NY, US (2003)
29. Schmidt, R.A., Lee, T.D.: Motor control and learning: a behavioral emphasis, 4th ed., pp. vi, 535. Human Kinetics, Champaign, IL, US (2005)
30. MiniMed™ 770G System. Medtronic Diabetes, 10 September 2020. http://www.medtronicdiabetes.com/products/minimed-770g-insulin-pump-system. Accessed Oct. 05, 2020
31. Diabetes Service. Air Liquide Healthcare UK, 4 February 2019. https://www.airliquidehealthcare.co.uk/diabetes-service. Accessed Oct. 05, 2020
32. Forlenza, G.P., et al.: Successful at-home use of the tandem control-IQ artificial pancreas system in young children during a randomized controlled trial. Diabetes Technol. Ther. **21**(4), 159–169 (2019). https://doi.org/10.1089/dia.2019.0011
33. Digital health. https://www.who.int/westernpacific/health-topics/digital-health. Accessed 9 March 2021
34. Farahani, B., Firouzi, F., Chang, V., Badaroglu, M., Constant, N., Mankodiya, K.: Towards fog-driven IoT eHealth: promises and challenges of IoT in medicine and healthcare. Futur. Gener. Comput. Syst. **78**, 659–676 (2018). https://doi.org/10.1016/j.future.2017.04.036
35. van Gemert-Pijnen, J.E.W.C., et al.: A holistic framework to improve the uptake and impact of eHealth technologies. J. Med. Internet Res. **13**(4), e111 (2011). https://doi.org/10.2196/jmir.1672

36. Imbesi, S., Mincolelli, G.: Design of smart devices for older people: a user centered approach for the collection of users' needs. In: Intelligent Human Systems Integration 2020, pp. 860–864. Cham (2020). https://doi.org/10.1007/978-3-030-39512-4_131
37. De Vito Dabbs, A., et al.: User-centered design and interactive health technologies for patients. Comput. Inform. Nurs. **27**(3), 175 (2009). https://doi.org/10.1097/NCN.0b013e31819f7c7c
38. Witteman, H.O., et al.: User-centered design and the development of patient decision aids: protocol for a systematic review. Syst. Rev. **4**(1) (2015). https://doi.org/10.1186/2046-4053-4-11
39. 'Android Developers'. Android Developers. https://developer.android.com/design. Accessed 23 October 2020
40. Chatzipavlou, I.A., Christoforidou, S.A., Vlachopoulou, M.: A recommended guideline for the development of mHealth apps. mHealth **2** (2016). https://doi.org/10.21037/mhealth.2016.05.01
41. Keogh, A., Dorn, J.F., Walsh, L., Calvo, F., Caulfield, B.: Comparing the usability and acceptability of wearable sensors among older Irish adults in a real-world context: observational study. JMIR mHealth uHealth **8**(4), e15704 (2020). https://doi.org/10.2196/15704
42. Lee, S.M., Lee, D.: Healthcare wearable devices: an analysis of key factors for continuous use intention. Serv. Bus. **14**(4), 503–531 (2020). https://doi.org/10.1007/s11628-020-00428-3
43. Ferguson, C., Hickman, L.D., Turkmani, S., Breen, P., Gargiulo, G., Inglis, S.C.: "Wearables only work on patients that wear them": barriers and facilitators to the adoption of wearable cardiac monitoring technologies. Cardiovascular Digital Health J. **2**(2), 137–147 (2021). https://doi.org/10.1016/j.cvdhj.2021.02.001
44. Friedman, C.P., Owens, D.K., Wyatt, J.C.: Evaluation and technology assessment. In: Shortliffe, E.H., Perreault, L.E. (eds.) *Medical Informatics: Computer Applications in Health Care and Biomedicine*, pp. 282–323. Springer, New York, NY (2001). https://doi.org/10.1007/978-0-387-21721-5_8
45. Davis, F.D.: Perceived usefulness, perceived ease of use, and user acceptance of information technology. MIS Q. **13**(3), 319–340 (1989). https://doi.org/10.2307/249008
46. Herrmann, L.K., Kim, J.: The fitness of apps: a theory-based examination of mobile fitness app usage over 5 months. mHealth **3** (2017). https://doi.org/10.21037/mhealth.2017.01.03
47. ISO/DIS 9241-11.2(en), Ergonomics of human-system interaction—Part 11: usability: definitions and concepts. https://www.iso.org/obp/ui/#iso:std:iso:9241:-11:dis:ed-2:v2:en. Accessed 27 April 2021
48. Bergquist, R., Vereijken, B., Mellone, S., Corzani, M., Helbostad, J.L., Taraldsen, K.: App-based self-administrable clinical tests of physical function: development and usability study. JMIR mHealth uHealth **8**(4), e16507 (2020). https://doi.org/10.2196/16507
49. Nouri, R., Niakan Kalhori, S.R., Ghazisaeedi, M., Marchand, G., Yasini, M.: Criteria for assessing the quality of mHealth apps: a systematic review. J. Am. Med. Inform. Assoc. **25**(8), 1089–1098 (2018). https://doi.org/10.1093/jamia/ocy050
50. BinDhim, N.F., Hawkey, A., Trevena, L.: A systematic review of quality assessment methods for smartphone health apps. Telemed. e-Health **21**(2), 97–104 (2014). https://doi.org/10.1089/tmj.2014.0088
51. Jake-Schoffman, D.E., et al.: Methods for evaluating the content usability, and efficacy of commercial mobile health apps. JMIR mHealth uHealth **5**(12), e8758 (2017). https://doi.org/10.2196/mhealth.8758
52. Paglialonga, A., Lugo, A., Santoro, E.: An overview on the emerging area of identification, characterization, and assessment of health apps. J. Biomed. Inform. **83**, 97–102 (2018). https://doi.org/10.1016/j.jbi.2018.05.017
53. Sensors Overview. Android Developers. https://developer.android.com/guide/topics/sensors/sensors_overview?hl=it. Accessed 25 June 2021
54. Bluetooth Low Energy. Android Developers. https://developer.android.com/guide/topics/connectivity/bluetooth/ble-overview?hl=it. Accessed 25 June 2021
55. C. for D. and R. Health, 'Device Software Functions Including Mobile Medical Applications', FDA, 9 September 2020. https://www.fda.gov/medical-devices/digital-health-center-excell

ence/device-software-functions-including-mobile-medical-applications. Accessed 2 April 2021
56. 'EUR-Lex- - L:2017:117:TOC - EN - EUR-Lex'. https://eur-lex.europa.eu/legal-content/EN/TXT/?uri=OJ:L:2017:117:TOC. Accessed 2 April 2021
57. Keutzer, L., Simonsson, U.S.: Medical device apps: an introduction to regulatory affairs for developers. JMIR mHealth uHealth **8**(6), e17567 (2020). https://doi.org/10.2196/17567
58. Shull, P.B., Jirattigalachote, W., Hunt, M.A., Cutkosky, M.R., Delp, S.L.: Quantified self and human movement: a review on the clinical impact of wearable sensing and feedback for gait analysis and intervention. Gait Posture **40**(1), 11–19 (2014). https://doi.org/10.1016/j.gaitpost.2014.03.189
59. Singh, I.: Assessment and management of older people in the general hospital setting. Challenges Elder Care (2016). https://doi.org/10.5772/64294
60. Mudge, A.M., O'Rourke, P., Denaro, C.P.: Timing and risk factors for functional changes associated with medical hospitalization in older patients. J. Gerontol. A Biol. Sci. Med. Sci. **65**(8), 866–872 (2010). https://doi.org/10.1093/gerona/glq069
61. Mlinac, M.E., Feng, M.C.: Assessment of activities of daily living, self-care, and independence. Arch. Clin. Neuropsychol. **31**(6), 506–516 (2016). https://doi.org/10.1093/arclin/acw049
62. Albert, M.S., et al.: The diagnosis of mild cognitive impairment due to Alzheimer's disease: recommendations from the National Institute on Aging-Alzheimer's Association workgroups on diagnostic guidelines for Alzheimer's disease. Alzheimers Dement **7**(3), 270–279 (2011). https://doi.org/10.1016/j.jalz.2011.03.008
63. Liu, C.-J., Chang, W.-P., Chang, M.C.: Occupational therapy interventions to improve activities of daily living for community-dwelling older adults: a systematic review. Am. J. Occup. Ther. **72**(4), pp. 7204190060p1–7204190060p11 (2018). https://doi.org/10.5014/ajot.2018.031252
64. Katz, S., Downs, T.D., Cash, H.R., Grotz, R.C.: Progress in development of the index of ADL. Gerontologist **10**(1), 20–30 (1970). https://doi.org/10.1093/geront/10.1_part_1.20
65. Mahoney, F.I., Barthel, D.W.: Functional evaluation: the Barthel index. Md. State Med. J. **14**, 61–65 (1965)
66. Keith, R.A., Granger, C.V., Hamilton, B.B., Sherwin, F.S.: The functional independence measure: a new tool for rehabilitation. Adv. Clin. Rehabil. **1**, 6–18 (1987)
67. Desai, A.K., Grossberg, G.T., Sheth, D.N.: Activities of daily living in patients with dementia: clinical relevance, methods of assessment and effects of treatment. CNS Drugs **18**(13), 853–875 (2004). https://doi.org/10.2165/00023210-200418130-00003
68. Jekel, K., et al.: Mild cognitive impairment and deficits in instrumental activities of daily living: a systematic review. Alzheimers Res. Ther. **7**(1), 17 (2015). https://doi.org/10.1186/s13195-015-0099-0
69. Graessel, E., Viegas, R., Stemmer, R., Küchly, B., Kornhuber, J., Donath, C.: The Erlangen test of activities of daily living: first results on reliability and validity of a short performance test to measure fundamental activities of daily living in dementia patients. Int. Psychogeriatr. **21**(1), 103–112 (2009). https://doi.org/10.1017/S1041610208007710
70. Freedson, P., Bowles, H.R., Troiano, R., Haskell, W.: Assessment of physical activity using wearable monitors: recommendations for monitor calibration and use in the field. Med. Sci. Sports Exerc. **44**(1 Suppl 1), S1–S4 (2012). https://doi.org/10.1249/MSS.0b013e3182399b7e
71. Ehn, M., Eriksson, L.C., Åkerberg, N., Johansson, A.-C.: Activity monitors as support for older persons' physical activity in daily life: qualitative study of the users' experiences. JMIR mHealth uHealth **6**(2), e8345 (2018). https://doi.org/10.2196/mhealth.8345
72. Schrack, J.A., et al.: Assessing the "physical cliff": detailed quantification of age-related differences in daily patterns of physical activity. J. Gerontol. A Biol. Sci. Med. Sci. **69**(8), 973–979 (2014). https://doi.org/10.1093/gerona/glt199
73. Roeing, K.L., Hsieh, K.L., Sosnoff, J.J.: A systematic review of balance and fall risk assessments with mobile phone technology. Arch. Gerontol. Geriatr. **73**, 222–226 (2017). https://doi.org/10.1016/j.archger.2017.08.002

74. Nevitt, M.C., Cummings, S.R., Kidd, S., Black, D.: Risk factors for recurrent nonsyncopal falls. A prospective study. JAMA **261**(18), 2663–2668 (1989)
75. Podsiadlo, D., Richardson, S.: The timed "Up & Go": a test of basic functional mobility for frail elderly persons. J. Am. Geriatr. Soc. **39**(2), 142–148 (1991). https://doi.org/10.1111/j.1532-5415.1991.tb01616.x
76. Lord, S.R., Rogers, M.W., Howland, A., Fitzpatrick, R.: Lateral stability, sensorimotor function and falls in older people. J. Am. Geriatr. Soc. **47**(9), 1077–1081 (1999). https://doi.org/10.1111/j.1532-5415.1999.tb05230.x
77. Berg, K.O., Wood-Dauphinee, S.L., Williams, J.I., Maki, B.: Measuring balance in the elderly: validation of an instrument. Can. J. Public Health **83**(Suppl 2), S7-11 (1992)
78. Peters, D.M., Fritz, S.L., Krotish, D.E.: Assessing the reliability and validity of a shorter walk test compared with the 10 m walk test for measurements of gait speed in healthy, older adults. J. Geriatr. Phys. Ther. **36**(1), 24–30 (2013). https://doi.org/10.1519/JPT.0b013e318248e20d
79. Bohannon, R.W.: Reference values for the five-repetition sit-to-stand test: a descriptive meta-analysis of data from elders. Percept. Mot. Skills **103**(1), 215–222 (2006). https://doi.org/10.2466/pms.103.1.215-222
80. Jonkman, N.H., van Schooten, K.S., Maier, A.B., Pijnappels, M.: eHealth interventions to promote objectively measured physical activity in community-dwelling older people. Maturitas **113**, 32–39 (2018). https://doi.org/10.1016/j.maturitas.2018.04.010
81. Nunes, F., Silva, P.A., Cevada, J., Correia Barros, A., Teixeira, L.: User interface design guidelines for smartphone applications for people with Parkinson's disease. Univ Access. Inf. Soc. **15**(4), 659–679 (2016). https://doi.org/10.1007/s10209-015-0440-1
82. Gabyzon, M.E., Chiari, L., Laufer, S., Corzani, M., Danial-Saad, A.: Evaluation of touch technology for the aging population. In: 2019 International Conference on Virtual Rehabilitation (ICVR), July 2019, pp. 1–6. https://doi.org/10.1109/ICVR46560.2019.8994539
83. Bravell, M.E., Zarit, S.H., Johansson, B.: Self-reported activities of daily living and performance-based functional ability: a study of congruence among the oldest old. Eur. J. Ageing **8**(3), 199–209 (2011). https://doi.org/10.1007/s10433-011-0192-6
84. Bhidayasiri, R., Martinez-Martin, P.: Chapter Six—Clinical assessments in Parkinson's disease: scales and monitoring. In: Bhatia, K.P., Chaudhuri, K.R., Stamelou, M. (eds.) International Review of Neurobiology, vol. 132, pp. 129–182. Academic Press (2017). https://doi.org/10.1016/bs.irn.2017.01.001
85. Monje, M.H.G., Foffani, G., Obeso, J., Sánchez-Ferro, Á.: New sensor and wearable technologies to aid in the diagnosis and treatment monitoring of Parkinson's disease. Annu. Rev. Biomed. Eng. **21**(1), 111–143 (2019). https://doi.org/10.1146/annurev-bioeng-062117-121036
86. Rovini, E., Maremmani, C., Cavallo, F.: How wearable sensors can support Parkinson's disease diagnosis and treatment: a systematic review. Front. Neurosci. **11**, 555 (2017). https://doi.org/10.3389/fnins.2017.00555
87. Giuffrida, J.P., Riley, D.E., Maddux, B.N., Heldman, D.A.: Clinically deployable Kinesia technology for automated tremor assessment. Mov. Disord. Official J. Mov. Disord. Soc. **24**(5), 723–730 (2009). https://doi.org/10.1002/mds.22445
88. Pulliam, C.L., Heldman, D.A., Orcutt, T.H., Mera, T.O., Giuffrida, J.P., Vitek, J.L.: Motion sensor strategies for automated optimization of deep brain stimulation in Parkinson's disease. Parkinsonism Relat. Disord. **21**(4), 378–382 (2015). https://doi.org/10.1016/j.parkreldis.2015.01.018
89. Morris, T.R., et al.: A comparison of clinical and objective measures of freezing of gait in Parkinson's disease. Parkinsonism Relat. Disord. **18**(5), 572–577 (2012). https://doi.org/10.1016/j.parkreldis.2012.03.001
90. Moore, S.T., MacDougall, H.G., Ondo, W.G.: Ambulatory monitoring of freezing of gait in Parkinson's disease. J. Neurosci. Methods **167**(2), 340–348 (2008). https://doi.org/10.1016/j.jneumeth.2007.08.023
91. Palmerini, L., Rocchi, L., Mellone, S., Valzania, F., Chiari, L.: Feature selection for accelerometer-based posture analysis in Parkinson's disease. IEEE Trans. Inf Technol. Biomed. **15**(3), 481–490 (2011). https://doi.org/10.1109/TITB.2011.2107916

92. Mellone, S., Tacconi, C., Chiari, L.: Validity of a Smartphone-based instrumented timed up and go. Gait Posture **36**(1), 163–165 (2012). https://doi.org/10.1016/j.gaitpost.2012.02.006
93. Linares-del Rey, M., Vela-Desojo, L., Cano-de la Cuerda, R.: Mobile phone applications in Parkinson's disease: a systematic review. Neurología (English Edition) **34**(1), 38–54 (2019). https://doi.org/10.1016/j.nrleng.2018.12.002
94. Lopane, G., Mellone, S., Corzani, M., et al.: Supervised versus unsupervised technology-based levodopa monitoring in Parkinson's disease: an intrasubject comparison. J. Neurol. **265**(6), 1343–1352 (2018). https://doi.org/10.1007/s00415-018-8848-1
95. Arora, S., et al.: Detecting and monitoring the symptoms of Parkinson's disease using smartphones: a pilot study. Parkinsonism Relat. Disord. **21**(6), 650–653 (2015). https://doi.org/10.1016/j.parkreldis.2015.02.026
96. Lakshminarayana, R., et al.: Using a smartphone-based self-management platform to support medication adherence and clinical consultation in Parkinson's disease. NPJ Parkinson's Disease **3**(1) (2017). https://doi.org/10.1038/s41531-016-0003-z
97. Gatsios, D., et al.: Feasibility and utility of mHealth for the remote monitoring of Parkinson Disease: ancillary study of the PD_manager randomized controlled trial. JMIR mHealth uHealth **8**(6), e16414 (2020). https://doi.org/10.2196/16414
98. Cano-de-la-Cuerda, R., et al.: Theories and control models and motor learning: clinical applications in neurorehabilitation. Neurología (English Edition) **30**(1), 32–41 (2015). https://doi.org/10.1016/j.nrleng.2011.12.012
99. Sánchez Rodríguez, M.T., Collado Vázquez, S., Martín Casas, P., Cano de la Cuerda, R.: Neurorehabilitation and apps: a systematic review of mobile applications. Neurologia (Barcelona, Spain) **33**(5), 313–326 (2018). https://doi.org/10.1016/j.nrl.2015.10.005
100. Intiso, D., et al.: Rehabilitation strategy in the elderly. J. Nephrol. **25**(Suppl 19), S90-95 (2012). https://doi.org/10.5301/jn.5000138
101. American College of Sports Medicine: In: Ehrman, J.K., Liguori, G., Magal, M., Riebe, D. (eds.) ACSM's Guidelines for Exercise Testing and Prescription (2018)
102. Segev-Jacubovski, O., Herman, T., Yogev-Seligmann, G., Mirelman, A., Giladi, N., Hausdorff, J.M.: The interplay between gait, falls and cognition: can cognitive therapy reduce fall risk? Exp. Rev. Neurother. **11**(7), 1057–1075 (2011). https://doi.org/10.1586/ern.11.69
103. Nelson, M.E., et al.: Physical activity and public health in older adults: recommendation from the American College of Sports Medicine and the American Heart Association. Med. Sci. Sports Exerc. **39**(8), 1435–1445 (2007). https://doi.org/10.1249/mss.0b013e3180616aa2
104. Boulton, E., et al.: Implementing behaviour change theory and techniques to increase physical activity and prevent functional decline among adults aged 61–70: the PreventIT project. Prog. Cardiovasc. Dis. **62**(2), 147–156 (2019). https://doi.org/10.1016/j.pcad.2019.01.003
105. Taraldsen, K., et al.: Protocol for the PreventIT feasibility randomised controlled trial of a lifestyle-integrated exercise intervention in young older adults. BMJ Open **9**(3), e023526 (2019). https://doi.org/10.1136/bmjopen-2018-023526
106. Lees, A.J., Hardy, J., Revesz, T.: Parkinson's disease. Lancet (London, England) **373**(9680), 2055–2066 (2009). https://doi.org/10.1016/S0140-6736(09)60492-X
107. Sprenger, F., Poewe, W.: Management of motor and non-motor symptoms in Parkinson's disease. CNS Drugs **27**(4), 259–272 (2013). https://doi.org/10.1007/s40263-013-0053-2
108. Lyons, K.E., Pahwa, R., Troster, A.I., Koller, W.C.: A comparison of Parkinson's disease symptoms and self-reported functioning and well being. Parkinsonism Relat. Disord. **3**(4), 207–209 (1997). https://doi.org/10.1016/s1353-8020(97)00021-7
109. Bloem, B.R., van Vugt, J.P., Beckley, D.J.: Postural instability and falls in Parkinson's disease. Adv. Neurol. **87**, 209–223 (2001)
110. Seppi, K., et al.: The movement disorder society evidence-based medicine review update: treatments for the non-motor symptoms of Parkinson's disease. Mov. Disord. Official J. Mov. Disord. Soc. **26**(Suppl 3), S42-80 (2011). https://doi.org/10.1002/mds.23884
111. Goetz, C.G., Pal, G.: Initial management of Parkinson's disease. BMJ (Clinical research ed.) **349**, g6258 (2014). https://doi.org/10.1136/bmj.g6258

112. Abbruzzese, G., Marchese, R., Avanzino, L., Pelosin, E.: Rehabilitation for Parkinson's disease: current outlook and future challenges. Parkinsonism Relat. Disord. **22**(Suppl 1), S60-64 (2016). https://doi.org/10.1016/j.parkreldis.2015.09.005
113. Nonnekes, J., Nieuwboer, A.: Towards personalized rehabilitation for gait impairments in Parkinson's disease. J. Parkinsons Dis. **8**(Suppl 1), S101–S106. https://doi.org/10.3233/JPD-181464
114. Bloem, B.R., de Vries, N.M., Ebersbach, G.: Nonpharmacological treatments for patients with Parkinson's disease. Mov. Disord. **30**(11), 1504–1520 (2015). https://doi.org/10.1002/mds.26363
115. Lee, S.J., Yoo, J.Y., Ryu, J.S., Park, H.K., Park, H.K., Chung, S.J.: The effects of visual and auditory cues on freezing of gait in patients with Parkinson disease. Am. J. Phys. Med. Rehabil. **91**(1), 2–11 (2012). https://doi.org/10.1097/PHM.0b013e31823c7507
116. Morris, M.E.: Locomotor training in people with Parkinson disease. Phys. Ther. **86**(10), 1426–1435 (2006). https://doi.org/10.2522/ptj.20050277
117. Morris, M.E., Iansek, R., Galna, B.: Gait festination and freezing in Parkinson's disease: pathogenesis and rehabilitation. Mov. Disord. **23**(Suppl 2), S451-460 (2008). https://doi.org/10.1002/mds.21974
118. Ferrazzoli, D., Ortelli, P., Madeo, G., Giladi, N., Petzinger, G.M., Frazzitta, G.: Basal ganglia and beyond: the interplay between motor and cognitive aspects in Parkinson's disease rehabilitation. Neurosci. Biobehav. Rev. **90**, 294–308 (2018). https://doi.org/10.1016/j.neubiorev.2018.05.007
119. Redgrave, P., et al.: Goal-directed and habitual control in the basal ganglia: implications for Parkinson's disease. Nat. Rev. Neurosci. **11**(11), 760–772 (2010). https://doi.org/10.1038/nrn2915
120. Shine, J.M., et al.: Abnormal patterns of theta frequency oscillations during the temporal evolution of freezing of gait in Parkinson's disease. Clin. Neurophysiol. **125**(3), 569–576 (2014). https://doi.org/10.1016/j.clinph.2013.09.006
121. Arnulfo, G., et al.: Phase matters: a role for the subthalamic network during gait. PLOS ONE **13**(6), e0198691, giu 2018. https://doi.org/10.1371/journal.pone.0198691
122. Pozzi, N.G., et al.: Freezing of gait in Parkinson's disease reflects a sudden derangement of locomotor network dynamics. Brain **142**(7), 2037–2050 (2019). https://doi.org/10.1093/brain/awz141
123. Sánchez-Ferro, Á., Maetzler, W.: Advances in sensor and wearable technologies for Parkinson's disease. Mov. Disord. **31**(9), 1257 (2016). https://doi.org/10.1002/mds.26746
124. Ginis, P., et al.: Feasibility and effects of home-based smartphone-delivered automated feedback training for gait in people with Parkinson's disease: a pilot randomized controlled trial. Parkinsonism Relat. Disord. **22**, 28–34 (2016). https://doi.org/10.1016/j.parkreldis.2015.11.004
125. Ginis, P., Heremans, E., Ferrari, A., Dockx, K., Canning, C.G., Nieuwboer, A.: Prolonged walking with a wearable system providing intelligent auditory input in people with Parkinson's disease. Frontiers Neurol. **8** (2017). https://doi.org/10.3389/fneur.2017.00128
126. Ginis, P., Heremans, E., Ferrari, A., Bekkers, E.M.J., Canning, C.G., Nieuwboer, A.: External input for gait in people with Parkinson's disease with and without freezing of gait: one size does not fit all. J. Neurol. **264**(7), 1488–1496 (2017). https://doi.org/10.1007/s00415-017-8552-6
127. Ahn, D., et al.: Smart gait-aid glasses for Parkinson's disease patients. IEEE Trans. Biomed. Eng. **64**(10), 2394–2402 (2017). https://doi.org/10.1109/TBME.2017.2655344
128. Chong, R., Hyun Lee, K., Morgan, J., Mehta, S.: Closed-loop VR-based interaction to improve walking in Parkinson's disease. J. Nov. Physiother. **1**(1) (2011). https://doi.org/10.4172/2165-7025.1000101
129. Espay, A.J., et al.: At-home training with closed-loop augmented-reality cueing device for improving gait in patients with Parkinson disease. J. Rehabil. Res. Dev. **47**(6), 573–581 (2010)
130. Mancini, M., Smulders, K., Harker, G., Stuart, S., Nutt, J.G.: Assessment of the ability of open- and closed-loop cueing to improve turning and freezing in people with Parkinson's disease. Sci. Rep. **8**(1) (2018). https://doi.org/10.1038/s41598-018-31156-4

131. Keus, S., et al.: European physiotherapy guideline for Parkinson's disease. KNGF/ParkinsonNet, the Netherlands (2014)
132. Nieuwboer, A., Rochester, L., Müncks, L., Swinnen, S.P.: Motor learning in Parkinson's disease: limitations and potential for rehabilitation. Parkinsonism Relat. Disord. **15**, S53–S58 (2009). https://doi.org/10.1016/S1353-8020(09)70781-3
133. Casamassima, F., Ferrari, A., Milosevic, B., Ginis, P., Farella, E., Rocchi, L.: A wearable system for gait training in subjects with Parkinson's disease. Sensors **14**(4), 6229–6246 (2014). https://doi.org/10.3390/s140406229
134. Ferrari, A., Ginis, P., Nieuwboer, A., Greenlaw, R., Muddiman, A., Chiari, L.: Handling gait impairments of persons with Parkinson's disease by means of real-time biofeedback in a daily life environment. In: Chang, C.K., Chiari, L., Cao, Y., Jin, H., Mokhtari, M., Aloulou, H. (eds.) Inclusive Smart Cities and Digital Health, vol. 9677, pp. 250–261. Springer International Publishing, Cham (2016). https://doi.org/10.1007/978-3-319-39601-9_22
135. Wiederhold, B.K.: Time to port augmented reality health apps to smart glasses? Cyberpsychol. Behav. Soc. Netw. **16**(3), 157–158 (2013). https://doi.org/10.1089/cyber.2013.1503
136. McNaney, R., et al.: Exploring the acceptability of google glass as an everyday assistive device for people with Parkinson's. In: Proceedings of the 32nd Annual ACM Conference on Human Factors in Computing Systems—CHI '14, Toronto, Ontario, Canada, pp. 2551–2554 (2014). https://doi.org/10.1145/2556288.2557092
137. Imbesi, S., Corzani, M., Petrocchi, F., Lopane, G., Chiari L., Mincolelli, G.: User-centered design of cues with smart glasses for gait rehabilitation in people with Parkinson's disease: a methodology for the analysis of human requirements and cues effectiveness. In: Advances in Simulation and Digital Human Modeling, pp. 348–358. Cham (2021). https://doi.org/10.1007/978-3-030-79763-8_42
138. Vuzix Blade®. https://www.vuzix.com/products/blade-smart-glasses. Accessed 3 December 2020
139. Dorsey, E.R., et al.: Moving Parkinson care to the home. Mov. Disord. **31**(9), 1258–1262 (2016). https://doi.org/10.1002/mds.26744

IoT-Enabled Smart Elderly Living Environment and Their Autonomy for Ageing Well

An Experience of Co-Design with Elderly People in the HABITAT Project: Improving Older Users' Lifestyle with Assistive Home Systems

Giuseppe Mincolelli, Gian Andrea Giacobone, Michele Marchi, Filippo Petrocchi, and Silvia Imbesi

Abstract The ageing trend involving populations all over the world is focusing Design Research's attention on smart devices addressed to older people with specific needs. The project HABITAT, carried out by a multidisciplinary research team with the participation of several companies, aimed to develop and test a smart platform composed of smart interoperable objects able to adapt themselves to satisfy the user's necessities. The final objective of the project was the realization of an assistive, safe and reconfigurable environment, able to enhance the person's autonomy in daily activities, postponing the personal necessity of assistance or hospitalization. The project was designed following a User Centered approach involving older users, their relatives and care-givers, and some stakeholders, in the different stages of the design process. Co-Design workshops were practiced to improve the project usability by designing with users' solutions able to satisfy their needs and requirements.

Keywords User centered design · Co-Design · Design for the elderly · Smart system · Smart devices · Assistive environment · Smart device · Internet of Things · HABITAT project

---

G. Mincolelli · G. A. Giacobone · M. Marchi · F. Petrocchi · S. Imbesi (✉)
Inclusive Design Research Unit, Department of Architecture, University of Ferrara, Ferrara, Italy
e-mail: silvia.imbesi@unife.it

G. Mincolelli
e-mail: giuseppe.mincolelli@unife.it

G. A. Giacobone
e-mail: gianandrea.giacobone@unife.it

M. Marchi
e-mail: michele.marchi@unife.it

F. Petrocchi
e-mail: filippo.petrocchi@unife.it

© The Author(s), under exclusive license to Springer Nature Singapore Pte Ltd. 2022
S. Scataglini et al. (eds.), *Internet of Things for Human-Centered Design*,
Studies in Computational Intelligence 1011,
https://doi.org/10.1007/978-981-16-8488-3_12

1 Introduction

Today's world is getting older and older. The aging of the baby boomer generation (Those born between 1946 and 1964) combined with the increased longevity and the decrease of birth rate has created a world more and more populated by a new aged population [1].

In Europe, according to WHO the number of people aged 65 and older is forecast to almost double between 2010 and 2050 and the number of people aged 85 years and older is projected to rise from 14 to 19 million by 2020 and to 40 million by 2050 [2].

This is not just a European but a worldwide problem. In the USA the ageing society comes with several issues that need to be solved by the local authorities. This is the reason why the federal government will spend over two third of its budget on citizens over 65 years old over the next decade [3]. A similar situation is also present in China where the number of older seniors is increasing. According to the United Nations Population Division, in 2000 the people over 65 years old were the 7.0% share of total population with 88 million while in the future there will be an increase of the older people of 10% reaching the amount of 247 million by 2030 [4]. In Australia also, it is expected a rise of older seniors from a current scenario of 13% of the population to a projected 25% in 2051 [1].

This rise of the ageing society involves several problems: According to Jaul and Barron [5] an 85 and older population comes with several problems that can be divided into these categories: normal aging, common diseases, functional, cognitive/psychiatric and social changes. Normal Aging impairments involve Sensory changes (Hearing loss, visual acuity, vestibular function), Muscle Strength and Fat changes (such as: sarcopenia and strength decline), immunosenescence (weaker capacity of the body to fight infection) and urologic changes (Not sterile bladder).Concerning the common and somatic disease, Cardiovascular disease is the most common cause of death among seniors followed by Hypertension, Cancer, Osteoarthritis, Diabetes mellitus, Osteoporosis and multiple chronic conditions. Regarding the physical impairments, elderly mostly suffer of: reduction in the walking speed, often even more reduced by another disease; Mobility disability which often is associated with social isolation, falls and depression; Disabilities in activities in daily living (such as Bathing, use of the toilet); Falls as major morbidity and disability among older adults; Frailty as a special vulnerability to stressors; Incontinence; on the psychological and cognitive side, elderly people suffer from: Cognitive aging (such as Mid-short-term memory loss, word finding difficulty and slower processing speed), Dementia and Depression. Finally, it is important to add the social and environmental impairments with Marriage as important factor to avoid social isolation and a consequent mortality increase.

Considering the progressive increase of elderly people all over the world, the entire landscape of strategies, systems, services and products needs to be redesigned in order to maintain and enhance an inclusive society. This is the reason why several actions are taken into account by different organizations all over the world.

The World Health Organization has elaborated the "Healthy ageing" guideline in order to improve the self-sufficiency of older people to improve their quality of life, making them feel useful in the society and postponing the necessity of hospitalization [6].

Within the frame of Horizon 2020, the European Union has actually invested a great deal of resources in R&D projects regarding ICT for active aging and healthy ageing. The AAL Programme (Advancing Inclusive Health & care solutions for ageing in the new decade) is an example of a co-financed project by the European Commission (through Horizon 2020) and 17 countries until 2020 for an approximate budget of €700 million. Such a program aims to create a better quality of life for older people in the field of Healthy ageing technology and innovation [7].

In a scenario characterized by a progressive increase of elderly people and a consequent demand of innovation to solve the related problems, the Internet of Things technology (IoT) and Artificial Intelligence (AI) seem to be two possible drivers to boost the current shift from a more senior friendly society [8].

Formulated for the first time in 1999 by the English Kevin Ashton, co-founder of the Auto-ID Center in Massachusetts, the Internet of Things (IoT) refers to a process where potentially every object of everyday experience acquires its own identity in the digital world. The idea of IoT is based on "smart objects" interconnected by the internet that are able to exchange, own, collect and process information [9].

A peculiarity of these smart objects lies in their ability to autonomously operate in order to extend their performance by means of used and transmitted data. Furthermore, thanks to Artificial Intelligence, smart objects are also able to process data and implement them in the system to tailor the service to the needs of the user.

Concerning the elderly people, these smart objects can be very significant because they are designed not only for internet experts but also for people, like elderly, that usually are not so keen to use this technology.

This technology can be really significant for them to enhance their daily life from house management to their health monitoring and their social relation in the smart city.

2 The HABITAT Project

Previously described themes, as the ageing populations trend and technological innovations like the IoT, are the starting considerations of the HABITAT project (Home Assistance Basata su IoT per l'Autonomia di Tutti) [10]. HABITAT is a research project funded within the POR FESR 2014–2020 program of the Emilia Romagna Region [11], Italy, which started in April 2016 and was completed in 2019. Authors were part of the multidisciplinary team that faced this project aimed at designing and testing a system of smart objects for the realization of reconfigurable life spaces, for care and monitoring of the elderly in an independent living perspective.

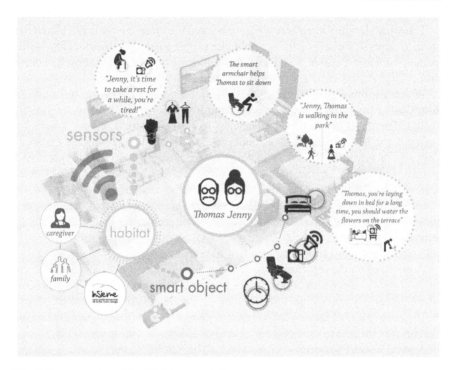

Fig. 1 Representation of HABITAT smart platform

HABITAT integrated innovative technologies as Radio Frequency Identification (RF-ID), wearable electronics, wireless sensor networks (WSN), artificial intelligence (AI). These were used in order to empower some traditional objects or furniture with smartness elements, turning them into smart objects able to interoperate for the realization of assistive environments addressed to older users [12].

Designed smart objects had the purpose to compose an IoT platform able to modify itself in order to adapt progressively to the users' needs, by monitoring usual behaviors and collecting data on the specific person.

Technological solutions adopted in this project aim to give a safe and assistive life space in a short- and long-term perspective to people with specific needs. This in order to allow the ageing person to continue carrying out autonomously his daily life activities, postponing the necessity of full time care-giving or hospitalization [13] (Fig. 1).

2.1 Partners and Purposes

The HABITAT research project was conducted by a multidisciplinary team composed by several institutions.

CIRI ICT (Interdepartmental Center for Industrial Research on Information and Communication Technologies) was the leading partner and had the role of project coordination and management. The participant provided realization criteria of the project scenarios, to realize the ICT infrastructure for the selected use case, and to develop the middleware platform for the management of services.

CIRI SDV (Interdepartmental Center for Industrial Research on Life's Sciences and Health Technologies) was responsible for the selection and the engineering of sensors and actuators. This partner was responsible for specification related to smart objects, for their prototypes and for the realization of algorithms based on data fusion techniques.

TekneHub is a laboratory of Ferrara's Technological Pole in Italy, with a background in product design, interaction design and design-driven innovation, with particular reference to accessibility and social inclusion. TekneHub had the role of designing and realizing working and interoperable devices' prototypes, of verifying the matching between users' requirements and design solutions adopted by the system. This partner had also the responsibility for the verification of the Technology Readiness Level (TRL) of 5 [14].

ASC InSieme is a public authority working for social services for the Union Valli Reno, Lavino and Samoggia, Bologna, Italy. ASC InSieme is involved in activities for social, welfare, health and education for four intervention areas: Children and Families, Adults, Elderly, Disability. In the HABITAT project they had to contribute to the collection of requirements and specifications for application in chosen project scenarios.

Romagna Tech is a member of the High Technology Network of Emilia Romagna Region working in the communication field in relation with industrial research, innovation, technology transfer and dissemination. In the HABITAT project they had the task of spreading and diffusion of the project's results.

Together with the described project partners, several companies of the Emilia Romagna Region were involved, due to their experience and knowledge in the realization of devices. Specifically, companies participating were Cte International (telecommunication), Ergotek (furniture industry), Uniset (telecommunication and electronic), Wiman (information technology), U-Watch (electronic) and mHealth Technologies (mobile health).

Within the HABITAT project, several devices were re-designed in order to interoperate in a smart platform, enriching them with sensors able to collect data on the user and giving them a natural interface for an effective communication with the older person [12].

The developed smart objects were:

- A wall light for indoor localization: A RFID system composed by a reader and multiple active tags to provide indoor localization facilities.
- An armchair to assess sitting posture in real-time, and detect parameters and movements of the users.
- A sort of belt for the collection of information on movements and postures.

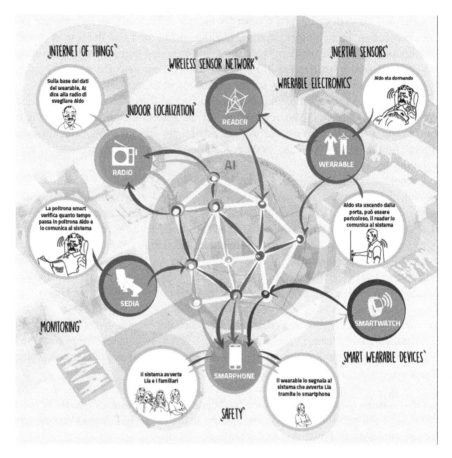

Fig. 2 Schematization of the HABITAT project's smart objects and system

- A wall panel and mobile devices as an interface between the smart system and the final user (Fig. 2).

3 Methodologies

For the purpose of being able to meet the objectives of the project HABITAT, a highly specialized and expert academic and industrial partnership had to be planned.

Specifically, the authors are part of TekneHub—the laboratory of Ferrara Technopole—and have dealt with the part regarding the product and interface design, the platform trial designed in assistive environments, and the definition of the final Technology Readiness Level of the demonstrator.

The first obstacle to tackle was represented by planning a common methodology among several partners. A working methodology that was not only shared by partners, but also able to smooth out and solve any disagreement typical of each sector of specialization, such as language and communication.

On the basis of the range and complexity of the involved users, in terms of needs, necessities and context, the shared methodology defined as User Centered Design was chosen to be applied [15].

Such methodology allows users to be placed at the center of the planning and strategic process; during each phase, the focus is on the user who is involved from the first moments of the project [16].

In the first phase of the research, the Teknehub laboratory was in charge of the analysis of users and needs.

The main users of the HABITAT project were self-sufficient and non-self-sufficient elderly people who live in their own homes and need to safeguard their autonomy, trying to avoid the hospitalization and assistance period. The secondary users and stakeholders taken into account in the project were professional and non-professional caregivers, family members of the elderly, health workers (social workers in public health services, nurses, physiotherapists, etc.), doctors, decision-makers in the social-health sector, etc.

The goal of this phase was to obtain a series of brief statements that best specified and contextualized the real needs of all the involved users [13].

Such activity was carried out thanks to participatory activities between academic partners and users: organization of focus groups, interviews, questionnaires, direct observations. The work led to the filing of about five hundred needs from all the users interviewed. After having listed hierarchically and by importance all these needs, we defined the needs analysis—containing about one hundred needs—which represented a fundamental element for developing the first project briefs.

At this moment, a further planning tool belonging to the design research was used: the Quality Function Deployment (QFD) [17]; a tool born in Japan that allows—by means of a calculation matrix—to relate qualitative data (expressed by needs) with quantitative data (expressed by the tangible characteristics of the smart objects to be created). This part of the work led to the creation of six QFD matrices, one for each smart object (Fig. 3).

The aim of this research phase was to be able to understand which measurable elements and characteristics were most important and influential for satisfying users' needs.

At the same time of this research phase, the first project concepts were developed, thanks to the support of partner companies, as well. The prototypes were then tested by the people who initially participated in the observation and analysis phase. This design tool, called Co-Design, has the merit of being able to tangibly improve the products and the perception of technology in the home environment for elderly people [18]. Therefore, the objective of this participatory methodology is not only a tangible result, but also to develop—specifically concerning elderly users—both empathy and recognition between smart objects and users; as well as to make people feel themselves less lonely, involving them in the creative process with the aim of triggering virtuous and resilient dynamics.

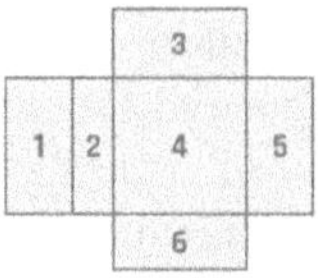

QUALITY FUNCTION DEPLOYMENT	RELEVANCE OF NEEDS	% RELEVANCE OF NEEDS	1. PRODUCT SPECIFICATION	2. PRODUCT SPECIFICATION	3. PRODUCT SPECIFICATION	4. PRODUCT SPECIFICATION	5. PRODUCT SPECIFICATION	6. PRODUCT SPECIFICATION	7. PRODUCT SPECIFICATION	8. PRODUCT SPECIFICATION	9. PRODUCT SPECIFICATION	10. PRODUCT SPECIFICATION	1. COMPETITOR	2. COMPETITOR	3. COMPETITOR	4. COMPETITOR	5. COMPETITOR
1. COSTUMER NEED	4	6%	0	9	0	0	0	3	1	0	0	3	2	1	3	3	3
2. COSTUMER NEED	1	1%	0	3	0	0	0	3	0	3	0	0	2	1	1	2	3
3. COSTUMER NEED	5	7%	0	3	3	0	1	3	1	3	3	1	5	3	4	2	4
4. COSTUMER NEED	3	4%	0	3	0	1	0	3	0	1	0	1	2	1	1	3	4
5. COSTUMER NEED	3	4%	0	3	0	9	0	3	0	1	1	3	2	3	3	3	4
6. COSTUMER NEED	2	3%	9	3	3	3	3	1	3	3	3	1	1	1	2	1	2
7. COSTUMER NEED	1	1%	0	3	3	1	1	3	1	3	3	1	1	2	2	3	1
8. COSTUMER NEED	2	3%	0	1	1	1	1	1	0	1	0	1	2	2	3	3	3
9. COSTUMER NEED	4	6%	3	3	3	3	3	1	3	3	3	1	3	3	2	4	5
10. COSTUMER NEED	5	7%	0	9	0	0	0	9	0	1	0	1	3	2	3	4	5
ABSOLUTE TECHNICAL IMPORTANCE			65	280	188	142	68	216	72	164	129	87					
% TECHNICAL IMPORTANCE			5%	20%	13%	10%	5%	15%	5%	12%	9%	6%					

Fig. 3 Structure of the QFD matrices used in the HABITAT project

4 Co-Design Activities

Considering the importance of developing an inclusive and accessible assistive home system for improving lifestyles of older people in their domestic environments, the Habitat project adopted the participatory Co-Design approach for performing two cooperative workshops in collaboration with the main end-users. This allowed the project to involve many older people, as main users, throughout the concept development process.

The scope of the two workshops was to contribute to generation of the final prototypes of the smart objects from the perspective of elderly people, which was significant in defining the morphological and technological aspect of every smart object of the entire home system. In that human-centered approach, the users played the role of experts [19] the idea generation while the design team acted as facilitators by supporting older people in giving shape to their feeling and their ideas, providing prototyping tools for ideation and expression [20].

Both Co-Design workshops were organized with the contribution of ASC Insieme, one of the partners of the Habitat project, which represents a public elderly day-care organization. In fact, all the participatory activities were held at the ASC Insieme's headquarter in Casalecchio di Reno, Bologna, Italy. In order to differentiate the audience and gather numerous insights from a wider perspective of the elderly's demands, the two workshops involved 12 elderly families over 65 years old, including self-sufficient and non-self-sufficient seniors. The families with non-self-sufficient seniors included either an informal caregiver, such as a relative, or a professional health operator. The active participation of older people was fundamental to define proper solutions that would solve the main problems and needs to be encountered at old age [21].

In the first workshop, the activities developed the early concepts of the Habitat home system, in particular defining their functionality and appearance. The idea-generation process was structured around three collaborative round tables, which were constituted of both elderly people and facilitators, each associated with a specific smart object resulting from the research.

By using a brainstorming section and by elaborating many user-journey maps with the participants, the Co-Design activities focused on investigating the elderly's primary needs and frustrations encountered during their everyday living experiences. Furthermore, the use of an empathy map collected the emotional aspects of all the participants, which, in turn, produced useful insights to improve the qualitative characteristics of the overall home system.

The collected data coming from those activities were translated in the form of low-fidelity prototypes (Fig. 1), which were subsequently used to assess the level of acceptance of every smart object. In particular, the new collaborative activities focused on evaluating the wearability of both the inertial and the tracking sensors, the comfort and functions of the smart chair, and the visual aspect of the Habitat's interface (Fig. 4).

At the end of the first workshop, the outcomes were utilized to improve and refine the early concepts. In fact, new updated mid-fidelity prototypes were developed

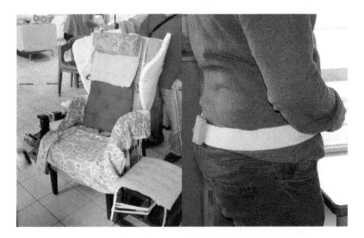

Fig. 4 Two low-fidelity prototypes developed with the older people during the participative prototyping session, in the first Co-Design workshop, at the ASC Insieme's day center, Casalecchio di Reno Bologna, Italy

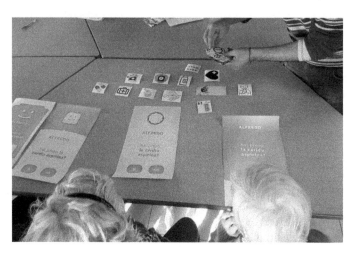

Fig. 5 Participants of the second co-design workshop while configuring, with the support of a moderator, the graphical elements of the Habitat's interface according to their necessities. ASC Insieme's day center, Casalecchio di Reno Bologna, Italy

according to the most important considerations drawn from older people's expectations. After this, those prototypes were analyzed—with the same elderly families of the first participatory activities—in the second Co-Design workshop, in order to evaluate correspondence of the new smart objects' improvements with the real expectations of the elderly.

The main activities involved observing older people while interacting with the prototypes to improve the functional and morphological properties of every expected smart object. This practice allowed the research team to discover some users' latent needs that could be elicited from their behavior [22] (Fig. 5).

A specific participatory activity evaluated also the usability and accessibility of the Habitat's interface. In fact, the design team proposed to the elderly different possible configurations of the interface and they asked them to identify those graphical elements (for example colors, icons and labels) that, for them, would make the contents or the visual notifications clearly readable and understandable for all (Fig. 2). The feedback was used to refine the graphical aspect and the main functions of the interface. Moreover, at the end of the second Co-Design workshop, any criticality indicated by the older people that, for them, was presented on each smart object, was examined and utilized to review the prototypes.

In order to estimate the technological maturity of the entire project, the teamwork developed a working version of Habitat system—based on all the users' consideration gathered in both Co-Design workshops—which was tested in a conclusive usability test [23] conducted by an external expert in a simulated environment and, again, with real older end-users to formally validate the TRL—technology readiness level [24] of the entire research project.

The final activities were held at one of the ASC Insieme's day-care centers in order to test the smart objects in a real space environment and they involved 19 people who had already been involved in the previous Co-Design phase. The heuristic evaluation analysis [25] and direct interviews were the two main methods adopted by the external expert to assess the Habitat system. In particular, the interviews were divided in two categories of users, self-sufficient and non-self-sufficient seniors, in order to acquire several opinions about the use and the experience of Habitat from two different user's perspectives. In fact, the direct interviews were structured by following this order: 7 self-sufficient seniors; 4 couples composed of caregivers and non-self-sufficient seniors; 2 caregivers; 2 non-self-sufficient seniors.

At the end of the entire testing session, all users were able to experience the Habitat system and report their considerations to the external expert who processed and collected every data into a final report, which, in turn, would be used as guidelines to make conclusive refinements to the final high-fidelity prototypes. The report also provided positive feedback for every smart object, which was significant—from the users' perspective—to confirm the high level of acceptance of the Habitat system.

Indeed, the testers considered both the inertial and the tracking sensors pleasant to wear and not invasive, the smart chair relaxing and comfortable, the indoor localization system well designed and suitable with the home furniture, and the interface easy-to-use, pleasant and not intrusive in the domestic environment.

Moreover, all smart objects were very appreciated for their high level of customization, in terms of colors, fabrics (in the case of the wearable sensors) and message dialog and notifications setting (regarding the digital interface).

5 Conclusions

The project was concluded in 2019 with the exposition of developed smart solutions in the fair Exposanità in Bologna, Italy. The research results have been disseminated through the publication of several scientific papers in specialized scientific journals and through participation in various conferences and their proceedings.

Feedbacks from users, stakeholders and the scientific community were encouraging, proving how the applied User Centered methodology is effective and flexible. This is mainly due to the possibility of using it in different contexts and with different kinds of users characterized by peculiar necessities not common to the majority of the population.

In conclusion, regarding the older people's involvement in the design process, the Co-Design activities permitted the conception and development of smart objects with the main end-users throughout the entire design development process. The active participation of the older people was fundamental to receive the right feedback to iteratively refine and improve the expected smart objects, based on the real end-users exigencies.

The chance of designing, testing and evaluating in collaboration with the end-users the various prototypes made the design team more aware of older users' ways of approaching and perceiving smart devices. This permitted the functionality and the appearance of every smart object to be more effective, suitable and close to the different needs—for instance habits, limitations or capabilities—expressed by the older people. The final considerations gathered from the usability test confirmed the objectives set at the beginning of the research project.

References

1. Fatima, K., Moridpour, S.: Measuring public transport accessibility for elderly. In: MATEC Web of Conferences, vol. 259, p. 03006. EDP Sciences (2019)
2. WHO. Active ageing policy framework (2012). Retrieved from https://www.who.int/ageing/publications/active_ageing/en/
3. Super, N.: Three trends shaping the politics of aging in America. Innov. Aging **4**(Suppl 1), 680 (2020)
4. Zheng, W., Yao, Y., Liu, Z., Lyu, Y.: Healthy ageing in China: expanding health protection for the middle-age and elderly [Ebook]. Swiss Re Institute (2020)
5. Jaul, E., Barron, J.: Age-related diseases and clinical and public health implications for the 85 years old and over population. Front. Public Health **5**, 335 (2017)
6. WHO. World Health Organization: World Report on Aging and Health. WHO Press, Geneve (2015)
7. AAL Programme (2020). Retrieved 14 April 2021, from http://www.aal-europe.eu/about/
8. Feng, Z., Liu, C., Guan, X., Mor, V.: China's rapidly aging population creates policy challenges in shaping a viable long-term care system. Health Aff. **31**(12), 2764–2773 (2012)
9. Ashton, K.: That 'internet of things' thing. RFID J **22**(7), 97–114 (2009)
10. Paolini, G., et al.: Human-centered design of a smart "wireless sensor network environment" enhanced with movement analysis system and indoor positioning qualifications. In: 2017 IEEE MTT-S International Microwave Workshop Series on Advanced Materials and Processes for RF and THz Applications (IMWS-AMP), 2017, pp. 1–3. https://doi.org/10.1109/IMWS-AMP.2017.8247434.
11. Emilia Romagna Region, POR-FESR 2016–2020. Retrieved 28 April 2021, from https://fesr.regione.emilia-romagna.it/por-fesr
12. Borelli, E., Paolini, G., Antoniazzi, F., Barbiroli, M., Benassi, F., Chesani, F., Chiari, L., Fantini, M., Fuschini, F., Galassi, A., Giacobone, G.A., Imbesi, S., Licciardello, M., Loreti, D., Marchi, M., Masotti, D., Mello, P., Mellone, S., Mincolelli, G., Raffaelli, C., Roffia, L., Salmon Cinotti, T., Tacconi, C., Tamburini, P., Zoli, M., Costanzo, A.: HABITAT: An IoT solution for independent elderly. Sensors **19**, 1258 (2019). https://doi.org/10.3390/s19051258
13. Mincolelli, G., Marchi, M., Imbesi, S.: Inclusive design for ageing people and the Internet of Things: understanding needs. In: Di Bucchianico, G., Kercher, P., (eds.) Advances in Design for Inclusion. AHFE 2017. Advances in Intelligent Systems and Computing, vol. 587. Springer, Cham (2018). https://doi.org/10.1007/978-3-319-60597-5_9
14. Mincolelli, G., et al.: Inclusive design of wearable smart objects for older users: design principles for combining technical constraints and human factors. In: Di Bucchianico G. (ed) Advances in Design for Inclusion. AHFE 2018. Advances in Intelligent Systems and Computing, vol. 776. Springer, Cham (2019). https://doi.org/10.1007/978-3-319-94622-1_31
15. ISO 13407, Human-centred design processes for interactive systems, ISO, 1999.
16. Mincolelli, G., Imbesi, S., Marchi, M.: Design for the active ageing and autonomy: the role of industrial design in the development of the "Habitat" IOT project. In: Di Bucchianico, G., Kercher, P., (eds.) Advances in Design for In-clusion. AHFE 2017. Advances in Intelligent Systems and Computing, vol 587, Springer (2018)

17. Mincolelli, G., Imbesi, S., Zallio, M.: Collaborative quality function deployment. a methodology for enabling co-design research practice. In: Di Bucchianico, G. (ed.) Advances in Design for Inclusion. AHFE 2019. Advances in Intelligent Systems and Computing, vol. 954. Springer, Cham (2020). https://doi.org/10.1007/978-3-030-20444-0_9
18. Imbesi, S., Mincolelli, G., Petrocchi, F.: How to enhance aging people's wellness by means of human centered and co-design methodology. In: Cassenti, D., Scataglini, S., Rajulu, S., Wright, J. (eds.) Advances in Simulation and Digital Human Modeling. AHFE 2020. Advances in Intelligent Systems and Computing, vol. 1206. Springer, Cham (2021). https://doi.org/10.1007/978-3-030-51064-0_28
19. Codarin, S., Giacobone, G.A.: User Redemption: l'evoluzione dei non-designer nella progettazione contemporanea. Officina* **27**, 54–57 (2019)
20. Sanders, E.B.-N., Stapper, P.J.: Co-creation and the new landscapes of design. Int. J. CoCreation Des. Arts **4**(1):Design Participation(-s): 5–18
21. Hendriks Niels, Slegers, K., Duysburgh, P.: Co-Design with people living with cognitive and sensory impairments. Int. J. CoCreation Des. Arts **11**(1), (2015). https://doi.org/10.1080/15710880701875068
22. Brown, T.: Change by design: how design thinking transforms organizations and inspires innovation. Harper Collins, New York (2015)
23. Mincolelli, G., Imbesi, S., Marchi, M., Giacobone, G.A.: New domestic healthcare. Co-designing assistive technologies for autonomous ageing at home. Int. J. Aspects Des. **22**(1), 503–516 (2019)
24. Héder, M.: From NASA to EU: the evolution of the TRL scale in public sector innovation. Innov. J. Public Sector Innov. J. **22**(2), 1–23 (2017)
25. Nielsen, J.: Usability Engineering. AP Professional, Cambridge (1993)

From Driver to Passenger: Exploring New Driving Experiences for Older Drivers in Highly Automated Vehicles

Gian Andrea Giacobone

Abstract The progressive advancement of highly automated vehicles is expected to make self-mobility more accessible and comfortable for the elderly population, because the potentialities of this technology allows older drivers to drive longer and safer. In that case, since autonomous driving is able to disengage drivers from the driving task, it opens a unique opportunity to develop new interactions that could completely change the use and the experience of traveling. Considering this scenario, the contribution explores the design space related to autonomous driving, specifically investigating new driving experiences that can be aligned with the older drivers' necessities, in order to support them in maintaining their self-independence and autonomy as long as possible. Therefore, the paper analyzes some case studies that focus on novel forms of in-car activities and transportation-related services, which, in turn, are trying to offer a new perspective on the use of highly automated technology. In particular, the first two examples focus on changing the perceived cost of traveling by exploring unedited and playful non-driving-related activities. Instead, the other cases focus on redefining the relationship with the space of traveling, by proposing new services that provide to older drivers new exploratory and shareable commuting experiences.

Keywords Autonomous driving · Vehicle automation · Smart mobility · Human–machine interaction · Human–machine interface · Older drivers

1 Introduction

In the last few years, rapid advances in technology have been causing radical changes in the automotive industry. This expects to envision new driving scenarios totally different from the current state-of-the-art, aiming at developing a safer, more comfortable and efficient urban transportation system for our society [1]. In fact, if, until the last two decades, drivers were fully responsible for driving and controlling all vehicle

G. A. Giacobone (✉)
Department of Architecture, University of Ferrara, Ferrara, Italy
e-mail: gcbgnd@unife.it

parameters—so as every behavior conditioned by poor control often led the outcomes to a road accident—nowadays, the human driving control is progressively assisted with sophisticated assistive driving technologies, named Advanced Driver Assistance Systems (ADAS), which help the driver to recover from their driving errors, namely the first causes that provoke road accidents [2, 3].

ADAS are interfaces that support users in the primary task of driving [4]. The Adaptive Cruise Control (ACC) [5], the Lane Keeping Assist System (LKAS) [6] and the collision avoidance assistance [7] are some of the main assistive driving technologies that are already available among various automakers. They are able to intervene directly on the driver's driving operations, to control the vehicle (for example steering, accelerating and breaking) and to prevent the human error during dangerous situations [8].

The main interest in adopting ADAS technology is due to the limited capacity of humans to maintain attention for long periods [9]. In fact, the attentional limitations could have adverse consequences for the drivers' driving performance, because most of the time they can lead to driver inattention. This is because the act of driving is inherently a highly complex skill [10] requiring the sustained monitoring of integrated perceptual and cognitive inputs for monitoring the surrounding environment [11] and for efficiently processing the different perception, decision and reaction operations necessary while driving [12].

Therefore, while ADAS are becoming an indispensable technology for increasing road safety, on the other hand, they are transforming the relationship between the human and the vehicle, resulting in changes regarding the responsibility of the driver [13]. In fact, the automation skill-based control of the vehicle is capable of making urban traveling safer and more efficient than human through its high level of driving precision [14], and this leads consequently to the situation where most parts of the driving tasks can be easily performed by the ADAS, addressing the driver's tasks only to the supervision of the vehicle system [15].

In this case, since the driver can be easily replaced by assistive driving technologies, the upcoming scenario opens new opportunities and benefits for new research studies in the field of human–machine interaction to rethink the entire driving experience.

2 The New Paradigm of Autonomous Driving

On the basis of the above considerations, ADAS technologies, concerning the safety and safeguarding of drivers' lives, have urged the Society of Automotive Engineering (SAE), an international standard developing organization, to define a consistent taxonomy of ADAS by categorizing the level of driving automation through a classification system based on the amount of driver intervention and attentiveness required [16]. Compressively, there are six levels of vehicle automation system, ranging from basic level 0, which refers to the manual driving where a conventional vehicle is driven by a driver without any artificial aid, through to the ultimate level 5, which refers to the full-automated driving where a driver-less car can monitor driving and performing all safety–critical driving controls, under all conditions and with no direct human input.

Autonomous vehicles, also called automated or self-driving vehicles [17], are the final vision of that classification system, in which the high level of automation intends to move the drivers completely out of the loop, progressively changing themselves from error-prone operators into normal passengers, in vehicles controlled by an infallible technology [18, 19]. In this upcoming scenario, the drivers have only the duty to enter the destination and, at most, select the target cruise speed and enjoy their journeys [13], inevitably revealing a new perspective for reconsidering the use and the experience of the automotive vehicles in the future.

Even though this new paradigm is currently a significant research topic that has opened, in the past years, a long debate about new opportunities, it also presents new challenges and questions that self-driving technology will introduce in the field of mobility and urban transportation [20, 21]. Specially, one of the main topics of autonomous driving is focused on the analysis and investigation of new types of interactions between humans and vehicles that will reconsider many aspects related to the role of the autonomous vehicle in the urban context. Some of those aspects refer to the characteristics of the vehicle itself, which will re-evaluate the value of both the time spent in the vehicle and the context in which the travel experience occurs, since the task of driving can be easily replaced with other activities [22].

Hence, autonomous driving is a significant opportunity to foster inclusion since the highly automated systems allow the vehicle to be more accessible to a wider group of people through the conceptual reshaping of the traditional driving experience. This is mainly related to the opportunity to transform driving as an individual, stressful and complex activity into a more relaxing and accessible travel experience. In conclusion, this transformation can provide passengers more comfort, well-being and even more socialization by developing new models of public transportation services that can increase people's autonomy and mobility [23].

3 Older Drivers and the Benefit of Autonomous Driving

One of the most important benefits associated with the adoption of autonomous vehicle is inclusion. In fact, the highly automated systems can offer great opportunities to all people who struggle with mobility, because they provide the ability to travel easily and independently without being able to drive. The most beneficiaries of these technologies are mostly people who cannot drive conventional cars for loss in confidence, for financial reason (for instance people who cannot afford the costs of car ownership), or for problems related to age or health, such as underage travelers, people with permanent or temporary disabilities and the elderly [24].

In the recent years, the last category has aroused great interest among the scientific community, because, due to the increased longevity of worldwide population combined with the decrease of birth rate—the number of people aged 60 years and older is expected to outnumber children younger than 5 years by 2050 [25]—nowadays, the world is increasingly populated by a new aged population [26]. In fact, as reported by United Nations [27], by 2050, the world's population aged 60 years and older is expected to total 2 billion, up from 900 million in 2015. Again, today, people who are aged 80 years or older are 125 million but by 2050, the number will increase to 434 million. For these reasons, the global aging is raising many fundamental questions for policy-makers, which in turn, is leading most of the country to change their sociological, political and economic systems to foster a more age-friendly global environment [25].

Considering aging from the mobility perspective, it is possible to note that the older is the worldwide population, the greater is the number of older drivers on the road. Therefore, investigating this phenomenon is critical to enhance elderly driving activities and to maintain their mobility, which it also impacts to their health and well-being [28]. In fact, the ability of driving allows older people to maintain their independence to move freely within their community environments [29] or to stay engaged in society by accessing social and leisure activities, and important facilities, such as public health and medical services [30]. While, on the contrary, continuing to drive in advanced age—even if some studies suggest that older drivers are not necessarily more dangerous than others [31]—can negatively affect road safety to everyone [32]. Some authors [33, 34] highlight that aging can cause an age-related sensory, cognitive and psychomotor decline, which is the main responsible for having a negative influence on the elderly's safe driving abilities, because it makes them more vulnerable to traffic crashes and collisions. Moreover, a recent study [35] has found that the number of older drivers on the road has increased in the last few years so does the accident rates compared to those provoked by younger drivers.

For this reason, it is important to guarantee a safe urban environment to older people to ensure healthy aging. In fact, driving safely produces many benefits both to mobility and self-independence, which consequently have a great impact even on their physical and psychological well-being [30].

Nevertheless, nowadays, there is not enough awareness on those themes, because many older people, instead of driving independently, prefer to reduce use of the car and the risk of creating accidents by adopting self-regulation strategies that limit themselves to being exposed to particular driving situation that are difficult, for them, to handle [36]. Indeed, the implication of adopting self-regulations in driving may cause drastic losses in personal mobility, which consequently may have negative impacts on the elderly's quality of life, because they lead to phenomena of isolation and, in turn, to many impairments of cognitive status and mental health [34] such as depressiveness [37] and reduced self-esteem [38].

3.1 Healthy and Active Aging for Enhancing Autonomy in Mobility

In order to tackle aging issues, it is important to ensure—even in the field of mobility—an environmental system that is able to foster new innovative solutions for healthy and active aging, aiming at extending life expectancy for all the elderly.

From this point of view, as reported by the WHO—World Health Organization's frameworks [39], producing a supportive environment is one of the potential solutions that enables older people to do what is important to them, despite losses in capacity. Rethinking a more efficient and accessible environment will benefit the independent living of older people, which would consequently improve their quality of life and would implement their physical and mental well-being [40], making them feel contributive and participative in society and postponing the necessity of hospitalization [41]. In order to achieve those goals, it is important guarantee to people to maintain their independence and autonomy as long as possible.

3.2 The Benefits of Autonomous Driving

Nowadays, from a mobility perspective, the development of ADAS technologies can empower the elderly through a supportive environment, specifically addressed to a more accessible mobility. In fact, as touched in the previous sections, the progressive advancement of highly automated vehicles will be, in the next future, a significant element that can support the society by ensuring the elderly to drive autonomously longer and safer [42].

As already investigated by other authors [43], the potential benefits offered by the functionalities of autonomous driving already enable older drivers to keep themselves active and mobile for longer, since ADAS are able to provide adequate driving aids that fill their driving difficulties during their everyday routines. From this point of view, full-automation expects to be a valid solution to ensure the elderly's self-mobility, because the highly automated technology promise self-independence, not only by increasing road safety [17, 44], but also by reducing stress associated to the driving task, which, in turn, will fundamentally change the entire travel experience through several possibilities and solutions. For instance, increasing comfort and facilitating the use of automated vehicles enable older users to travel to a variety of places comfortably but also in specific contextual conditions that they usually avoid, due to their driving ability decline. [45]. These benefits can be provided by offering new typologies of non-driving-related activities during the piloted journey [46]. Among those activities, it is possible to think of new forms of productivity, entertainment, gamification, as well as novel transportation-related or in-car services, which can change the value of time travel, producing, at the same time, a unique and relaxing transportation experience.

The latter also contributes to reshape the driving space to foster social interaction (for example, shared mobility services), to provide new services for commuting but mostly to reduce older people's social margination and loneliness, producing, at the same time, an alternative and comfortable vehicular environment for socializing [21, 47].

4 Case Studies of Inspiring Automated Driving Experiences

Currently, the research studies in human–machine interaction are putting a lot of attention on autonomous vehicles, because the rising of highly automated systems are expected to drastically change the way of interacting between the human and the car [48–50]. For this reason, this paper investigates the new potentialities of driver-less technology, examining those factors that are able to provide to older people accessible mobility, enhancing, at the same time, additional benefits to their independence and well-being.

The studies explore two meaningful macro aspects that characterize the new paradigm of highly automated systems, which—when they are well implemented—are able to enhance the quality of the entire travel experience: the first aspect refers to the time of interaction and the perceived cost of time traveling, which both contribute to develop new types of activities according to the traveling time spent in the vehicle; the second aspect regards the interaction with the space, which contributes to generate new ways of experiencing traveling in the urban context.

Therefore, according to the previous considerations, the contribution focuses on exploring the design space related to autonomous vehicles, specifically investigating on some examples of new driving experiences that give shape to new in-car interactions and services related to the necessities of older drivers. In particular, the paper analyzes some peculiar case studies that explore the implementation of non-driving-related activities through innovative and meaningful perspectives, aiming at initiating a public reflection on the opportunities that autonomous vehicles can offer to improve the quality of older people, beyond the mere aspect of technological performance. Considering the aforementioned levels of driving automation for on-road vehicles, introduced by SAE International [16], all case studies are based on the fourth and fifth levels of automation. This means a situation where the driving performance and the monitoring of the driving environment are totally under the control of the automated driving system.

4.1 Playful and Healthy Non-Driving-Related Activities

One of the main characteristics of highly automated technology is to redefine the perceived cost of time travel, because the characteristics of ADAS allow drivers to replace the task of driving with new typologies of non-driving-related activities [10] during the piloted journey. Although other studies on public transportation show that people generally prefer entertainment or work-related activities [51], the opportunity of exploring autonomous driving through new lenses—such as gamification—fosters the development of more pleasant and joyful interactions but also novel travel experiences based on the elderly's necessities, which refer also to health and leisure time.

Considering this, AutoJam and AutoGym are two interesting and inspiring research studies that focus on unconventional in-car activities. The two projects are parts of the design research series Autoplay, funded by Audi [52], and they explore new dynamics of interaction with passengers during the travel experience to open a reflection of new potential benefits of autonomous vehicles. In particular, AutoJam focuses on entertainment and creativity while AutoGym concentrates on personal health and well-being. Although the prototypes are originally intended for interacting with a general audience, their peculiarities open the chances to adapt all design solutions perfectly to the characteristics and necessities of the elderly.

4.1.1 An In-Car Music Experience

The prototype of AutoJam is an in-car music experience that combines music listening with the game of playing music. Music plays a central role in in-car entertainment. While listening to music is one of the few accepted entertainment activities during driving operations, because it establishes a unique emotional experience of driving [53]. Therefore, in a driver-less scenario, music can provide a more interactive experience by using the concept of gamification. In that case, AutoJam is based on a touch sensitive steering-wheel cover that enables users to play their favorite song as a member of the band, because it can be played as a drum machine. Instead of using a traditional visual display for interacting with the users, the vehicle communicates with them by involving their body through a touch-based interaction. The game provides three types of interaction according to three stages of a driving situation: the idle phase corresponds to a drum mode, the acceleration phase to a free-play mode and the cruise phase to a progress-mode. From the perspective of an older person, this gaming experience is really interesting, because it presents different benefits. The interactive system involves the users in an engaging experience that makes the trip more enjoyable even when stressful or frustrating situations occur, such as traffic. Music rhythm makes the users more aware of the car speed and the surrounding traffic, because it becomes a medium that informs the users of the driving situation. Regarding particular seniors with specific limitations (for example, those who are suffering from mild cognitive impairments), following music rhythms can be a great cognitive training activity and a healthy way to stay active, because the system stimulates people's motor and cognitive skills and also fosters a space of creativity and self-expression through gamification, challenges and a free-play mode. Instead, regarding self-sufficient seniors, the direct connection with the steering wheel provides great benefits to the situational awareness [54] of the inactive drivers, because it stimulates the users to maintain attention on the vehicle's driving operations. Considering this, although this system is conceived for the fourth or fifth level of vehicle automation, facilitating the relationship with the dynamics of driving through this interaction is an essential element for road safety also in the third level of automation, because it facilitates the human driver to take over control of the vehicle when the automated driving system requires to intervene.

4.1.2 An In-Car Fitness System

The second prototype that explores a non-driving-related activities through the use of gamification is the AutoGym project, an in-car fitness system that translates the experience of traveling, in particular the traffic, into an interactive physical exercise program [55]. Driving a car is not the healthiest mode of transportation, because it allows a very limited space for body movements that provide negative effects on the driver, resulting in sitting fatigue and postural defects [52]. On the contrary, doing exercises enables people to prevent negative side effects of inactivity and it can have also a beneficial impact of the general well-being and stress relieve [56]. In order to decrease issues related to the inactivity, the project explores an interactive system for in-car exercises that transform autonomous driving into an active and healthy in-car experience.

With this aim, Autogym motivates the users to perform mini exercises through a game-like interaction by using a spinning machine that can be used by hand. The system requires the user to predict the traffic situation and choose the length of the exercise based on this prediction. Considering this, the length of the exercise is related to a certain amount of spinning turns, which are determined by the driver's prediction. The goal is to complete the spinning turns within the predicted length of time. However, the resistance of the spinning machine varies according to the speed of the car, so the users can spin only when the vehicle drives slowly. For this reason, the users must anticipate the current traffic condition to select the correct time segment, in order to complete the selected workout in time.

In that case, referring to the older users, this prototype is undoubtedly a great opportunity to increase health and well-being among the users even during the travel experience because it provides a supportive environment that incites people to perform physical activity. That particular physical activity also promotes users to maintain a correct heads-up posture, which can reduce motion sickness, usually related to other common non-driving-related activities, such as reading a book or interacting with an electronic device. Moreover, the interactive system can increase trustiness in the automated driving system, because the relationship between physical exercise and driving activity confers to the users a feeling of control over the vehicle's driving operations [13]. This consequently enriches the situational awareness of the drivers, because the system pushes the inactive drivers to unconsciously monitor the automated driving system's performance and speed while they are engaged in the game. In addition, using the car's speed as a playable input during the workout segment can positively reframe the perception of traffic, ensuring a more pleasant and less stressful journey. Connecting users to the vehicle speed can also increase the feeling of autonomy and competency—typically related to the traditional driving experience—because the game, instead of adapting human's activity to the speed of the car, could transform it into a parameter for controlling the driving style of the car even in the full level of automation. This could enable a sort of dialogue with the automated driving system, allowing users to affect the car's behavior through their personal intentions.

4.2 Exploratory and Shareable Commuting Experiences

Another important fact is that highly automated technology is able to redefine the interactions between the vehicle and the context of traveling, specifically regarding commuting and socialization among passengers.

As already mentioned before, making mobility more accessible for older people helps them to increase their engagement in society [57], and to stay connected to their community [30]. Increased level of accessibility reduces also loneliness and social exclusion, increasing, at the same time, psychological well-being, independence and self-determination [58]. For many seniors with decreasing physical and cognitive abilities, mobility can be traditionally supported by using public transportation services as a valid alternative to the private car.

However, poor street and network design and limited transport services might potentially create a sense of anxiety and discomfort to seniors, which, in turn, decrease the perceived levels of transport accessibility [59]. Considering this scenario, the potential benefits of the elderly's mobility can be restricted due to the risk of social exclusion but extended by using the potentialities of the highly automated technology.

Since autonomous vehicles have the opportunity to relieve the older people from the task of driving, the sensation of being out of the loop can be experienced as a loss of control as well as a feeling of reduced competency and autonomy, because the users' intended journeys are completely managed by the highly automated system [60]. Furthermore, the assumption of using an autonomous vehicle for moving people efficiently from a place to another may risk producing new mobility services with characteristics very similar to those presented in traditional public transportation.

This may not resolve the perceived barriers that the elderly already experience in meeting their daily mobility needs while using public services. On the contrary, the value of autonomous driving could build a new perspective for commuting, which would generate a new urban system that would foster a space for conviviality and leisure time—due to the ability of the ASAD to drive a vehicle autonomously—without losing the feeling of independence of traditional vehicles that are usually affected by fixed schedules and routes of the conventional public transport.

Considering this, in the following section, the paper analyzes two project concepts that aim to redesign the experience of commuting by utilizing the potentialities of autonomous driving to make older people safer and more motivated in traveling, according to their necessities.

4.2.1 An Exploratory Navigation Application

A project example that focuses on the theme of commuting is the third prototypes of the AutoPlay series, named AutoRoute, which investigates the relationship between the vehicle and the urban context through a new exploratory travel service. Although the project refers mostly to the work-related activities, commuting can refer to any regular or often repeated traveling between two locations. In both cases, car-based commuting is often perceived as a daily hassle, because, for most of the drivers, it is a stressful routinized driving task [61]. However, autonomous vehicles have the chance to change the commuting experience fundamentally as the highly automated system can provide to the passenger extra time, not only for doing some non-driving-related activities, but also for self-reflection or relaxation.

For this reason, AutoRoute offers a playful navigation and screen-based application that frames commuting as an explorative and self-fulfilling activity, because it enables the users to route the autonomous vehicle through their personal reflections of preferences and point-of-interests. The system works as a two-stage process in the return trip: in the going phase, the users have the opportunity to predefine the route back by selecting interesting tags (such as surrounding point-of interests) and routing corresponding point-of-interests that they want to visit completely in an exploratory mode; in the return phase, based on the time-budget available to the user, the system calculates the best route depending on the point-of-interests that were selected in previous phase. If there are too many point-of-interests for the selected time-budget, the users are asked to review the trip. If the time is larger than the selected point-of-views, the users can immediately route new point-of interests on the go. In that case, the user can route or un-route some point-of-interests spontaneously while the highly automated system is driving, and then, the vehicle immediately adapts the trip to the new route.

Therefore, the project can offer to older people a new tool for redefining their own travel routines with the inspiration to undertake new ways. In fact, Auto Route promotes the exploration of new places or routes by suggesting new point-of-interests during the time trip. This feature can also be capable of increasing awareness about the commuting routine-nature, because it enables the users to avoid repetitive and stressful activities by replacing them with novel and relaxing trips. Moreover, the system offers the feeling of freedom and independence, because older people have the chance to potentially go everywhere and stop or return instantly by spontaneously re-routing their trip, according to their preferences. In that case, although the system is conceived for a fourth or fifth level of automation, it enables users to afford the feeling of independence, because it provides them with a sense of being in control of the vehicle by directly promoting spontaneous decisions—based on the driving context—that change the initial destination decided by the automated driving system.

4.2.2 A Commuting Service for Social Interactions

A second interesting example linked to commuting is Hōyō, a research project developed by the design researcher Alice Buso, in collaboration with Ford Motor Company. Although Hōyō is in a form of a concept, the project offers a promising scenario that rethinks the interaction of the vehicle with the space of the urban context. The project is similar to AutoRoute but it is more addressed in stimulating social relations within citizens.

The project, indeed, envisions a scenario of shared automated transport, based on an on-demand-service. Hōyō offers to older people the freedom to choose their journey according to their preferences, sharing, at the same time, the travel experience with other people who have common interests.

Selecting the trip mates can be performed by a peculiar interface, which, instead of being located in the vehicle, as a normal dashboard, is a pocket and transportable device that can travel with older people as a wearable item. In that way, the device enables users to predefine their trips before interacting directly with the tangible space of the vehicle, which, in turn, extends the experience also within the domestic environment. Older people, indeed, can set up their trips comfortably at home while the intelligent system provides some reminders (such as advising to do not forget personal objects), or useful information (for instance, weather forecast), according to their needs. Hōyō acts also as a pass to open and access into the booked vehicle, in order to increase the feeling of privacy and security among all passengers. When entering in the vehicle, the device can be paired with the vehicle, in order to adapt the functionalities of the car to the elderly's needs, such as playing a specific typology of music, setting a particular light ambient, or providing visual information about the trip. At the end of the journey, users can rate their travel mates according to their preferences so that Hōyō enables them to repeat the experience on the next travel, with the same people who received higher scores.

Therefore, this project provides to older people autonomy and feeling of control on the vehicle, because the traveling system can be easily set up by users based on their intentions. The project also produces a supportive space for conservation that facilitates social interactions among people with common interests, safely and comfortably. This helps older people to stay psychologically active, as the system increases the opportunity to reduce social exclusion, loneliness and depressiveness by supporting them in meeting and socializing with new people. In addition, the system acts as a personal companion, because—according to their needs—it empowers older people's independence by supporting them throughout their travel experience with reminders or suggestions about their journey.

5 Conclusion

As described in the previous sections, the progressive world aging society and the consequent increase of the elderly population are showing the necessity to redesign the current mobility according to the needs and expectations of older population. Among the various new technologies that can assist aging, the development of ADAS systems and the rising of autonomous driving are becoming significant elements that are giving to the current transport system a new perspective. That technology, indeed, can enhance mobility to older people, by providing them, not only a more efficient and safe transportation system, but also several benefits that increase comfort, well-being and social inclusion.

In fact, nowadays, the highly automated systems create new chances to completely redesign the user experience of the vehicle, which, in turn, can support mobility for the elderly by maintaining their self-independence and autonomy as long as possible. This is because, the vehicle—once relieved the elderly from the task of driving—is able to change the way of interacting between the human and the car by providing new non-driving-related activities that enhance a more comfortable and less stressful quality of the entire travel experience and, at the same time, offer new possibilities to increase physical and psychological health of people.

Considering this, the case studies presented in this paper, are great examples of alternative uses of autonomous driving. In fact, the future of fully autonomous driving might suggest a scenario in which inactive passengers only need to enter the destination making their independency of feeling of autonomy quite obsolete qualities. Instead, within the described examples, driver-less technology is able to stimulate active and healthy aging by exploring more active typologies of non-driving-related activities and offers new scenarios of urban mobility that can increase social inclusion, but also the feeling of autonomy and competency by facilitating the relationship between the vehicle's behaviors and the user's actions.

In addition, all projects try to translate the common belief of the car as an extension of the office, by providing meaningful activities beyond entertainment or work. In fact, the first two examples offer two unedited activities that suggest and motivate older people to perform psychological and physical activities while traveling. The second examples propose new traveling experiences that can be used to transform the routine of commuting into an explorative navigation experience or into a space that facilitates social interactions among people. In every case, the examples benefit from situational awareness of the inactive driver, because the users are constantly encouraged to interact with the external context and/or the vehicle's dynamics of driving. This keeps the users unconsciously monitoring the behaviors of the vehicle—even though it is already capable of driving itself—that makes them ready to intervene in case of exceptional take-over-control.

Therefore, highly automated systems present, nowadays, great chances to open a novel design space for experimenting new useful and meaningful interactions that can produce a more age-friendly future for older people. For this reason, the presented automated driving experiences can be a valid starting point to promote further research investigations on autonomous driving beyond the mere aspect of technological or functional performance aiming at discovering new significant activities that enhance accessibility and, at the same time, support a healthy aging by preserving the elderly's autonomy, health and well-being.

References

1. Milakis, D., van Arem, B., van Wee, B.: Policy and society related implications of automated driving: a review of literature and directions for future research. J. Intell. Transp. Syst. **21**, 324–348 (2017). https://doi.org/10.1080/15472450.2017.1291351
2. Stanton, N.A., Salmon, P.M.: Human error taxonomies applied to driving: a generic driver error taxonomy and its implications for intelligent transport systems. Saf. Sci. **47**, 227–237 (2009). https://doi.org/10.1016/j.ssci.2008.03.006
3. Lu, M., Wevers, K., Van Der Heijden, R.: Technical feasibility of advanced driver assistance systems (ADAS) for road traffic safety. Transp. Plan. Technol. **28**, 167–187 (2005). https://doi.org/10.1080/03081060500120282
4. Eskandarian, A.: Fundamentals of driver assistance. In: Eskandarian, A. (ed.) Handbook of Intelligent Vehicles, pp. 491–535. Springer, London (2012). https://doi.org/10.1007/978-0-85729-085-4_19
5. Naranjo, J.E., Gonzalez, C., Garcia, R., DePedro, T.: ACC+Stop&Go maneuvers with throttle and brake fuzzy control. IEEE Trans. Intell. Transp. Syst. **7**, 213–225 (2006). https://doi.org/10.1109/TITS.2006.874723
6. Wu, S.-J., Chiang, H.-H., Perng, J.-W., Chen, C.-J., Wu, B.-F., Lee, T.-T.: The heterogeneous systems integration design and implementation for lane keeping on a vehicle. IEEE Trans. Intell. Transp. Syst. **9**, 246–263 (2008). https://doi.org/10.1109/TITS.2008.922874
7. Eidehall, A., Pohl, J., Gustafsson, F., Ekmark, J.: Toward autonomous collision avoidance by steering. IEEE Trans. Intell. Transp. Syst. **8**, 84–94 (2007). https://doi.org/10.1109/TITS.2006.888606
8. Meschtscherjakov, A., Perterer, N., Trösterer, S., Krischkowsky, A., Tscheligi, M.: The neglected passenger—how collaboration in the car fosters driving experience and safety. In: Meixner, G., Müller, C. (eds.) Automotive User Interfaces, pp. 187–213. Springer, Cham (2017). https://doi.org/10.1007/978-3-319-49448-7_7
9. Driver, J.: A selective review of selective attention research from the past century. Br. J. Psychol. **92**, 53–78 (2001)
10. Ho, C., Spence, C.: The Multisensory Driver: Implications for Ergonomic Car Interface Design (Human Factors in Road and Rail). CRC Press, Boca Raton (2008)
11. Hills, B.L.: Vision, visibility, and perception in driving. Perception **9**, 183–216 (1980). https://doi.org/10.1068/p090183
12. Green, M.: How long does it take to stop? Methodological analysis of driver perception-brake times. Transp. Hum. Factors. **2**, 195–216 (2000). https://doi.org/10.1207/STHF0203_1
13. Terken, J., Levy, P., Wang, C., Karjanto, J., Yusof, N.M., Ros, F., Zwaan, S.: Gesture-based and haptic interfaces for connected and autonomous driving. In: Nunes, I.L. (ed.) Advances in Human Factors and System Interactions, pp. 107–115. Springer, Cham (2017). https://doi.org/10.1007/978-3-319-41956-5_11
14. Cummings, M.M.: Man versus machine or man + machine? IEEE Intell. Syst. **29**, 62–69 (2014). https://doi.org/10.1109/MIS.2014.87
15. Bengler, K.: Driver and driving experience in cars. In: Meixner, G., Müller, C. (eds.) Automotive User Interfaces, pp. 79–94. Springer, Cham (2017). https://doi.org/10.1007/978-3-319-49448-7_3
16. Engineers, S.: Taxonomy and Definitions for Terms Related to On-Road Motor Vehicle Automated Driving Systems (2014). https://doi.org/10.4271/j3016_201401
17. Fagnant, D.J., Kockelman, K.: Preparing a nation for autonomous vehicles: opportunities, barriers and policy recommendations. Transp. Res. Part A Policy Pract. **77**, 167–181 (2015). https://doi.org/10.1016/j.tra.2015.04.003
18. Mirnig, A.G., Trösterer, S., Meschtscherjakov, A., Gärtner, M., Tscheligi, M.: Trust in automated vehicles. i-com. **17**, 79–90 (2018). https://doi.org/10.1515/icom-2017-0031
19. Giacobone, G.A.: Auto Indipendente: l'Interazione Applicata al Veicolo Urbano [Independent car: the interaction applied to the urban vehicle]. Officina*. **23**, 68–71 (2018)

20. Gavanas, N.: Autonomous road vehicles: challenges for urban planning in European cities. Urban Sci. **3**, 61 (2019). https://doi.org/10.3390/urbansci3020061
21. Lipson, H., Kurman, M.: Driverless: Intelligent Cars and the Road Ahead. The MIT Press, Cambridge (2016)
22. Meyer, J., Becker, H., Bösch, P.M., Axhausen, K.W.: Autonomous vehicles: the next jump in accessibilities? Res. Transp. Econ. **62**, 80–91 (2017). https://doi.org/10.1016/j.retrec.2017.03.005
23. Pickford, A., Chung, E.: The shape of MaaS: the potential for MaaS lite. IATSS Res. **43**, 219–225 (2019). https://doi.org/10.1016/j.iatssr.2019.11.006
24. Bradley, M., Langdon, P.M., Clarkson, P.J.: An inclusive design perspective on automotive HMI trends. In: Antona, M., Stephanidis, C. (eds.) UAHCI 2016: Universal Access in Human-Computer Interaction. Users and Context Diversity, pp. 548–555. Springer, Cham (2016). https://doi.org/10.1007/978-3-319-40238-3_52
25. World Health Organization: Global Strategy and Action Plan on Ageing and Health. WHO Press, Geneve (2017)
26. Fatima, K., Moridpour, S.: Measuring public transport accessibility for elderly. MATEC Web Conf. **259**, 1–5 (2019). https://doi.org/10.1051/matecconf/201925903006
27. United Nations: World Population Ageing 2019: Highlights. UN Press, New York (2019)
28. Metz, D.: Mobility of older people and their quality of life. Transp. Policy **7**, 149–152 (2000). https://doi.org/10.1016/S0967-070X(00)00004-4
29. Webber, S.C., Porter, M.M., Menec, V.H.: Mobility in older adults: a comprehensive framework. Gerontologist **50**, 443–450 (2010). https://doi.org/10.1093/geront/gnq013
30. Stanley, J.K., Hensher, D.A., Stanley, J.R., Vella-Brodrick, D.: Mobility, social exclusion and well-being: exploring the links. Transp. Res. Part A Policy Pract. **45**, 789–801 (2011). https://doi.org/10.1016/j.tra.2011.06.007
31. Hakamies-Blomqvist, L., Raitanen, T., O'Neill, D.: Driver ageing does not cause higher accident rates per km. Transp. Res. Part F Traffic Psychol. Behav. **5**, 271–274 (2002). https://doi.org/10.1016/S1369-8478(03)00005-6
32. Li, S., Blythe, P., Guo, W., Namdeo, A.: Investigation of older drivers' requirements of the human-machine interaction in highly automated vehicles. Transp. Res. Part F Traffic Psychol. Behav. **62**, 546–563 (2019). https://doi.org/10.1016/j.trf.2019.02.009
33. Ball, K., Owsley, C., Stalvey, B., Roenker, D.L., Sloane, M.E., Graves, M.: Driving avoidance and functional impairment in older drivers. Accid. Anal. Prev. **30**, 313–322 (1998). https://doi.org/10.1016/S0001-4575(97)00102-4
34. Karthaus, M., Falkenstein, M.: Functional changes and driving performance in older drivers: assessment and interventions. Geriatrics **1**, 12 (2016). https://doi.org/10.3390/geriatrics1020012
35. Cox, A.E., Cicchino, J.B.: Continued trends in older driver crash involvement rates in the United States: data through 2017–2018. J. Safety Res. (2021). https://doi.org/10.1016/j.jsr.2021.03.013
36. Charlton, J.L., Oxley, J., Fildes, B., Oxley, P., Newstead, S., Koppel, S., O'Hare, M.: Characteristics of older drivers who adopt self-regulatory driving behaviours. Transp. Res. Part F Traffic Psychol. Behav. **9**, 363–373 (2006). https://doi.org/10.1016/j.trf.2006.06.006
37. Fonda, S.J., Wallace, R.B., Herzog, A.R.: Changes in driving patterns and worsening depressive symptoms among older adults. J. Gerontol. Ser. B Psychol. Sci. Soc. Sci. **56**, S343–S351 (2001). https://doi.org/10.1093/geronb/56.6.S343
38. Musselwhite, C.B.A., Haddad, H.: Exploring older drivers' perceptions of driving. Eur. J. Ageing **7**, 181–188 (2010). https://doi.org/10.1007/s10433-010-0147-3
39. World Health Organization: Active Ageing: A Policy Framework. WHO Press, Geneve (2014)
40. Fernández-Ballesteros, R.: Active Aging: The Contribution of Psychology. Hogrefe & Huber Publishers, Boston (2008)
41. World Health Organization: World Report on Ageing and Health. WHO Press, Geneve (2015)
42. Li, S., Blythe, P., Guo, W., Namdeo, A., Edwards, S., Goodman, P., Hill, G.: Evaluation of the effects of age-friendly human-machine interfaces on the driver's takeover performance

in highly automated vehicles. Transport. Res. F: Traffic Psychol. Behav. **67**, 78–100 (2019). https://doi.org/10.1016/j.trf.2019.10.009
43. Bellet, T., Paris, J.-C., Marin-Lamellet, C.: Difficulties experienced by older drivers during their regular driving and their expectations towards advanced driving aid systems and vehicle automation. Transport. Res. F: Traffic Psychol. Behav. **52**, 138–163 (2018). https://doi.org/10.1016/j.trf.2017.11.014
44. Curto, S., Severino, A., Trubia, S., Arena, F., Puleo, L.: The effects of autonomous vehicles on safety. In: Simos, T., Kalagiratou, Z., Monovasilis, T. (eds.) International Conference Of Computational Methods In Sciences And Engineering ICCMSE 2020, p. 110013. AIP Publishing, Melville (2021). https://doi.org/10.1063/5.0047883
45. Eby, D.W., Molnar, L.J., Zhang, L., St. Louis, R.M., Zanier, N., Kostyniuk, L.P., Stanciu, S.: Use, perceptions, and benefits of automotive technologies among aging drivers. Inj. Epidemiol. **3**, 28 (2016). https://doi.org/10.1186/s40621-016-0093-4
46. Pfleging, B., Rang, M., Broy, N.: Investigating user needs for non-driving-related activities during automated driving. In: Häkkila, J., Ojala, T. (eds.) Proceedings of the 15th International Conference on Mobile and Ubiquitous Multimedia, pp. 91–99. Association for Computing Machinery, New York (2016). https://doi.org/10.1145/3012709.3012735
47. Lewin, T.: Speed Read Car Design: The History Principles and Concepts Behind Modern Car Design. Motorbooks, Minneapolis (2017)
48. Meschtscherjakov, A., Ratan, R., Tscheligi, M., McCall, R., Szostak, D., Politis, I., Krome, S.: 2nd workshop on user experience of autonomous driving. In: Osswald, S., Pearce, B., Szostak, D., Kun, A.L., Boyle, L.N., Miller, E., Wu, Y. (eds.) Proceedings of the 6th International Conference on Automotive User Interfaces and Interactive Vehicular Applications—AutomotiveUI '14, pp. 1–3. Association for Computing Machinery, New York (2014). https://doi.org/10.1145/2667239.2667425
49. Kun, A.L., Boll, S., Schmidt, A.: Shifting gears: user interfaces in the age of autonomous driving. IEEE Pervasive Comput. **15**, 32–38 (2016). https://doi.org/10.1109/MPRV.2016.14
50. Chuang, L.L., Manstetten, D., Boll, S., Baumann, M.: 1st workshop on understanding automation. In: Boll, S., Löcken, A., Schroeter, R., Baumann, M., Alvarez, I., Chuang, L., Feuerstack, S., Jeon, M., Broy, N., Hooft van Huysduynen, H., Osswald, S., Politis, I., Large, D. (eds.) Proceedings of the 9th International Conference on Automotive User Interfaces and Interactive Vehicular Applications Adjunct, pp. 1–8. Association for Computing Machinery, New York (2017). https://doi.org/10.1145/3131726.3131729
51. Lyons, G., Jain, J., Holley, D.: The use of travel time by rail passengers in Great Britain. Transp. Res. Part A: Policy Pract. **41**, 107–120 (2007). https://doi.org/10.1016/j.tra.2006.05.012
52. Krome, S., Holopainen, J., Greuter, S.: AutoPlay: unfolding motivational affordances of autonomous driving. In: Meixner, G., Müller, C. (eds.) Automotive User Interfaces, pp. 483–510. Springer, Cham (2017). https://doi.org/10.1007/978-3-319-49448-7_18
53. Bull, M.: Automobility and the power of sound. Theory Cult. Soc. **21**, 243–259 (2004). https://doi.org/10.1177/0263276404046069
54. Endsley, M.R.: Toward a theory of situation awareness in dynamic systems. Hum Factors. **37**, 32–64 (1995). https://doi.org/10.1518/001872095779049543
55. Krome, S., Goddard, W., Greuter, S., Walz, S.P., Gerlicher, A.: A context-based design process for future use cases of autonomous driving. In: Burnett, G., Gabbard, J., Green, P., Osswald, S., Eren, A., Antrobus, V. (eds.) Proceedings of the 7th International Conference on Automotive User Interfaces and Interactive Vehicular Applications, pp. 265–272. Association for Computing Machinery, New York (2015). https://doi.org/10.1145/2799250.2799257
56. Taylor, A.H., Dorn, L.: Stress, fatigue, health, and risk of road traffic accidents among professional drivers: the contribution of physical inactivity. Annu. Rev. Public Health **27**, 371–391 (2006). https://doi.org/10.1146/annurev.publhealth.27.021405.102117
57. Faber, K., van Lierop, D.: How will older adults use automated vehicles? Assessing the role of AVs in overcoming perceived mobility barriers. Transp. Res. Part A: Policy Pract. **133**, 353–363 (2020). https://doi.org/10.1016/j.tra.2020.01.022

58. Bascom, G.W., Christensen, K.M.: The impacts of limited transportation access on persons with disabilities' social participation. J. Transp. Health **7**, 227–234 (2017). https://doi.org/10.1016/j.jth.2017.10.002
59. Metz, D.: Transport policy for an ageing population. Transp. Rev. **23**, 375–386 (2003). https://doi.org/10.1080/0144164032000048573
60. Eckoldt, K., Knobel, M., Hassenzahl, M., Schumann, J.: An experiential perspective on advanced driver assistance systems. IT—Inf. Technol. **54**, 165–171 (2012). https://doi.org/10.1524/itit.2012.0678
61. Krome, S., Walz, S.P., Greuter, S.: Contextual inquiry of future commuting in autonomous cars. In: Kaye, J., Druin, A., Lampe, C., Hourcade, J.P., Terveen, L., Morris, S. (eds.) Proceedings of the 2016 CHI Conference Extended Abstracts on Human Factors in Computing Systems, pp. 3122–3128. Association for Computing Machinery, New York (2016). https://doi.org/10.1145/2851581.2892336

Remote Caring for Older People: Future Trends and Speculative Design

Oya Demirbilek

Abstract The present chapter explores IoT trends and applications' current and speculative futures to support older people living independently. It focuses on the bathroom area, one of the most dangerous domestic places for ageing bodies. The chapter first presents literature on IoT devices and older people ageing in place, discussing their relationship, the blurring into cyborg territories and the ramifications. Next, technology uptake is discussed, with an example from a previous research study. Next, healthy ageing, active ageing, and quality of life are discussed through the medical and social models of health, and a new model of technological enhancement and monitoring is proposed. The vulnerabilities of older people and IoT's risks and ethical implications are also covered, followed by current IoT trends and applications for accessible bathrooms, with pros and cons for each. The following section introduces speculative design approaches exploring the possibilities and implications on the future of caring for older people, illustrated with three examples: two speculative projects and one science fiction movie. The final section discusses the inclusive nature of caring and the importance of inclusive design approaches to designing and implementing IoT healthcare products and remote-age-care systems for older people and their families/caregivers.

Keywords IoT healthcare for older people · Speculative design · Remote care for older people · Future of aged care

1 Introduction

Globally, billions of *Internet of Things* (IoT) and surfaces, from tiny to large, are connected to the Internet, have sensors, and collect and share real-time data. The predicted number of connected IoT devices by 2025 is 75 billion [1]. These devices and systems offer apparent benefits for large industries and companies, for which the top considerations are efficiency, agility, and targeted marketing. This chapter looks

O. Demirbilek (✉)
School of Built Environment, University of New South Wales, Sydney, Australia
e-mail: o.demirbilek@unsw.edu.au

© The Author(s), under exclusive license to Springer Nature Singapore Pte Ltd. 2022
S. Scataglini et al. (eds.), *Internet of Things for Human-Centered Design*,
Studies in Computational Intelligence 1011,
https://doi.org/10.1007/978-981-16-8488-3_14

at the benefits and detriments for older people and ways to make remote healthcare and support work for them and their caregivers.

The chapter has four parts. The first section looks at the literature on IoT and older people ageing in place, discussing the relationship between older people and IoT devices, how IoT extends the human body into cyborg territories and the ramifications. Technology uptake is then discussed, with an example from a research study done a few years ago with older people on future bathrooms. Next, healthy ageing, active ageing, and quality of life are discussed through the medical and social models of health, and a new model of technological enhancement and monitoring is proposed for healthcare supported by IoT. This section also covers the vulnerabilities of older people and the risks and ethical implications of IoT for them.

The second section presents current IoT trends and applications that can complement an accessible bathroom and support older people and their caregivers, with pros and cons for each. The third section introduces speculative design approaches to explore and understand the possibilities and implications of technologies on the future of caring for older people. This section is illustrated with three examples: two speculative projects and one science fiction movie, all three looking at what caring for older people is from different angles and exploring the relationships between technology, IoT, AI, and older people. The fourth section discusses the inclusive nature of caring and the importance of inclusive design approaches to designing and implementing IoT healthcare products and remote-age-care systems for older people and their family/caregivers, as both parties go through a range of emotional states.

1.1 The Merging of Commercial and Consumer IoT

Consumer IoT devices offer good opportunities within the domestic environment aside from the evident privacy and safety risks. Further to giving home dwellers a better understanding of how their homes operate, adjusting energy usage settings, or streaming music from smart speakers, IoT devices can also help family members, carers, and doctors provide remote care for older people living on their own. It does that by allowing the latter group to live independently for longer and avoid or delay the dreaded move to a nursing home [2, 3]. In an ideal scenario, those devices can ease communication between health practitioners, family/carers and older people and help support and monitor older people so that they can get on with their lives. Mobile health (m-health) is described as the use of mobile and wireless technologies such as smartphones, sensor devices, personal digital assistants, and other wireless devices to monitor and improve health outcomes [4, 5].

IoT m-health technology has the potential to empower its various stakeholders to make informed decisions [6]. Commercial IoT has already started to assist medical professionals and enhance the healthcare industry by monitoring the well-being of patients and speeding the access to a wealth of patients' data. This data can help provide better opportunities for patients' healthcare as they merge with consumer IoT and allow self-monitoring via connected sensor devices. Such devices collect and allow for manipulating large quantities of data, also known as Big Data, related to human activity, behaviour, performance, and interactions with devices. In healthcare, this data is sent to primary health care individuals and professionals and helps provide feedback, individualised treatment and care plans, reminders for medication, recommendations, and coaching, back to the users. For example, IoT devices with sensors and robotic components can send alerts to family members and primary caretakers in cases when patients would forget to take their medication, have a fall, or stay inactive for too long in one space [6, 7].

Health Big Data also offers medical practitioners and academics the capability to perform large scale research on emerging phenomena and identify correlations, provided that human research ethics conditions are met. Human research ethics requires that all participants give their informed consent regarding their participation in the research, recording their data, and transparency regarding what will be done with this recorded data. In addition, health Insurance companies are also very interested in this health data.

The growing range of IoT devices is fuelling an increasing group of connected patients and care recipients, which will see the merging of commercial and consumer IoT products and services. From 2015 to early 2021, there have been 53,054 healthcare apps available globally at Google Play and over 318,000 health apps available in app stores worldwide, with varying degrees of success. To be more precise, very few such apps are successful, and most would only be used for a short period [8, 9]. Medical-grade wearable IoT products are among the most promising IoT healthcare applications, empowering people by allowing them to have an active role in monitoring their health by tracking their vital signs, sleep, and activity data. As a result, patients are empowered and made more aware of their health status. This awareness helps them become collaborators with healthcare practitioners on their health outcomes, take a more active role in their care plan, and make decisions [10]. In other words, IoT healthcare devices have the affordance to make patients more proactive about their health.

These devices can support the remote care of older people if they are designed to be appropriate to their needs and lifestyle [11]. For example, IoT with sensor technology has been identified to support ageing in place in the following three ways [12]: (1) Health status monitoring [13–16]; (2) Emergency detection [17]; (3) Health status change notifications to healthcare providers [18]. The devices come in various shapes and forms, such as light fixtures, domestic appliances, voice assistance, and medical wearables. They are composed of sensors, cameras for video monitoring, and microphones, and these can accurately track heart rate, pulse, blood pressure, activity or lack of activity, steps, tremor, body composition (hydration levels and muscles and bones balance) or body posture.

1.2 Extending the Human Body

When technology is designed to enhance people's health and activities via close connections with the human body, this extends the body's capabilities and morphs into something else. One definition of the term cyborg (cybernetic organism) is an individual with organic, mechanical and biomechatronic body parts to enhance senses, physical abilities, and body movement beyond typical human limits. We can already see varying levels of applications of this definition, with people having pacemakers or cochlear implants or even those using exoskeleton suits or even contact lenses. However, the story becomes complicated when implants or assistive devices become connected to the Internet. The first legally recognised human-cyborg is Neil Harbisson, an artist and a transspecies rights activist with an electronic antenna device implanted in his skull, protruding over his head. This implant is to help him extend his colour perception through vibrations, as he was born with Achromatopsia (colour blindness). Harbisson identifies himself as a cyborg as he sees his antenna as an organ, an extension of his body, and not a device.

Most IoT devices, smartphones, and health wearables enhance people's abilities in some ways, allowing them to extend their physical, mental, and physiological abilities into and through the devices [19], augmenting them and making them become temporary cyborgs. This very combination is now rapidly expanding the boundaries of the self and our humanness, raising important ethical and philosophical questions, especially when much Big Data is constantly collected, shared, and processed. People using these IoT devices should be the rightful owners of the private and personal data generated from their everyday actions and bodily status. They should have the right to own and control this data and decide who else to share it with, how often, and when to share it. This situation requires us to amend and adapt our legislation accordingly, to extend privacy and human rights to encompass the IoT devices by which people choose to extend themselves physically, mentally, and socially [19]. This is even more important for an ageing population, where older people would be more vulnerable to the possible misuse of their data and violation of their dignity and privacy.

2 IoT and Older People

One important megatrend that will shape our future is that the world's population is ageing due to increasing longevity and decreasing fertility rates. By 2030, a World Health Organisation report estimates that the number of people over 60 will be 1.4 billion [20]. In 2012, this number was 8% of the total population, and in 2030, it will double and be close to 17% of the total global population [21]. In Australia, the percentage of people over 65 is estimated to reach 22% by 2056 [22].

Living life independently and as healthy as possible is necessary for an ageing population living longer and growing fast in numbers. In addition to the growing ageing population, the average household sizes decrease as more and more people live alone [23]. These two trends have brought a need for most people to "age in place", intending to remain as active, healthy, safe, and independent as possible for as long as they can. However, accessibility issues within the home, compounded with communication and connection issues between older people and their family members, carers, and health care providers, can exacerbate older people's daily life experiences.

2.1 Technology Uptake

Older people's attitudes and beliefs are somewhat different for technology adoption and use, and they can be slower or more reluctant in adopting new technologies and devices [24]. The Senior Technology Acceptance and Adoption Model (STAM), developed for mobile phone technology [25], assumes that users either adopt or reject technology. Several studies looked at ways to reduce barriers and improve the acceptance and use of technology for older people [26–30]. Moreover, older people seem to be given technology by their children or their primary carers. As such, they would not have an appropriation phase [31] where they would decide to select and make purchasing decisions. Instead, perceived usefulness and social influence from family, carers, and friends would primarily determine their intention to use the technology.

Concerning technology uptake for older people, ease of learning has been identified as a critical determinant of the actual use and a primary factor in acceptance or rejection, without even going through a use phase. A bad experience can lead to the perception that the technology is challenging to use, resulting in direct rejection. Furthermore, informing older people to help them increase their understanding of IoT technology, their potential benefits, and how to protect themselves and avoid the risks has been identified as necessary for their adoption of new technology [24, 32, 33].

Comparable to the above, our findings with a research project we did a few years ago with a small group of older people indicated similar results. The findings challenged the assumption that older people would fear technology or not use it [34]. In particular, the research findings showed that our group of older people were keen to accept change, especially about new bathroom technology. This acceptance, however, only surfaced after we demonstrated the potentials and possibilities of a range of materials and technologies during an intensive co-design workshop with the older participants. In the subsequent workshops, our participants came up with more daring and exciting ideas to use technology. For example, one idea was to have smart mirrors that could help track and monitor the appearance of skin moles over time, a topic especially relevant for Australia. Some other proposed ideas were to have a large air dryer in the shower and dry before stepping out of the shower and voice-controlled water flow and temperature control in the shower [34].

2.2 Healthy Ageing, Active Ageing, and Quality of Life

Health and quality of life are interrelated for older people [35, 36]. Focusing on the quality of life seems to be more beneficial than focusing on healthy ageing, as the latter tends to be more related to the *medical model* of health. In the medical model, the older person's body would be considered "the problem needing fixing" and would be the passive recipient of treatments due to deteriorating physical, cognitive, or mental health and increasing dependence. This model, depicted in Fig. 1a, is directed at the medical professions and focuses on relieving symptoms, curing, and making the person physically fit and able.

In addition, quality of life would relate more to the *social model* of health, originating as the social model of disability [38]. In this model, health and physical impairments would be affected by a range of external barriers such as social, attitudinal (deliberate or unintentional), cultural, and environmental (physical barriers), and economic factors. In the original model, disability is viewed as socially constructed. The social model accepts that people are diverse with different needs and that individual people would not be able to participate in everyday activities of the society in the same way as everybody else due to physical and social barriers [39]. In this model, depicted in Fig. 1b, the arrows represent all the external factors mentioned above that are considered potential problem areas affecting health and well-being [40], making them design, attitude, or policy problems. The social model is not about fixing the person. Instead, it is about fixing external causes of health damage or impairment by designing inclusive and accessible environments and policies.

The technological enhancement and monitoring model depicted in Fig. 1c) represents the situation where the person's health, behaviour, and activity data are collected

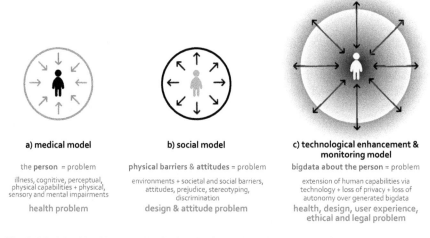

Fig. 1 Models of healthcare: **a** Medical model, **b** social model (both **a** and **b** adapted from McCain [37]), and, **c** technological enhancement and monitoring model (by the Author)

and analysed by various stakeholders, quantified, and monitored by the person, healthcare practitioners, and potentially unwanted third parties. This model combines the two previous ones, (a) and (b), focusing on the health-related data retrieved from the person. The impacts extend beyond the body's boundaries and the immediate environments. The person is now a proactive recipient of treatments. However, ensuring the privacy and security of this data and the transparency of what will happen to it become the main problems. This new model also highlights how the current situation with IoT health devices creates ethical and legal problems intertwined with issues related to health, IoT device design, and user experience.

2.3 Vulnerability

The World Health Organisation (WHO) predicts that by 2050, 80% of older people globally will live in low- and middle-income countries [41]. The growing number of older people has also increased the number of people with mobility issues, with roughly 2 in 5 people with disability being 65 years or older. Globally, the estimation is that there are around 1.27 billion people with disabilities, which equates to 1 in 5 people [42]. This large yet underrepresented group includes older people and people with various disabilities. In addition, most of them will have carers, close friends, and family with emotional attachment, which adds a further 2.3 billion people [42] whom accessibility issues indirectly impact. These figures reinforce the needs for inclusive design approaches to be embedded in all research and design development processes.

Living longer is among humanity's most outstanding achievements, with over half of current younger generations predicted to live to be 103 years old, making our time the century of centenarians [43]. However, living longer is also one of humanity's most significant challenges, as older people have one or more health conditions or chronic diseases and are often more vulnerable in one or more of the following three areas [44]:

1. Health and physical capability, as older people are more likely to have chronic conditions and disability, increasing their dependence and the cost of care and living.
2. Cognitive aptitude,
3. Social network and support that is reducing with time.

Disability is defined as caused by mismatched interactions between humans and environments [45]. This mismatch also happens amidst a market saturated with IoT health-related and medical devices. Most of these devices would be needlessly acquired or would not be used safely and efficiently as intended or not used at all, or even may not have been satisfactorily tested and evaluated for specific health outcomes [46]. Older people above 85 years of age are also the most vulnerable to abuse and exploitation as there would be worsening in all the three areas mentioned above [44]. Furthermore, the older people who could benefit most from digital technology have also been found not to use it [47]. Additionally, there is no evidence that more useable and intuitive IoT health products positively affect the quality of life of older people [48].

2.4 IoT Risks and Ethical Implications

Principle 9 of the Declaration of Helsinki (amended in 2013) states: "It is the duty of physicians who are involved in medical research to protect the life, health, dignity, integrity, right to self-determination, privacy, and confidentiality of personal information of research subjects." [49]. Therefore, all potential issues must be thoroughly considered when researching and designing healthcare medical IoT wearables. There are hardware, software, and network-related issues around the accuracy and robustness of IoT wearables. The limited battery power and accuracy of the data are just two of the potential issues. As mentioned earlier, there are also issues related to the safety and privacy of collecting, transmitting, and using the data collected from IoT devices, especially for a more vulnerable older generation. An article of the World Economic Forum [50] points to the following three main risk areas:

(1) Firstly, the privacy-related risks for vast amounts of personal user data to be combined in novel ways, allowing on the one hand to enhance user experiences, and on the other, for corporations or for other unwanted manipulative third parties to learn a great deal about individuals' private lives and behaviours.
(2) Secondly, the provision of a means to undermine the Internet with malware.
(3) Thirdly, the increased risks of privacy and physical threats, malevolently or not, with IoT devices within smart cities, where the entire digital ecosystem is interconnected, linking the online and the physical world, making it vulnerable to errors and manipulation.

3 IoT Applications in an Accessible Bathroom

The bathroom is a very private and personal space. However, it is also a dangerous area, especially for older people, with many emergency visits to the hospital resulting from falls in the bathroom [51, 52]. Falls in the bathroom are particularly dangerous, due to the high concentration of hard surfaces and fittings, with a high probability for injury and even mortality [53]. In particular, the bathtub and the shower are hazardous areas, and most falls for older people happen near the toilet. Among the reasons for falls in the bathroom are wet floors, small spaces to manoeuvre, bending and lifting required in accessing the bathtub, shower or toilet, glare from lighting and shiny surfaces, or vision-related trips and falls caused by not enough light [51].

The risk of falls makes bathroom safety one of the top concerns in making a home more accessible to allow ageing in place. The increasing group of older people and people with disabilities need to modify existing homes, especially bathrooms, to make them more accessible and less dangerous to help them live independently for longer. The following section presents a range of IoT devices that can complement an accessible bathroom and support older people and their caregivers.

3.1 IoT Products for the Bathroom

The growing demand for products and environments accessible for all and that can support and enhance life for ageing in place has created research and design opportunities in these areas. Some of the outcomes have resulted in an expanding range of IoT products turning domestic environments into smart homes and allowing family members and healthcare professionals to provide remote support for older people. Prominent examples of recent IoT products for the bathroom are illustrated in Fig. 2 and described below.

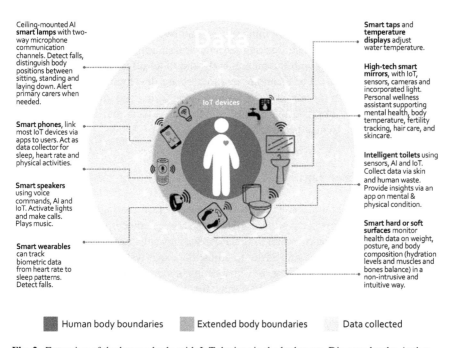

Fig. 2 Extension of the human body with IoT devices in the bathroom. Diagram by the Author

3.1.1 Smart Lamps

These are ceiling-mounted smart lamps with Artificial Intelligence (AI) that look like regular light fixtures and have two-way microphone communication channels. They have motion sensors and can be used in all rooms and detect if an older person needs help if they fall, distinguishing postures between sitting, standing, and laying down. They also track activity and can provide light, tips, or warnings in case of danger. In addition, these lamps also have smoke and air quality detection sensors and can be programmed to send alerts to ask for help when needed [54].

3.1.2 Smart Toilets

Intelligent toilets use sensors, AI and IoT to track and analyse mental and physical conditions. For instance, a wellness toilet in development collects data via skin and human waste, allowing people to monitor their current health and receive insights via an app on their smart devices [55–57]. Smart toilets include self-cleaning ones with electronic water and ultraviolet light, toilet seats with an integrated bidet attachment to improve hygiene, heating, soothing music, and overflow protection. Some even include built-in speakers and docking systems for smartphones or tablets. Due to its intimate relationship with the human body, the toilet offers potentials for many healthcare applications. For example, researchers are developing a toilet seat that monitors heart health for non-invasive in-home monitoring and diagnosis of cardiovascular disease to improve the quality of life for patients and facilitate a more proactive approach to healthcare [58].

3.1.3 Smart Water Taps

Digital faucets can now come with anti-fingerprint surface coatings and have touch-only or touch-free sensor activation. Taps can also come with temperature gauges and efficiency sensors to control water usage. Besides, they can have digital programable displays to make it visible and easier to adjust the exact water temperature, as this is crucial to help avoid scalding, as older people's skin is thinner and burns more quickly. These taps are useable and accessible for everyone, especially for people with dexterity issues. A second advantage is that they save water, hence are sustainable [59].

Issues related to smart taps are that they require power, and their battery will run out in a year, needing replacement. If the taps are connected to the power, they become unusable during a power cut. Sensor taps can also self-activate due to reflections on shiny surfaces. Lastly, due to the internal design and materials, some types of sensor taps can harbour bacteria and need regular maintenance, disinfecting and cleaning.

3.1.4 Smart Mirrors

IoT high-tech smart mirrors have sensors, high-quality cameras, incorporated lights and can be operated by touchscreen controls, remotes, or voice commands. These mirrors can become personal healthcare and wellness assistants and trainers, supporting a wide range of things, including mental health, body temperature, fertility tracking, hair care, skincare, and make-up support, to name a few [60]. Smart mirrors can also be connected to security systems and check security cameras or the front door. Furthermore, smart mirrors are not confined to the bathroom and expand in interactive home gym applications and fitness industries. These physical exercise mirrors will make it possible to take private lessons or participate in real-time classes with other people from around the globe [61, 62].

As attractive as these new gadgets may seem, there are issues related to smart mirrors that still need unpacking from the perspective of everyday users. The main issues are whether people feel comfortable having cameras in their bathroom or while exercising and whether sound-activated or touch commends would work for everyone. Other worries are the potential to become another means for businesses to capture more data on private lives and be vulnerable to hacking and misuse. However, issues do not stop there and include the many ways these mirrors can and will potentially alter how we relate socially to each other, ourselves, our body image, the environment, and technology.

3.1.5 Smart Fabric Products

The term smart fabric refers to a range of fabric products with integrated active functionality that extends the convenience and functionality of textile materials. The difference with smart wearables is that they are encased in clothing material, whereas smart fabrics have their functionality integrated and woven into the fabric [63]. For example, a smart bathroom mat that looks like a standard plush fabric mat can automatically capture and monitor health data on weight, posture, body hydration levels, and muscle and bone balance in an easy and non-intrusive way. This mat collects information with medical-grade pressure sensing technology, sends the data to an app that makes the information easy to understand [64].

4 Speculations on the Future

A *speculative design* approach suggests that design research and design processes can look beyond finding applications for technologies. This approach can be a great way to explore and understand possibilities and implications related to the impact of emerging technologies and design [65]. *Critical design* is an attitude that uses speculative design outcomes to question and challenge assumptions about the role that products and technology have in people's life and explores people's relationship to technology [65].

Speculative design approaches use design skills and tools to provoke discussions and help us think critically about the future by imagining and depicting possible futures, as if these were real, with the good and the bad. The outcomes of speculative design provide a guide for a preferable future and more ethical and responsible ways to design the future by drawing attention to likely social, moral, ethical, and political complications and by visualising what the possible consequences of those could be. To this end, speculative project outcomes often trigger more questions than providing answers.

Science fiction (Sci-Fi), a form of speculative fiction, has already been doing the above in written stories and films based on scientific discoveries and technological advancements by exploring interactions between science, design and depicting realistic possible futures. Sci-Fi movies have popularised and normalised future technologies and helped establish their feasibility, as in the example of the 1981 film *Thresholds*, where a permanent heart implant was introduced and saved the life of a female protagonist [66]. Sci-Fi is especially relevant to healthcare and medicine, and it has in many instances opened the door for medical and technological innovations [67–70].

Below are three examples of speculations on the future. Two are speculative projects, and one is a science fiction movie. These examples explore relationships between technology, IoT, AI and older people. All the examples look at what caring is from different angles.

4.1 When IoT Devices Are an Imposition

Uninvited Guests is a short film by Superflux Laboratory [71] that explores IoT devices, intrusion on privacy and the concept of the *quantified self*, a term coined by Wired Magazine editors Gary Wolf and Kevin Kelly in 2007. The Quantified Self is about people tracking information and data about themselves (biological, physical, and behavioural) and their environments [72]. This short film has been widely discussed and given as an example of unintended consequences of remote healthcare for older people, behaviour monitoring and possible frictions between humans and IoT health-related devices [73–79]. The hero, Thomas, is 70-years old and is living independently. The topic is about Thomas dealing with a set of tracking and monitoring IoT devices given to him by his children, supposedly to help him live a healthier life. The devices are bright fluorescent green and look alien to Thomas' domestic environment. These devices are more to help his children keep a remote eye on their ageing parent without having to be there, as in the findings from a recent PhD study on IoT to support ageing in place [80]. All these devices are connected to the older person's smartphone and his children's phones, sending him constant warnings and messages on what to do or not do. The set of devices includes:

- a fork that tracks his diet by measuring calories, salt, and fat in foods,
- a walking cane that tracks his steps and recommends daily step counts,
- a medication box that monitors medication intake, and
- a bed that tracks when he goes in and out of bed.

The short film has three stages. The first stage, where the hero tries to comply with the new rules and impositions brought up by the devices and struggles to keep up. In the second stage, he ignores the devices and receives constant alerts and calls from his children nudging him to comply. Finally, in the third stage, Thomas outsmarts the devices and fools the sensors, allowing him to live how he pleases and calm his children with fake data, receiving stars and "well done" messages on his smartphone from the apps linked with the devices. The film is a reminder that technologies seldom function as intended, as people adapt and modify their use of products in unintended ways to suit their preferences. In addition, the film poses questions on how life could be in a not-so-distant future where smart IoT devices would provide remote care for older people and how older people could keep their privacy and sense of independence to enjoy life the way they prefer. Above all, the film asks what care and caring really mean and for whom. This approach brings a new angle to the term Quantified Self, and the author proposes *Quantified Remote Caring* for it.

4.2 A Take on Serviced Apartments for Older People

Another example of a speculative future for older people living alone and ageing in place is the *Amazin* concept apartments that integrate consumption via smart systems. Amazin is the name given to a fictional tech company inspired by Amazon, and the project is based on smart city developments and Amazon's *Amazon Go Groceries Just Walk Out Shopping* store in Seattle [81, 82]. This conceptual project is by Future Facility [83], commissioned by the Design Museum for the New Old exhibition in 2017 [84, 85] that offers technology as a service rather than products. These apartments consist of smart interiors with serviced IoT appliances embedded into the walls as part of the architecture and positioned at a standing height, with simple, intuitive, and straightforward designs. The wall appliances self-replenish and self-maintain, designed to "facilitating domestic dignity" [82]. They are connected to a service, ensuring that the fridge is continuously replenished and maintained. The washing machine is always ready to work and has detergent and softener in it. The dryer is maintained and cleaned, and drinking water continuously flows from the tap when needed.

The goal is to provide worry-free domestic independence for older people via property development that removes any stress related to purchasing appliances and the associated domestic upkeep burdens and provides convenience via discreet maintenance and supply services. The servicing and maintenance are done from the back of each appliance, accessed via a corridor placed right behind the appliance wall, to maintain older people's privacy, cause minimal disruption, and balance the compromise of the data shared in exchange for this convenience. The project assumes that older people's quality of life would improve with carefully designed self-supplied domestic appliances that do not require any maintenance and servicing and are a permanent part of the home. This speculative project offers a glimpse of what a convenient independent domestic life could look like for older people yet leaves the problems associated with data exploitation open for discussion and interpretation.

4.3 Frank and the Robot

This example is from a near-future Sci-Fi movie, *Robot and Frank* [86], where technology is depicted as humanised and subtle. The movie tells the story of the bond between Frank, an older person with dementia and a retired burglar living alone, and a caregiver robot that does household chores and provides healthcare and health advice. Frank has a daughter and a son. Both his children are busy with their own lives yet want to ensure their father is doing well. The robot is given as a gift to Frank by his son to help him have a routine to cope better on his own and allow the son to spend more time with his young family, relieving him from spending his weekends travelling to and from his father's home. The robot is white and has friendly, harmless, and human features without a face. It can also learn via AI, recording everything in its "memory", make calls to family or carers, and is programmed to do anything required to keep its owner mentally healthy and physically fit. The robot only becomes attractive to Frank when he realises that he can train it to perform burglary, as this is the one thing that seems to keep his mind alive and healthy. Frank brightens up during his preparations for a heist with the robot, and his dementia seems to subside. Through the evolving relationship between Frank and the robot, the movie addresses the care and caregiving issues. This movie also illustrates how people can potentially use AI programable technologies in unexpected ways and questions what "normal" expectations and routines for ageing should be, or whether there should be any expectation or routine at all.

5 Inclusive Nature of Caring

A baseline definition of care would be that it is a positive, compassionate attitude that requires emotional connection and investment in the well-being of the person cared for [87]. This caring attitude is inclusive and empathic and requires reciprocity of dependencies [88]. For example, people who genuinely care for their ageing parents and relatives will gift technological devices to them to help track their activities, monitor health-related data, and be alerted in case of an emergency. This *Quantified Remote Caring*, in a way, is a well-intentioned good thing yet is only concerned with physical and physiological issues and cannot compensate for the loss of social contact and the feelings of guilt for less time spent with older parents or relatives. Are we at risk of losing our humanity and being "impoverished without our old people, for only by contact with them can we come to know ourselves", as Littman and Myerhoff propose [89]?

On the other hand, besides the various difficulties older people have in maintaining their independence, they also deal with psychological issues, such as loneliness and the need for belonging. Therefore, IoT healthcare devices can only work if this allows them to feel connected and cared for instead of feeling monitored and controlled [90].

Accessibility is about designing products usable by everybody, and an inclusive design approach is a mindset that requires learning from and addressing user diversity to include as many people and viewpoints as possible. If we solve an issue for people affected by a specific condition, the solutions will work for a larger group, if not everyone. Inclusive design approaches to IoT healthcare products and remote-agecare systems can help develop compassionate empathy and respect for older people. We need to feel compassionate empathy towards ageing and older people wanting to live independently. This compassion enables to act and help by developing design solutions that would be ethical and work for as many people as possible, ideally for all, including family members and carers.

6 Conclusion

Designing and building delightful IoT solutions accessible to all is half of the story. "Ageing issues are not referable to the physical sphere only" [83]. Older peoples' dreams, need for purpose, and social lives are equally important as their health and mobility for their well-being. Remote caring does not replace social interactions. IoT products cannot fix loneliness and replace missing social company, not to mention the possible feelings of anxiety and stress caused by constant monitoring and alerts. This anxiety and stress can occur both in older people and in their family/caregivers, as both parties can have to go through a lot of data and information, some of which potentially triggering unnecessary worry or panic.

Future speculations on IoT healthcare devices and systems can only be codesigned collectively with older people and their close family and carers for a sound rethink and reimagination of how we can all "age in place" with reasonable care and support. Technology on its own does not solve things; people do. Considering that socialisation is a crucial component of healthy ageing, IoT healthcare devices should be designed to allow for healthy and meaningful connectedness between older people, their family, carers, and friends for such collaboration to happen at larger scales. Furthermore, such devices should be simple and intuitive to use, with minimal setup burden [90].

It is important to remember that if and when older people decide which device or product to adopt, use, or purchase, they will prioritise their dignity over convenience [91]. Besides, "Nobody likes to admit they are getting older and need help." [92]. Healthcare IoT devices are a new technology for most older people and should be designed by carefully considering their lifestyles, needs, and wants [28]. Such devices and systems should also be as unobtrusive as possible [93] to better support family members and carers to help older people get on with their lives by using monitoring to connect with them and detect any changes that could require intervention. To this end, we need to imagine and explore the future we all want to live in and make sure it happens, as designing for older people is "designing for our future selves" [94, 95]. This task requires us to imagine and speculate on possible futures based on current technological and scientific developments and make a preferable future happen.

References

1. Maayan, G.D.: The IoT Rundown For 2020: Stats, Risks, and Solutions, security-today.com/articles/ (2020)
2. Riedl, M., Mantovan, F., Them, C.: Being a nursing home resident: a challenge to one's identity. Nurs. Res. Pract. (2013)
3. Fiveash, B.: The experience of nursing home life. Int. J. Nurs. Pract. **4**(3), 166–174 (1998)
4. Almotiri, S.H., Khan, M.A., Alghamdi, M.A.: Mobile health (m-health) system in the context of IoT. In: IEEE 4th International Conference on Future Internet of Things and Cloud Workshops. FiCloudW, pp. 39–42 (2016)
5. Rekha H.S., Nayak, J., Sekhar, G.T.C., Pelusi, D.: Impact of IoT in healthcare: improvements and challenges. In: Das, K., Mishra, B.S.P., Das, M. (eds.) The Digitalization Conundrum in India. India St. Bus. Econ. Springer, pp. 73–107 (2020)
6. Kranz, M.: Fourth industrial revolution: 6 ways the Internet of Things is improving our lives, World Economic Forum (2018)
7. Kvedar, J.C., Colman, C., Cella, G.: The Internet of Healthy Things, 1st edn. Partners Healthcare Connected Health, Boston, MA (2015)
8. Statista.: Number of mHealth apps available in the Google Play Store from 1st quarter 2015 to 1st quarter 2021 (2021). https://www.statista.com/statistics/779919/health-apps-available-google-play-worldwide/
9. Aitken, M., Clancy, B., Nass, D.: The growing value of digital health: evidence and impact on human health and the healthcare system. IQVIA Inst. Hum. Data Sci. **1** (2017)
10. Bastiaens, H., Van Royen, P., Pavlic, D.R., Raposo, V., Baker, R.: Older people's preferences for involvement in their own care: a qualitative study in primary health care in 11 European countries. Patient Educ. Counselling **68**(1), 33–42 (2007)
11. Miskelly, F.G.: Assistive technology in elderly care. Age Ageing. **30**, 455–458 (2001)
12. Rantz, M.J., Skubic, M., Miller, S.J., Galambos, C., Alexander, G., Keller, J., Popescu, M.: Sensor technology to support aging in place. JAMDA **14**(6), 386–391 (2013); In Carnemolla, P.: Ageing in place and the IoT—how smart home technologies, the built environment and caregiving intersect. Vis. Eng. **6**(1), 1–16 (2018)
13. Peetoom, K.K., Lexis, M., Joore, M., Dirksen, C.D., De Witte, L.P.: Literature review on monitoring technologies and their outcomes in independently living elderly people. Disabil. Rehabil **10**(4), 271–294 (2015)
14. Kaye, J.A., Maxwell, S.A., Mattek, N., Hayes, T.L., Dodge, H., Pavel, M., Jimison, H.B., Wild, K., Boise, L., Zitzelberger, T.A.: Intelligent systems for assessing aging changes: home-based, unobtrusive, and continuous assessment of aging. J. Gerontol. B **66**(1), i180–i190 (2011)
15. Dodge, H.H., Mattek, N.C., Austin, D., Hayes, T.L., Kaye, J.A.: In-home walking speeds and variability trajectories associated with mild cognitive impairment. J. Neurol. **78**(24), 1946–1952 (2012)

16. Cesta, A., Cortellessa, G., Rasconi, R., Pecora, F., Scopelliti, M., Tiberio, L.: Monitoring elderly people with the robocare domestic environment: interaction synthesis and user evaluation. Comput. Intell. **27**(1), 60–82 (2011)
17. Gill, A.Q., Phennel, N., Lane, D., Phung, V.L.: IoT-enabled emergency information supply chain architecture for elderly people: the Australian context. Inf. Syst. **58**, 75–86 (2016)
18. Kleinberger, T., Jedlitschka, A., Storf, H., Steinbach-Nordmann, S., Prueckner, S.: An approach to and evaluations of assisted living systems using ambient intelligence for emergency monitoring and prevention. In: International Conference on UAHCI, pp. 199–208 (2009)
19. Balkan, A.: Privacy and ethical design. SEE Conf. (2016)
20. Lloyd-Sherlock, P., Kalache, A., Kirkwood, T., McKee, M., Prince, M.: WHO's proposal for a decade of healthy ageing. The Lancet **394**(10215), 2152–2153 (2019)
21. Barac, M., Hunter, W., Parkinson, J.: Silver linings: the active third age and the city, Riba, Uk (2013)
22. Australian Institute of Health and Welfare: Older Australia at a glance. Web report, Cat. No. AGE 87 (2018)
23. Bradbury, M., Peterson, M.N., Liu, J.: Long-term dynamics of household size and their environmental implications. Popul. Environ. **36**, 73–84 (2014)
24. Niehaves, B., Plattfaut, R.: Internet adoption by the elderly: employing IS technology acceptance theories for understanding the age-related digital divide. Eur. J. Inf. Syst. **23**(6), 708–726 (2014)
25. Renaud, K., van Biljon, J.: Predicting technology acceptance by the elderly: a qualitative study. SAICSIT (2008)
26. Grguric, A.: ICT towards elderly independent living. Research and Development Centre, Ericsson Nikola Tesla (2012)
27. Sánchez-Rico, A., Garel, P., Notarangelo, I., Quintana, M., Hernández, G., Asteriadis, S., Popa, M., Vretos, N., Solachidis, V., Burgos, M.: ICT services for life improvement for the elderly. Stud. Health Technol. Inform. **242**, 600–605 (2017)
28. Fischer, S.H., David, D., Crotty, B.H., Dierks, M., Safran, C.: Acceptance and use of health information technology by community-dwelling elders. Int. J. Med. Inform. **83**, 624–635 (2014)
29. Ijsselsteijn, W., Nap, H.H., de Kort, Y., Poels, K.: Digital game design for elderly users. In: Conference on Future Play, pp. 17–22 (2007)
30. Gaßner, K., Conrad, M.: ICT enabled independent living for elderly. A status-quo analysis on products and the research landscape in the field of Ambient Assisted Living (AAL). Inst. Innov. Technol. (2010). (Steinplatz 1, 10623, Berlin, EU-27, VDI, pp. 22–34)
31. Silverstone, R., Haddon, L.: Design and the domestication of information and communication technologies: technical change and everyday life. In: Silverstone, R., Mansell, R. (eds.), Communication by Design: The Politics of Information and Communication Technologies. OUP, pp. 44–74 (1996)
32. Gelderblom, H., van Dyk, T., van Biljon, J.: Mobile phone adoption: do existing models adequately capture the actual usage of older adults? In: Research Conference on SAICSIT, pp. 67–74 (2010)
33. Neves, B.B., Amaro, F.: Too old for technology? How the elderly of Lisbon use and perceive ICT. J. Community Inform. **8**, 1–12 (2012)
34. Mintzes, A., Demirbilek, O.R., Sweatman, P., Davey, S., Birdge, C.: Co-design report, livable Bathrooms for older people (2015). https://www.unsworks.unsw.edu.au/permalink/f/5gm2j3/unsworks_modsunsworks_38431
35. Iwasa, H., Kawaai, C., Gondo, Y., Inagaki, H., Suzuki, T.: Subjective well-being as a predictor of all-cause mortality among middle-aged and elderly people living in an urban Japanese community: a seven-year prospective cohort study. Geriatr. Gerontol. Int. **6**, 216–222 (2006)
36. Cohen, R., Bavishi, C., Rozanski, A.: Purpose in life and its relationship to all-cause mortality and cardiovascular events: a meta-analysis. Psychosom. Med. **78**(2), 122–133 (2016)
37. McCain, H.: Medical model of disability versus social model of disability, living with disability and chronic pain, citizens for accessible neighbourhoods (CAN), July 15, (2017). https://canbc.org/blog/medical-model-of-disability-versus-social-model-of-disability/. Accessed 8 Mar 2020

38. Baldwinson, T.: UPIAS—The union of the physically impaired against segregation (1972–1990): a public record from private files. TBR Imprint (2019)
39. Woodward, K.: Feeling frail and national statistical panic: Joan Didion in Blue Nights and the American economy at risk. Age Cult. Humanit. Interdisc. J. **2**, 347–367 (2015)
40. Netuveli, G., Blane, D.: Quality of life in older ages. Br. Med. Bull. **85**, 113–126 (2008)
41. World Health Organisation: Ageing and health, WHO (2018). https://www.who.int/news-room/fact-sheets/detail/ageing-and-health
42. Donovan, R.: Return on disability: translate different into value: 2016 Annual Report: The Global Economics of Disability (2016)
43. Donovan, R.: Silver linings: the active third age and the city, Riba, Uk (2013)
44. Seniors First BC, Vulnerability. http://seniorsfirstbc.ca/for-professionals/vulnerability/
45. Shum, A., Holmes, K., Woolery, K., Price, M., Kim, D., Dvorkina, E., Dietrich-Muller, D., Kile, N., Morris, S., Chou, J., Malekzadeh, S.: Inclusive design toolkit, Microsoft Design (2016)
46. World Health Organization: Medical devices: managing the mismatch: An outcome of the Priority Medical Devices project, WHO, (2010)
47. Dascălu, M., Rodideal, A., Popa, L.: Romania, elderly people who most need ICT are those who are less probable to use it. Soc. Work Rev. **17**, 81–95 (2018)
48. Bong, W.K., Bergland, A., Chen, W.: Technology acceptance and quality of life among older people using a TUI application. Int. J. Env. Res. Publ. Health **16**(23), 4706 (2019)
49. Declaration of Helsinki. World Medical Association (WMA) Declaration of Helsinki. Ethical Principles for Medical Research Involving Human Subjects
50. Jordan, A.: Why securing the internet of things is crucial to the fourth industrial revolution. World Economic Forum (2019). https://www.weforum.org/agenda/2019/04/why-securing-the-internet-of-things-is-crucial-to-the-fourth-industrial-revolution/
51. Wringler, W., Prieto, N.: Top 5 things to consider when designing an accessible bathroom for wheelchair users, Easterseal Indata Project, (2014). https://www.eastersealstech.com/2014/06/11/top-5-things-consider-designing-accessible-bathroom-wheelchair-users/
52. Stevens, J.A., Mahoney, J.E., Ehrenreich, H.: Circumstances and outcomes of falls among high-risk community-dwelling older adults. Injury Epid. **1**(1), 1–9 (2014)
53. Schellenberg, M., Inaba, K., Chen, J., Bardes, J.M., Crow, E., Lam, L., Benjamin, E., Demetriades, D.: Falls in the bathroom: a mechanism of injury for all ages. J. Surg. Res. **234**, 283–286 (2019)
54. Gebhart, A.: Nobi will watch over your grandparents, literally, from a ceiling mounted Smart lamp, C|Net, (2021). https://www.cnet.com/home/smart-home/nobi-will-watch-over-your-grandparents-literally-from-a-ceiling-mounted-smart-lamp
55. PR Newswire, Cision, CES 2021, TOTO offers CLEANOVATION as key strategy for new normal way of life and highlights entry into wellness sector, (2021, Nov). https://www.prnewswire.com/news-releases/at-ces-2021-toto-offers-cleanovation-as-key-strategy-for-new-normal-way-of-life-and-highlights-entry-into-wellness-sector-301204893.html
56. Park Sm., Won, D.D., Lee, B.J., et al.: A mountable toilet system for personalized health monitoring via the analysis of excreta. Nat. Biomed. Eng. **4**, 624–635 (2020). https://www.nature.com/articles/s41551-020-0534-9
57. Toi Labs. https://www.toilabs.com/
58. Conn, N.J., Schwarz, K.Q., Borkholder, D.A.: In-home cardiovascular monitoring system for heart failure: comparative study. JMIR Mhealth Uhealth **7**(1), e12419, (2019)
59. Oras, Intelligent faucet solutions are part of today's smart home. https://stories.oras.com/en/intelligent-faucet-solutions-are-part-of-todays-smart-home
60. PR Newswire, Cision, CES 2021: CareoOS earns third CES innovation award three years in a row, Themis Smart Mirror (2021). https://www.prnewswire.com/news-releases/ces-2021-careos-earns-third-ces-innovation-award-three-years-in-a-row-this-time-for-its-themis-smart-mirror-301202995.html
61. Mirror: hiding in plain sight. https://www.mirror.co/
62. Hua, K.: Panasonic's new smart mirror shows you your flaws and helps you fix them. Forbes, (Oct. 7, 2016). https://www.forbes.com

63. Simon, C., Potter, E., McCabe, M., Baggerman, C.: Smart fabrics technology development, Final report. A NASA Innovation Fund Project, Johnson Space Center (2010, 8 Oct)
64. Mateo. https://www.mateo.ai/#features
65. Dunne, A., Raby, F.: Speculative everything: design, fiction, and social dreaming. MIT Press (2013)
66. Kirby, D.: The future is now: diegetic prototypes and the role of popular films in generating real-world technological development. Soc. St. Sci. **40**(1), 41–70 (2010)
67. Klugman, C.M.: From cyborg fiction to medical reality. Lit. Med. **20**(1), 39–54 (2001)
68. Petersen, A., Anderson, A., Allan, S.: Science fiction/science fact: medical genetics in news stories. New Genet. Soc. **24**(3), 337–353 (2005)
69. Hockstein, N.G., Gourin, C.G., Faust, R.A., Terris, D.J.: A history of robots: from science fiction to surgical robotics. J. Robot. Surg. **1**(2), 113–118 (2007)
70. Tsekleves, E., Darby, A., Whicher, A., Swiatek P.: 2017. Co-designing design fictions: a new approach for debating and priming future healthcare technologies and services. Arch. Des. Res. **30**(2), 5–21 (2017)
71. Superflux Lab: Uninvited guests. The ThingTank Project (2015). https://superflux.in/index.php/work/uninvited-guests/
72. Swan, M.: The quantified self: Fundamental disruption in big data science and biological discovery. Big Data. vol. 1, 2, pp. 85–99 (2013, Jun)
73. Vandenberghe, B., Slegers, K.: Designing for others, and the trap of HCI methods and practices. In: 2016 CHI Conference Extended Abstracts on Human Factors in Computing Systems (2016)
74. Helms, K.: Leaky objects: Implicit information, unintentional communication. In: 2017 ACM Conference Companion Publication on Designing Interactive Systems, pp. 182–186 (2017)
75. Raijmakers, B., Scheepers, R., Visser, F.S.: 18. Myfutures: imagining speculative care and support futures in the Netherlands. Letters to the Future (2018)
76. Ocnarescu, I., Cossin, I.: The contribution of art and design to robotics. In: International Conference on Social Robotics, pp. 278–287 (2019)
77. Bidasaria, R.: How many sides does a circle have? Perceptions and polemic around Critical Design. Royal College of Art (2019) rashmibidasaria.com
78. Bowen, J., Hinze, A.: Smarter software engineering methods for smart environments. In: EICS Workshops, pp. 3–9 (2019)
79. Pau, S., Hall, A.: Beyond speculation: using imperfect experts for designing the collective futures of healthcare for space. In: 6th International Conference on Design4Health, vol. 3, pp. 45–54, (2020)
80. Choi, Y.K.: Examining the feasibility of Internet of Things technologies to support ageing-in-place. Ph.D. diss. (2018)
81. amazon.com: Amazon Go and Amazon Go Grocery. https://www.amazon.com/b?node=16008589011
82. Kafka, G.: Amazin Apartments: How the internet of things will alter our homes (2017, Mar). https://www.metropolismag.com/ideas/amazin-apartments-how-internet-things-will-alter-homes/
83. Mincolelli G., Imbesi S., Marchi M., Giacobone G.A.: New domestic healthcare. Co-designing assistive technologies for autonomous ageing at home. Des. J. **22**(1), 03–516 (2019)
84. Future Facility. http://futurefacility.co.uk/grasping-the-future/thedesignmuseum/
85. New Old: Designing for our future selves. The design Museum, exhibition curated by Myerson, J., Hamlyn, H., the Royal College of Art, (January 2017). https://designmuseum.org/whats-on/pop-up-exhibitions/new-old
86. Schreier, J., Ford, C., Niederhoffer, G., Bisbee, S., Bisbee, J.K., Acord, L., Rifkin, D.: Robot & Frank. Sony Pictures Home Entertainment (Firm) (2013)
87. Kittay, E.F.: The ethics of care, dependence, and disability. Ratio Juris **24**(1), 49–58 (2011)
88. Noddings, N.: Caring: a relational approach to ethics and moral education. UCP (2013)
89. Littman, L., Myerhoff, B.: Inventing, in Woodward, K.M., (ed.) Figuring Age: Women, Bodies, Generations, vol. 23, p. 166. IU Press (1999)

90. Moss, D.: Smart aging—The impact of IoT on the elderly and caregivers alike. Medicine X, Public Presentation. Stanford University (September 2016). https://www.youtube.com/watch?v=H00TqDbBKL4
91. Wright A.: Old age is over: why are products for older people so ugly? MIT Technology Review (2019). https://www.technologyreview.com/2019/08/21/133320/why-are-products-for-older-people-so-ugly/
92. Abrahms S.: New technology could allow you or your parents to age at home, AARP (2014). https://www.aarp.org/home-family/personal-technology/info-2014/is-this-the-end-of-the-nursing-home.2.html
93. Almeida, A., Mulero, R., Rametta, P., Urošević, V., Andrić, M., Patrono, L.: A critical analysis of an IoT—aware AAL system for elderly monitoring. Futur. Gener. Comput. Syst. **97**, 598–619 (2019)
94. Coleman, R., Pullinger, D.J.: Designing for our future selves. Appl. Ergon. **24**(1), 3–4 (1993)
95. Benktzon, M.: Designing for our future selves: the Swedish experience. Appl. Ergon. **24**(1), 19–27 (1993)

Innovative Street Furniture Supporting Electric Micro-mobility for Active Aging

Theo Zaffagnini, Gabriele Lelli, Ilaria Fabbri, and Marco Negri

Abstract The promotion of active aging and healthy mobility among seniors is a global challenge. The recent diffusion of e-bikes, mobility scooters, and electric tricycles has disclosed new opportunities for older adults to get around with less effort and much later in life than they previously imagined. As electric micro-mobility makes it easier for older people to stay active and reduce isolation, they might, in turn, require cities and communities to implement better, more people-centric infrastructure to support them, delivering great benefits for residents and commuters of all ages, as well. Within this framework, this chapter presents objectives and preliminary outcomes of an applied research on IoT-based urban services, commissioned by one of the leading Italian utility operatings in environmental field, and dealing with the design and installation of a network of Smart Hubs, accessible and versatile street furniture combining electric charging station with a wide range of other urban services. Smart Hubs' network represents a cutting edge IoT application providing a smarter user experience for all city users, especially the elderly. The inclusive design approach combines physical and digital elements to improve well-being and offers innovative urban services. The chapter will point out how brand new IoT-based solutions and the global diffusion of electric micro-mobility have the potential to rewrite the consolidate distribution, density and features of services found in a traditional bike-friendly city, as they enable commuters and citizens, even those that can no longer cycle on a regular bike or comfortably moving around by foot, to reach longer

---

T. Zaffagnini (✉)
Architectural Technology, Architecture Department, University of Ferrara, Ferrara, Italy
e-mail: theo.zaffagnini@unife.it

G. Lelli
Architecture and Urban Design, Architecture Department, University of Ferrara, Ferrara, Italy
e-mail: gabriele.lelli@unife.it

I. Fabbri · M. Negri
International Doctorate in Architecture and Urban Planning (IDAUP), Architecture Department, University of Ferrara, Ferrara, Italy
e-mail: ilaria.fabbri@unife.it

M. Negri
e-mail: marco.negri@unife.it

© The Author(s), under exclusive license to Springer Nature Singapore Pte Ltd. 2022
S. Scataglini et al. (eds.), *Internet of Things for Human-Centered Design*,
Studies in Computational Intelligence 1011,
https://doi.org/10.1007/978-981-16-8488-3_15

distances in a shorter amount of time. Beyond the design of a new street furniture supporting personal electric vehicles, the research investigates the most effective aggregation of different public amenities and facilities (public restrooms, hydration stations, benches and others) and figures out the possible impacts of these smart living environments throughout the city on seniors' mobility and autonomy.

Keywords Urban Health · Urban design · IoT · Smart city · Sustainable mobility

1 Introduction

Urban mobility plays a fundamental role in the promotion of elderly healthcare. The main elements of this field—i.e. public space network, means of transportation, transport behaviors—affect not only the urban environment but also individual behaviors and social relationships.

All these issues, which account as non-clinical factors for 80% of people's health condition [1], can be referred to the Dahlgren and Whitehead rainbow [2], one of the most relevant frameworks about the social determinants of health. Urban mobility acts on all the Dahlgren–Whitehead rainbow layers, which set up the genetic and environmental factors that influence physical and mental health starting from the individual's ability to influence these factors. Between the individual lifestyle factors—the inner Dahlgren–Whitehead rainbow layer—we can include the choice of means of transportation and related mobility patterns have a direct impact on the other rainbow layers as their influence on social and community networks and on the level of accessibility to urban services.

These factors have been taken up in several in-depth studies and policies related to active aging, one of the most relevant issues in elderly healthcare. Health21, the European policy framework for the promotion and protection of health in the twenty-first century includes in its targets healthy ageing "as reflected in increases in life expectancy, disability-free life expectancy, and the proportion of older people who are healthy and at home"; "reducing non-communicable diseases" and "a healthy and safe physical environment" [3]. The importance of transportation in achieving Health 21 policy goals and its role in improving the social determinants of health has been highlighted in several documents and reports—cf. on impacts [4, 5]—which promote active and public transport as they provide physical exercise, reduce fatal accidents, increase social interaction, and decrease air pollution. Furthermore, WHO and European Commission [6, 7] has defined transport and mobility as one of the main domains to achieve an age-friendly city, providing a series of indicators to measure the impact of planned interventions to improve the social and physical environment. In this context, acting on the core factors of urban mobility—i.e. means of transportation and urban services—can provide significant improvements on supporting active living and maintaining elderly connections to social networks and urban services.

The digital revolution and particularly the widespread use of connected devices has created new networks of objects—Internet of Things (IoT)—leading to a radical change in all sectors, including those of healthcare and urban mobility. New opportunities of action with smart objects have changed the mobility sector from a car-based paradigm to a transversal one more focused on mobility service and user experience—Mobility as a Service (MaaS).

These improvements unlocked the spread of new approaches to urban mobility services more suited to the mobility demand and mode of transport. Sharing mobility has emerged as one of the most effective urban mobility services in both urban and suburban areas, enabling new optimizing the demand for mobility and improving the efficiency of the whole transportation system. The flexibility of sharing mobility platforms has also favored the use of new means of transportation, lighter and less polluting. One of the most interesting segments is electric micro-mobility—i.e. e-moped, e-scooter, e-bike—a hybrid transport system alternative to car sharing in urban and suburban areas, accessible to all age groups and able to combine the positive effects of active mobility while reducing the physical effort required. While most EU cities have already adopted e-car sharing systems, e-bike solutions are increasingly growing: for instance, Sharing Cities, one of the major EU sharing platforms on smart cities solutions, identified e-bike sharing schemes as one of the best practices supporting the shift to low carbon shared mobility solutions. Milan, London, and Lisbon are just some of the cities that have adopted electric bike sharing schemes to support sustainable and active mobility.

On the other hand, the availability of new digital technologies—artificial intelligence/AI, IoT networks, smart sensors—has changed healthcare services toward a more integrated and personalized system that supports people's autonomy and gathers personalized health datasets to assess people's lifestyle. The use of digital devices, smart objects, and smart services can unlock new health data, a key element for digital health services, supporting a continuous care system that overcomes the current hospital-centered common vision. According to the main policy framework [7], one of the core issues is to create an integrated health and care ecosystem, where Silver Economy and e-health are blended and ICT products and services are integrated to allow a cross-border use of health services. A patient-based model of health and care that takes greater account of the patient's social relationships, the quality of the physical environment, and the degree of accessibility to essential urban services.

Within this context, urban mobility services constitute one of the main IoT interfaces in the urban environment, contributing to active aging policies and urban accessibility. This chapter presents the objectives and preliminary outcomes of Smart Hubs, applied research on IoT-based urban services, particularly the ones related to elderly healthcare and active aging. Firstly, will be introduced the methodological pipeline in which the project has been developed. Then there will be a selected literature review on e-bikes and international case studies, linking them to the chapter issues. These findings will frame the Smart Hub project, described regarding the product issues and its relationships with the urban environment. The conclusions will outline the early findings of the project and their possible impacts on the creation of smart living environments fitted for the elderly.

2 Methodology

The applied research presented in this chapter regards the installation of innovative street furniture already developed as a prototype and named Smart Hub. The testing activities are made within the AIR BREAK project, a UIA initiative focused on the promotion and co-production of innovative air quality solutions to transform degraded areas into healthy living environments [8].

According to the project schedule and deliverables, the project activities considered for this contribution are mainly the site selection and the co-design process. These are completed with a literature review focused on the healthcare benefits that e-mobility systems could provide for the elderly and how these issues are related to the urban environment. The literature findings will enable us to put in perspective the project aims and its preliminary outcomes.

Regarding the selected activities, a first issue to point out is the fact that the Smart Hubs will be tested in 4 areas near the city center, selected according to the project needs and urban context characteristics. This would provide an opportunity to collect more feedback and information—which means more valuable data for research and project development—and to refer them to specific site issues e.g. demographic structure, environmental quality, or cycling network offer.

A second element to point out is the support of a co-design lab; a series of participatory events to involve users, stakeholders, experts, and local communities on three main objectives. First of all, sharing ideas about complementary services and features that could be installed or implemented in the Smart Hubs, both the four planned within AIR BREAK the project and the future ones. The second objective is to co-design the Smart Hubs character relating to the different urban contexts where they will be installed, involving locals to respond to the context needs and promote virtuous synergies. Finally, involving economic stakeholders and local communities to envision innovative business models which can contribute to Smart Hubs dissemination within the city, delivering tailored smart solutions according to local contexts and needs. The co-design process is structured in five steps (Fig. 1): preliminary presentation, first focus group, workshop on Smart Hub services, second focus group, public presentation of the results. The quantitative research techniques used for the co-design lab aim to deepen different aspects of user feedback. While the two focus groups stimulate interaction between participants, encouraging the sharing of ideas and new insights, the workshop seeks to co-define specific features of the project—i.e. sensors and services—with users and stakeholders. The combination of these methods supports the creation of valuable interactions and the deepening of user needs, key elements to improve system features such as usability, accessibility, and security.

All these activities share several elements with the User-Centered Design (UCD) framework (Fig. 2). In particular, the diversity of collected data consents different types of evaluations about both user experience widening the possible contributions on urban health. Thus, the heuristic evaluations about the project would impact

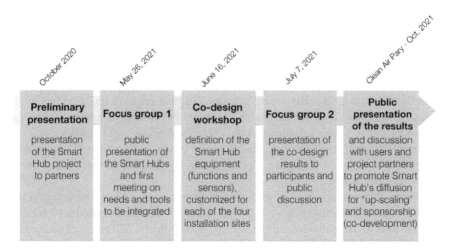

Fig. 1 Calendar of the co-creation process "designing together smart hubs"

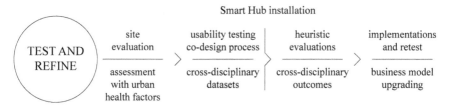

Fig. 2 Test and refine process edited from the usability.gov UCD map [9]

several urban health domains, from specific kinds of users—e.g. elderly—to environmental factors. Thus, the UCD framework would be used combining different fields of research to obtain new implementations of the whole project.

3 Literature Review

Researchers developed a wide range of scientific contributions to assess the e-bike phenomena, highlighting their contributions to decrease traditional cycling barriers, especially the level of physical effort required for the non-motorized vehicles and the average travel speed. The use of e-bikes is functional in hilly or windy environments and for users with limited physical impairments; moreover, electric bike sharing systems can improve connectivity [10, 11] not only in urban areas but also in rural territories with an underdeveloped public transportation system [12].

These characteristics have contributed to the increasing success of the e-bike, producing a substitution effect from other transportation modes in several countries.

In China, the use of e-bike has been widespread since the 90 s, where it is used by elderly and non-elderly people for commuting, establishing as an effective alternative to public transport and private cars as it is more convenient in terms of time and money [13–15]. In Europe, most of the scientific literature comes from northern countries such as Belgium, the Netherlands, and Sweden and confirmed the e-bikes' contributions to significantly reduce car trips [16] and improve traffic and environmental conditions. With the increasing popularity of e-bikes among the elderly and commuters [17], follow-up research [18, 19] highlighted the potential downsides of the unselective substitution of existing transport modes with e-bikes. These studies suggest more targeted engagement policies, mainly focused on users who benefit most from this solution.

Within this research field, several studies have been conducted focusing on the most frequent motivations for using an e-bike and the health benefits of e-bikes for the elderly. An extended survey in older e-bike riders [20] assesses their main motivations related to this transport choice. The survey showed how most of the respondents had already been regular cyclists and how the main motivations were related to riding with less effort and replacing car trips with other transportation modes. Another recent publication [21] confirmed these outcomes, finding that the main motivations for riding e-bikes are the possibility to conquer longer distances or steeper climbs and their improvement of physical and mental health.

Because of the features of this transport mode, the e-bike health impact depends on the mobility patterns it substitutes. On the one hand, when the e-bike replaces conventional bicycles, health benefits may decrease [22] or otherwise be challenged [23]. On the other hand, the shift from motorized vehicles leads to less air pollution, reduced traffic congestion, a more active mobility pattern. Regarding safety aspects, the higher speeds of e-bikes cause more risks compared to conventional bicycles. Although riding an e-bike is likely to cause more severe injuries and increase fatality risk, the elderly e-cyclists speed can be compared to the speed of cyclists in middle adulthood on a conventional bicycle [24].

Follow-up research by Van Cauwenberg et al. [25] analyzes how e-bike promotes healthy mobility among older adults aged more than 65 years. Survey results indicate that seniors use e-bikes for both transportation and recreation, helping to maintain the social relationships that are a central issue of healthy aging. The contribution of this mobility choice to sustainable mobility lies mostly in the fact that e-bike maintains cycling even for older adults and enables moderate-intensity physical activity.

A recent extended review of existing literature [26] confirmed that seniors, out-of-shape people, or people with physical impairments as those who can benefit most from the e-bike, balancing safety concerns with health and environmental benefits. Moreover, the same research detailed the factors influencing the health of e-bike users finding that e-bike is more indicated for people with a low or average level of health and that e-bikers aged between 50 and 64 years have more consistent health gains than younger cohorts. Regarding the trip length, the study indicates how health gains for this cohort are minor in a 5–10 km trip starting to be more and more significant from this distance.

These researches highlight how the promotion of urban bicycling and e-mobility leads to an effective improvement of urban health, considering both physical health and the social, economic, and environmental factors underlying the social determinants of health and active aging models.

Bringing these considerations back into the urban environment, if we consider the smart city as an "effective integration of physical, digital, and human systems in the built environment to deliver a sustainable, prosperous, and inclusive future for its citizens" [27] it can be argued that a real smart city has to take into account the active aging and healthy city concepts. The correlations between these concepts and the urban environment have been studied mostly in the field of transportation and urban planning. The five Ds model—density, diversity, design, destination accessibility, and distance to public transit—tries to define five key elements of urban form generally associated with walking and cycling [28, 29].

If density, destination accessibility, and urban design are strictly associated with high levels of walking, cycling can be intended as a more complex phenomenon that depends both on urban design and socio-economic factors as the perception of the bicycle as a "budget" transportation mode or as a "default" mode socially accepted by the whole population. Several Chinese studies made a quantitative analysis between cycling and urban environment characteristics, finding that a medium distance to the city center, finding that the e-bike is more widely used in areas not too far from the city center, with high occupancy density, use mix and with limited public transport offerings [30, 31]. The European context also seems to confirm these findings, correlating higher levels of bicycle use with urban areas well connected to other parts of the city and with a high density of points of interest [32]. Specifically, the research shows that the most influential factors for bicycle use are flat terrain, proximity to retail services, high population density, and good road network connectivity.

All these findings match with public health strategies for designing healthy environments. Mobility and accessibility are a fundamental part of the Urban Health promotion [33], as it can be easily traced in at least four of the thirteen Urban Health Strategies selected from a wide literature review that examined the correlations between urban health and physical environment [34]. The improvement of bike sharing systems, which we could extend to electric bike sharing systems because of the above mentioned research, is considered one of the key actions for the reduction of vehicular traffic, namely one of the urban health strategies indicated by the authors. According to the research findings, working on bike sharing schemes is correlated to several Health Outcomes such as Urban Heat Island, air and pollution and noise, safety and security, and the attractiveness of places. By demonstrating the key role of the urban environment to move from a medical model to a social model of Public Health, this study highlights how these strategies must be considered from the earliest stages of urban planning by involving professionals and communities to implement shared and verifiable urban health strategies.

Another relevant public health strategy related to these issues is the Healthy Streets approach [35], a human-centered framework aiming to improve urban health factors in the road network. This approach has been adopted, among others, in the Transport of London policies and design guidelines as a useful tool to evaluate the road network system—especially the urban road network—and address the design phase with an evidence-based approach focused on urban health promotion and social inclusion. The Healthy Street framework can be represented by the Healthy Streets indicators, ten evidence-based domains on what makes streets healthier and more inclusive.

Within this framework, which includes not only physical interventions but also those on mobility behaviors and urban services, we can find several indicators that are particularly interesting for this discussion. The first one is "clean air", which collects the measures related to the reduction of air pollution sources, especially from motor vehicles. Then "shade and shelter", grouping all actions for increasing shade and shelter spots within the streetscape—particularly important if we consider the aging population and climate change trends—and "places to stop and rest", dealing with opportunity to create inclusive streets with resting places for ill, injured, older or very young people. The Healthy Streets indicators, and particularly the previous ones, can be seen as potential benchmarks for urban smart services that promote active mobility through healthy environments.

This review highlighted the significant contribution of electric micro-mobility, especially e-biking, to the creation of smart healthy environments. A strategic contribution, given that this transportation mode is more and more used due to its ability to balance physical effort and environmental gains and has the greatest benefits in the older segments of the population. In this sense, the creation of innovative urban services in this field contributes not only to improve the attractiveness of this transportation mode but also to upgrade the environmental factors that influence public health. The above mentioned researches, crossing sustainable mobility, urban design, and urban health—especially Urban Health Strategies and Healthy Streets research—highlight how urban services are an essential element for the creation of an inclusive, smart, and healthy city that uses technology to improve urban health conditions across all ages.

4 E-mobility Infrastructure in Italy

The deployment of charging infrastructure and charging points is a crucial step for the spreading of e-mobility. Despite the consistent growth between 2015 and 2020, Italy still has a lower deployment than other EU Member States such as Germany, France, and the Netherlands which together account for the large majority of all charging points in Europe [36]. To exploit the benefits of this new transportation mode, urban e-mobility hubs are indicated as core elements that combine multiple charging solutions to support e-mobility while improving public space [37].

The most important players at the national scale—e.g. Enel X, Hera, IrenGo—have deployed primarily networks for Battery Electric Vehicles (BEVs), with more than one hundred thousand public and private charging points located mainly in the major cities. Despite this, RePower, another national e-mobility player, made a slightly different choice: while investing in corporate charging points for electric cars, it developed a network of charging points for e-bikes in northern Italy. A choice in line with the current offer of charging points, which are placed for a large majority in central and northern Italy. The charging network is composed mainly of urban stations, usually integrated with the local BSS, and other corporate stations—e.g. BikeEnergy and Alto Adige e-bike—placed in touristic areas to improve e-bike tourism. The market and stakeholder findings highlight how in Italy, cities are already structured to deploy e-bike charging infrastructure, with the opportunity to combine urban services to multiple charging points creating brand-new smart service hubs in cities.

The diffusion of charging points has also brought new design products acting on urban services and urban design issues. Among these products, two of the most relevant are Enel X Juicepole/Juicebox and RePower E-lounge, both awarded in 2020 with the Compasso d'Oro ADI, one of the most important awards in the field of product design.

Enel X Juicepole/Juicebox, designed by Koz Susani Design studio, conceived a discreet and simple object, with compact dimensions to reduce its visual impact which recalls pedestrian poles. The user interface has been condensed on top with a touchscreen hi-tech "head", while the body hosts charging sockets and the cladding, which can be replaced with different materials to better fit within the city landscape. RePower E-lounge, designed by Antonio Lanzillo and partners, is a public bench embedded with a wi-fi router and electric sockets for charging e-bikes, smartphones, and other technological devices. Anchored to the ground with metal plates, the bench is divided into two parts. The first one, in painted metal, contains the wiring and electrical outlets, and the second one, in solid wood, is shaped like a bike rack. The use of natural materials such as wood and metal recalls the concept of sustainable mobility and invites people to use the object as a resting place while recharging their bikes or electric devices.

These products represent two different ways to conceive e-mobility charging points in the urban context. While Juicepole/Juicebox is dedicated to BEV charging, E-lounge stands as one of the few solutions designed for e-bikes. Merging urban furniture, electric recharge, and public connectivity, e-lounge combines different mobility services with the social and visual needs of public space to offer a design product that aims to increase urban space value.

5 Smart Hub Street Furniture

In Ferrara, Smart Hub is one of the main deliverables of AIR BREAK, together with other key actions: the installation of new IoT air quality stations, a smart cycle path connecting the city center with the outskirts, the planting of more than 2.000 trees and shrubs in urban areas, the installation of innovative urban services dedicated to e-mobility. All these solutions have been planned to reach the AIR BREAK project goal, which is the reduction of air pollution by 25% in 3 years in poor environmental quality areas. An ambitious challenge, which blends physical interventions in the city with a set of co-design labs to involve city users and stakeholders.

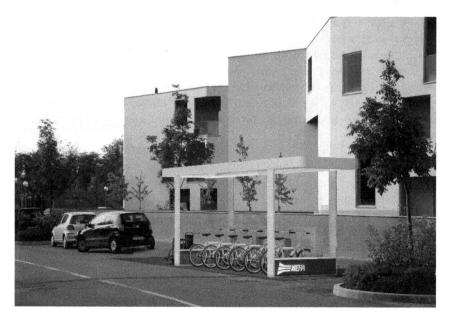

Fig. 3 Smart Hub tentative visualization in residential urban context

Regarding the design concept, Smart Hub proposes an innovative mobility concept combining IoT-based urban services with a contemporary design, suitable for different locations and seamlessly integrable into the urban space (Fig. 3). The solution is composed of a steel frame canopy, self-standing and easy to build, with a semi-transparent roof made of colored photovoltaic glass which shelters the e-bike charging point and other IoT urban services. In order to be compatible with most urban sites, the overall width of the shelter fits parallel parking lots and can also be adjusted for wider public space facing a road. The charging station, connected to the electric supply networks, can benefit from the solar panels on its roof. Along with charging for batteries and theft-proof bike stands, Smart Hub provides seating, a bike repair station, sensors, and cameras. Additional functions, such as inductive cell phone charging spots and parcel locker, can be easily added with incremental updates. Most of these features are IoT systems that share data related to the urban environment and city users' behaviors: smartphone, bike rack, locker, environmental sensors, security cameras. All this technological equipment will enable public administrations and utilities to collect urban data bringing together information sets rarely examined in combination, such as detailed travel patterns and the exposure to noise and air pollution. Sustainability issues that can be traced, in the project's intentions, not only in the main challenges of Smart Hub—e.g. sustainable mobility and urban health promotion—but also in construction materials: the steel structure is 100% recyclable, and the design options include the use of recycled wood composite slats and recycled plastic coverings.

Moreover, Smart Hubs features sum up several benefits for elderly healthcare. More than just bike shelters, Smart Hubs offer themselves as protected meeting points making streets a more comfortable environment for the elderly where they can take a break or socialize. The core services enable a more sustainable way to move within the city: e-bike stations providing not only health benefits but also contributing to other active aging factors such as social life and mental health; cameras increase public space security; environmental sensors monitor air pollutants and noise level. The system follows inclusive design principles, with heights and overall dimensions fitting wheelchair users and people with physical impairments and with material and edges designed for a safe and smooth user experience for all ages. In this sense, the installations carried out with the AIR BREAK project will allow to collect more data to validate these benefits, improving the design choices and adapting them to context needs.

Within this context, AIR BREAK planned the installation of Smart Hub in four strategic areas of Ferrara to promote sustainable mobility and to connect points of interest in the city (Fig. 4). The four areas are next to the rail station, the Technopole of Ferrara, the Darsena area, and the "Corti di Medoro" area. All of them, selected on their urban, environmental, and transport characteristics are located in the southwest of the city and near to the city center. The first location, near to the rail station, was selected because of its importance as a multimodal node for the area, for the potential synergy with the planned requalification project of Velostation in place of an existing bike rack area, and for the presence of both electrical and data connections which ease the installation process. The second location for Smart Hub is near to the Technopole of Ferrara, an area not far from the center crossing several points of interest—among these the Technopole and the Engineering University—and near to the smart bike path planned within the AIR BREAK project. The third location is the Darsena area (i.e. the docks) green area between Darsena street and Burana canal part of the main renovation project of the MOF area; its closeness to the rail station, to the city center, and the new smart cycle path make it a strategic location for the installation. The last selected area is "Corti di Medoro", a recently redeveloped housing complex at 10' by bike from the city center near to commercial activities and a sports center and with existing electrical and data connections.

The selection of Smart Hubs location highlights how urban networks—transport, data, electricity—represents a significant trade-off for installing urban services. This choice confirms the literature findings, which consider diversity and accessibility as key issues for cycling. In addition to that, another issue is that all the new hubs are close to urban regeneration areas, either already delivered—Corti di Medoro, Technopole of Ferrara—or in progress—Darsena and rail station. Within the AIR BREAK project, urban services are seen as enablers of healthy-based urban regeneration processes acting not through the redesign of the whole area but increasing the number of services and points of interest within the urban fabric. Starting from the traditional model of the bike-friendly city of Ferrara, which considers the historical city as the more fitted area in which to deploy sustainable mobility solutions, AIR BREAK aims to create new healthy urban environments through a series of material and immaterial interventions around the city center. The expected result is to improve

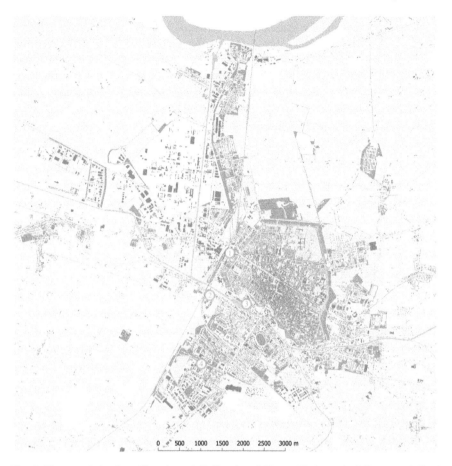

Fig. 4 The smart hub selected locations: 1. Rail station; 2. Ferrara Technopole; 3. Darsena; 4. Corti di Medoro

the regeneration process already planned to provide more efficient networks, more good data, more urban services. A new way to challenge communities and strategic urban projects for the improvement of urban health criteria for all ages.

6 Conclusions

The early outcomes of the project activities, which officially started in October 2020 with a public kick-off meeting [38], mainly concerned the inspection of selected areas to highlight critical installation issues and the first meetings of the co-design lab.

The first point confirms the relevance of urban regeneration interventions and the availability of cycling, electricity, and data infrastructures to better exploit the innovative potential of smart urban services based on IoT technologies. The site choice is consistent with the project goals and fosters an urban regeneration process that acts not only through building refurbishment but also through new distribution, density, and quality of urban services. A model that, as highlighted in the literature review, acts on urban health factors—especially the ones related to e-mobility issues—that produce the greatest health and environmental benefits for the elderly. The Smart Hub installations, scheduled for July 2022, will allow usability tests, survey the actual number of participants and structure them by age.

In the meantime, the co-design meetings started with the preliminary presentation of the smart hubs and the first focus group with stakeholders and experts. The first outcomes show considerable interest in relevant issues for elderly healthcare. In particular, the inclusion of sheltered spots and rest areas, which is one of the factors that influences positively Public Health strategies and the Healthy Streets approach, has been one of the most discussed issues in these meetings.

In conclusion, preliminary results seem to confirm the key role of point of interests—e.g. innovative street furniture—and regeneration processes to develop urban proximity and healthy-based urban environments. The first outcomes and feedbacks lead to services and features that would interest especially the elderly, as described before. The development of the project activities, with the main reports and deliverables published online,[1] will evaluate the impacts of the planned actions both on urban health factors and urban quality, assessing the different benefits of innovative street furniture for the city and its users.

Acknowledgements The patented prototype of smart bike shelter PUNTO NET BIKE (inventors: Enrico Piraccini, Simone Allegra, Gabriele Lelli, Ilaria Fabbri, Roberta Bandini) is currently under development as SMART HUB with Enrico Piraccini, Simone Allegra, Gabriele Lelli, Ilaria Fabbri, Roberta Bandini and Gabriele Mengozzi, Patrizia Mangifesta.

Within the AIR BREAK project, SMART HUB is one of the four main urban actions.

This chapter reports some of the activities of the UIA project "AIR BREAK-Co-producing healthy clean commuting air spots in town" ERDF. Hereafter the project credits.

AIR BREAK CREDITS

Project title: AIR BREAK—Co-producing healthy clean commuting air spots in town

UIA Urban Innovative Actions project—UIA 05-177.

Urban Authority coordinator: Municipality of Ferrara. Partners: University of Ferrara, Sipro Ferrara, Politecnico di Milano, Bruno Kessler Foundation, Dedagroup Public Services Srl, LabService Analytica, Hera spa.

Start date 01 /07 /2020

End date 30 /06/2023

FIGURES

Figures 1 and 4 are edited from online contents of the AirBreak website; Figs. 2 and 4 are made by the authors within the Next City Lab research group.

The authors are solely responsible for the content of this publication.

---

[1] https://airbreakferrara.net/air-breaking-news/.

References

1. Teutsch, S.M.: Getting to average life expectancy: it takes commitment. Am. J. Public Health **108**(1), 17–18 (2018)
2. Dahlgren, G., Whitehead, M.: In: Policies and Strategies to Promote Social Equity in Health. Institute for Futures Studies, Stockholm (1991)
3. WHO: Health 21. The health for all policy framework for the WHO European Region. Copenhagen: World Health Organization, Regional Office for Europe (1999)
4. Wilkinson, R., Marmot, M.: In: Social Determinants of Health: The Solid Facts. World Health Organization Office for Europe, Geneva (2003)
5. WHO: Global strategy and action plan on ageing and health. World Health Organization, Geneva (2017)
6. WHO: Measuring the age-friendliness of cities: a guide to using core indicators. World Health Organization, Kobe (2015)
7. WHO 2017: Global strategy on digital health 2020–2025. World Health Organization, Geneva (2021)
8. AIR BREAK—Co-producing healthy clean commuting air spots in town. Retrieved April 8th, (2021). https://uia-initiative.eu/en/uia-cities/ferrara-0
9. User-Centered Design Process Map. Retrieved April 8th (2021). https://www.usability.gov/how-to-and-tools/resources/ucd-map.html
10. Ji, S., Cherry, C.R., Han, L.D., Jordan, D.A.: Electric bike sharing: simulation of user demand and system availability. J. Clean. Prod. **85**, 250–257 (2014). https://doi.org/10.1016/j.jclepro.2013.09.024
11. Langford, B.C., Cherry, C., Yoon, T., Worley, S., Smith, D.: North America's first E-Bikeshare: a year of experience. Transp. Res. Rec. **2387**(1), 120–128 (2013)
12. Bruzzone F., Scorrano F., Nocera S.: The combination of e-bike sharing and demand-responsive transport systems in rural areas: a case study of Velenje. Res. Transp. Business Manage. 100570 (2021). https://doi.org/10.1016/j.rtbm.2020.100570
13. Cherry, C.R., Yang, H., Jones, L.R., He, M.: Dynamics of electric bike ownership and use in Kunming China. Transp. Policy **45**, 127–135 (2016). https://doi.org/10.1016/j.tranpol.2015.09.007
14. Ye, Y., Xin, F., Wei, L.: Characteristics of the electric bicycle: a comparative analysis with bicycles and public transit. In: CICTP 2014, pp. 3450–3458. (2014)
15. Xin, F., Chen, Y., Wang, X.: In: Research on Electric Bicycle Users' Travel Mode Choice Behavior Based on Prospect Theory (2017)
16. Winslott, H.L., Svensson, Å.: E-bike use in Sweden—CO_2 effects due to modal change and municipal promotion strategies. J. Clean. Prod. **141**, 818–824 (2017)
17. CONEBI: European Bicycle Market—2016 Edition.Industry and Market Profile, Brussels (2016)
18. De Haas, M., Kroesen, M., Chorus, C., Hoogendoorn-Lanser, S., Hoogendoorn, S.: E-bike user groups and substitution effects: evidence from longitudinal travel data in the Netherlands. Transportation (2021). https://doi.org/10.1007/s11116-021-10195-3
19. Sun, Q., Feng, T., Kemperman, A., Spahn, A.: Modal shift implications of e-bike use in the Netherlands: moving towards sustainability?. Transp. Res. Part D Transp. Environ. **78**, 102202 (2020)
20. Johnson, M., Rose, G.: Extending life on the bike: electric bike use by older Australians. J. Transp. Health **2**(2), 276–283 (2015). https://doi.org/10.1016/j.jth.2015.03.001
21. The European e-bike market is booming, latest industry figures show – and there is potential for more. Retrieved April 8th, 2021 (2020). https://ecf.com/news-and-events/news/european-e-bike-market-booming-latest-industry-figures-show-%E2%80%93-and-there
22. Kroesen, M.: To what extent do e-bikes substitute travel by other modes? evidence from the Netherlands. Transp. Res. Part D: Transp. Environ. **53**, 377–387 (2017)
23. Simsekoglu, Ö., Klöckner, C.A.: The role of psychological and sociodemographic factors for electric bike use in Norway. Int. J. Sustain. Transp. **13**(5), 315–323 (2019)

24. Vlakveld, W.P., Twisk, D., Christoph, M., Boele, M., Sikkema, R., Remy, R., Schwab, A.L.: Speed choice and mental workload of elderly cyclists on e-bikes in simple and complex traffic situations: a field experiment. Accid. Anal. Prev. **74**(2015), 97–106 (2014). https://doi.org/10.1016/j.aap.2014.10.018
25. Van Cauwenberg, J., De Bourdeaudhuij, I., Clarys, P., de Geus, B., Deforche, B.: E-bikes among older adults: benefits, disadvantages, usage and crash characteristics. Transportation **46**(6), 2151–2172 (2019). https://doi.org/10.1007/s11116-018-9919-y
26. Hasnine, M.S., Dianat, A., Habib, K. N.: Investigating the factors affecting the distance travel and health conditions of e-bike users in Toronto. Transport. Res. Interdisciplinary Perspect. **8**, 100265 (2020). https://doi.org/10.1016/j.trip.2020.100265
27. BSI British Standards Institution: PAS 180:2014: Smart cities—Vocabulary (2014).
28. Ewing, R., Cervero, R.: Travel and the built environment. a meta analysis. J. Am. Plann. Assoc. **76**, 265–294 (2010). https://doi.org/10.1080/01944361003766766
29. Zhang, Y., Li, C., Ding, C., Zhao, C., Huang, J.: The built environment and the frequency of cycling trips by urban elderly: insights from zhongshan China. J. Asian Architect. Build Eng. **15**(2016), 511–518 (2016)
30. Ding, C., Cao, X., Dong, M., Zhang, Y., Yang, J.: Non-linear relationships between built environment characteristics and electric-bike ownership in Zhongshan, China. Transp. Res. Part D: Transp. Environ. **75**, 286–296 (2019)
31. Zhao, P.: The impact of the built environment on bicycle commuting: evidence from Beijing. Urban Stud. **51**, 1019–1037 (2014)
32. Nielsen, T.A.S., Olafsson, A.S., Carstensen, T.A., Skov-Petersen, H.: Environmental correlates of cycling: evaluating urban form and location effects based on Danish micro-data transport. Res. Part Transp. Environ **22**(2013), 40–44 (2013). https://doi.org/10.1016/j.trd.2013.02.017
33. Capolongo, S., Lemaire, N., Oppio, A., Buffoli, M., Roue Le Gall, A.: Action planning for healthy cities: the role of multi-criteria analysis, developed in Italy and France, for assessing health performances in land-use plans and urban development projects. Epidemiologia e Prevenzione **40**, 257–264 (2016)
34. Capolongo, S., Buffoli, M., Brambilla, A., Rebecchi, A.: Strategie urbane di pianificazione e progettazione in salute, per migliorare la qualità e l'attrattività dei luoghi. TECHNE **19**, 271–279 (2020)
35. Transport for London: Guide to Healthy Streets indicators. Transport for London, London (2017)
36. European Court of Auditors: Infrastructure for charging electric vehicles: more charging stations but uneven deployment makes travel across the EU complicated. Retrieved April 8th, 2021 (2021). https://www.eca.europa.eu/Lists/ECADocuments/SR21_05/SR_Electrical_charging_infrastructure_EN.pdf
37. Transport & Environment: Recharge EU: how many charge points will Europe and its Member States need in the 2020s. Retrieved April 8th, 2021 (2020). https://www.transportenvironment.org/sites/te/files/publications/01%202020%20Draft%20TE%20Infrastructure%20Report%20Final.pdf
38. The meeting record is available at: https://www.facebook.com/comuneferrara/videos/kick-off-meeting-air-break/2793867910876988/

IoT-Enabled Assistance and Engagement

Understanding the Acceptance of IoT and Social Assistive Robotics for the Healthcare Sector: A Review of the Current User-Centred Applications for the Older Users

Elvira Maranesi, Giulio Amabili, Giacomo Cucchieri, Silvia Bolognini, Arianna Margaritini, and Roberta Bevilacqua

Abstract The population of elderly people has increased rapidly over the last decades in Europe, and today, Italy is the oldest European country. In this context, robotics and other emerging technologies are increasingly proposed as potential solutions to improve the autonomy and quality of life of the elderly. This chapter aims at investigating the acceptance of the most recent technological solutions, in the field of IoT and assistive and social robotic services for elderly people, taking into account the availability of results from both the design phase and clinical studies, to ensure and verify the usability and acceptability of the solutions. This review shows that there are several robots that have been developed to not only provide companionship to older adults, but also to cooperate with them during health and lifestyle activities, such as facilitating reminiscence through cognitive stimulation, remembering tasks to be done, monitoring vital signs and whether they fall down, while at the same time entertaining them. Despite the undeniable usefulness of SARs, developers are often forced to prioritize the improvement of specific technical features due to the unavailability of resources and the different degrees of flexibility and acceptability imposed by unstructured settings, as private homes. The analysed studies sought to explore the usability and acceptability of the latest technological solutions in the field of

---

E. Maranesi · G. Amabili · G. Cucchieri (✉) · S. Bolognini · A. Margaritini · R. Bevilacqua
Scientific Direction, IRCCS INRCA, Ancona, Italy
e-mail: g.cucchieri@inrca.it

E. Maranesi
e-mail: e.maranesi@inrca.it

G. Amabili
e-mail: g.amabili@inrca.it

S. Bolognini
e-mail: s.bolognini@inrca.it

A. Margaritini
e-mail: a.margaritini2@inrca.it

R. Bevilacqua
e-mail: r.bevilacqua@inrca.it

© The Author(s), under exclusive license to Springer Nature Singapore Pte Ltd. 2022
S. Scataglini et al. (eds.), *Internet of Things for Human-Centered Design*,
Studies in Computational Intelligence 1011,
https://doi.org/10.1007/978-981-16-8488-3_16

IoT and social assistive robotics for older people, taking into account the availability of results from both the design stages and clinical trials, ensuring a patient-centred approach to older people. Understanding how to integrate IoT and smart solutions into the care pathway as well as in the daily life of the end-users is another crucial aspect for research in the field, which will be addressed within this chapter.

Keywords Internet of Things · Human-centred design · Elderly · Social assistive robots · Acceptance

1 Introduction

According to World Population Prospects 2019 (United Nations, 2019), by 2050, 1 in 6 people in the world will be over 65 years old [1], and globally, the number of people aged 80 or over is expected to triple [2], as better living conditions and lower mortality rates have led to an exponential increase in life expectancy. At the same time, viewing ageing as an inexorable physical and cognitive decline has been questioned: considering advancing age associated with a generalized loss of skills is too simplistic [3]. Population ageing is a complex phenomenon that affects all aspects of society, and its consequences will be felt on the social, economic, and health environment [4]. In particular, the most problematic expression of the population ageing is the clinical condition of frailty understood as a geriatric condition characterized by a decline in physiological functions associated with age, which leads to a greater vulnerability for negative health outcomes, [5] given above all by the dementia pictures that affect the elderly. The most frequent are Alzheimer's Disease (AD), dementia with Lewy bodies and fronto-temporal dementia. As far as functional capacity is concerned, accidents and fractures in old age as a result of a fall are also relatively frequent: each year 28–35% of the elderly over 65 and 32–42% over 70 report at least one episode of a fall. Falls lead to a series of negative events: the elderly loses their autonomy, are forced to depend on their caregiver, become immobile, and may develop a depressive framework. Sometimes, hospitalization may be necessary and may produce comorbidities that could lead to death [3]. Finally, the social condition of loneliness and isolation in which the elderly often find themselves should be emphasized [6]. These conditions are associated with an approximately 50% increased risk of dementia and other serious medical conditions, an increased risk of premature death from all causes, a risk that may rival that of smoking, obesity, and physical inactivity, and a 29% increased risk of heart disease and a 32% increased risk of stroke [7]. Physical and sensory changes and chronic diseases lead to a reduction in the reserves available to the individual, which makes him more vulnerable to the environment and less able to manage certain daily tasks [3]. For all these reasons, much has been invested in the last decade in the search for technological solutions that could help the elderly to prevent the above. In particular, there has been a focus on the development of Social Assistive Robots (SARs). A social robot is defined as an embodied artificial agent with the characteristics of a human or an animal. It has been identified as an approach to meet the mental health needs of older adults through interaction or information exchange [8].

SARs could help people with health conditions maintain positive social life by supporting them in social interactions, providing the help (be it health care, companionship, coaching with respect to physical activity or other) that older people need and to do so by engaging humans socially. In healthcare, SARs are envisioned to play roles such as taking medical interviews, monitoring and keeping a record of symptoms, helping with pill sorting and medication schedules, guiding people through therapeutic tasks, providing companionship, acting as stress reducers and mood enhancers, and supporting social interactions between humans [9–12]. In addition, several studies [13–15] show that social robots seem to have a positive impact on agitation, anxiety, and quality of life in the elderly, although no statistical significance has been found. In addition to this, the use of SARs could also be useful for caregivers: working in care settings with a high prevalence of chronicity, terminality, can be emotionally exhausting, requiring good resilience and the implementation of appropriate forms of emotional self-protection. Social robots could alleviate this burden, by making the interaction between caregiver and the elderly more positive [9].

However, results from narrative reviews [16, 17] indicated that interactions with social robots could improve engagement, interaction, and stress indicators, as well as reduce loneliness and medication use for older people.

In this context, where robotics and other emerging technologies are increasingly proposed as potential solutions to improve the autonomy and quality of life of elderly people, it is evident the lack of an in-depth study on the acceptance of these devices by elderly people, which should instead be the core around which these robots are designed. Indeed, within the major risks of low technology uptake and low acceptability by elderly end-users, the focus on the disease characteristics rather than patient profile remains the most relevant barrier to the widespread adoption of Internet of Things (IoT) and smart technologies, such as SAR (s). Moreover, there are a variety of interconnected factors that influence the acceptance and quality of experience, from initial emotions and attitudes to people's perception of a technology. Understanding why older adults accept or reject a certain technology, such as assistive robots, is important both to improve their design, with a systematic and human-centred approach from this stage, and to develop strategies to maximize their adoption. Considering the effects of normal ageing (i.e. visual, tactile and auditory decline) in the design should facilitate older adults' ability to interact with this technology, highlighting its potential to improve their physical health and well-being, social connectedness and ability to live independently at home.

The aims of this narrative review are:

- to investigate the acceptance of the latest technological solutions, in the field of Internet of Things (IoT) and social assistive robotics for older people, taking into account the availability of results from both the design phases and clinical studies, to ensure and verify the usability and acceptability of the solutions;

- to understand how to integrate IoT and smart solutions in the care pathway and daily life of the end-users.

2 Materials and Methods

This study takes the form of a narrative review. The literature review was conducted in March 2021. Data were collected from PubMed, Scopus, and Elsevier databases by analysing manuscripts and articles from the last 10 years (from March 2011 to March 2021) in order to obtain the latest evidence from the field. Based on a consultation with the multidisciplinary team, papers addressing the acceptance of robotic devices were searched using the following search terms, and their combinations: social robotics AND old*, social robotics AND old* AND user acceptance, e-health AND old*, robot* AND old*. After the preliminary search, 283 articles were identified from PubMed, 0 from Scopus and 134 from Elsevier. The findings were analysed and screened by three experts in the team: a bioengineer, a clinical psychologist, and an electronic engineer. The first screening was based on analysis of the title and abstract, as well as deduplication of the findings. Another researcher confirmed the accuracy of the article selection and checked for possible omissions. After the first step, 28 articles were identified from PubMed, 0 from Scopus and 5 from Elsevier. After the screening based on the full text articles, the studies were selected as follows: 9 from PubMed, 0 from Scopus, and 1 Elsevier database.

3 Results

A total of 10 papers were included [18–27]. Table 1 shows the characteristics of the studies.

All studies focused on elderly persons with a mean age of 75.5 ($\pm$5.6) years. The number of participants involved in all studies was 349, ranging from 6 to 103. From the information obtained from some articles [19–21, 24–26], there were 105 males and 194 females. The participants considered are divided into three main categories: healthy elderly, elderly with dementia, and elderly with mild or moderate cognitive impairment. The testing period of the social robots ranged from 10 days to 32 weeks. The user acceptability of robots was tested both in the laboratory [18] and at home [19–27] of the subjects recruited for the studies. Figure 1 shows the different technologies used in the selected studies.

The study conducted by Wu et al. [18] in France, involved 11 volunteers aged 76–85 years. Almost all of them were university graduates; 6 had a diagnosis of mild cognitive impairment (MCI), and 5 were cognitively intact healthy persons (CIH). The Mann–Whitney U-test showed that the two groups only differed significantly in their experience with the computer. The robot used is called Kompai (Fig. 1 panel I) and can recognize speech, respond, and navigate environments. Participants were

Table 1 Descriptive analysis of the included studies

Authors and year	Participants in experimental group	Technology	Commercial	Prototype	Intervention	Results
Wu et al [18]	n = 11 older adults, 9 F/2 M Age: min 76, max 85, average 79.3 years MCI = 6 CIH = 5	Kompai	X		Participants interacted with an assistance robot in a Living Lab. After being shown how to use the robot, participants performed tasks to simulate the use of the robot in everyday life. Mixed methods were used in this study, including a robot acceptance questionnaire, semi-structured interviews, usability-performance measures and a focus group. Trial period: once a week for 4 weeks, 1 h for each session	The MCI subjects needed more time to learn how to use the robot. Both groups had similar scored in the robot acceptance questionnaire, showed low intention to use the robot and negative attitudes towards it. They did not perceive it as useful in their daily lives. Instead, they found it easy to use, fun and non-threatening. Furthermore, social influence was perceived as powerful on robot adoption. Direct experience with the robot did not change the way participants evaluated the acceptance, and several barriers were identified, including discomfort with the technology, feelings of stigma, ethical, and social issues
McGlynn et al. [19]	n = 30 older adults, 15 F/15 M Age: min 67, max 80, average 72.17 years MCI = 0 CIH = 30	Paro	X		This study assessed Paro's acceptance, perceived usefulness and ease of use with normally older adults. The robot was presented to participants in three ways: as a pet, a robot, or a toy. They were randomly divided into three groups. Pre- and post-interaction attitudes towards Paro were assessed by adapting the scales of perceived ease of use and perceived usefulness of the TAM. Participants were interviewed with eight questions about their pre-interaction opinions and perceptions of the robot and eight post-interaction questions. Trial period: 1 session for each participant	The main finding of the study was that healthy older people also perceive benefits in using Paro, and minimal differences were found in the different ways the robot was presented

(continued)

Table 1 (continued)

Authors and year	Participants in experimental group	Technology	Commercial	Prototype	Intervention	Results
Maartje et al. [20]	n = 6 older adults, 4 F/2 M Age: min 50, max 76, average 62 years MCI = 0 CIH = 6	Nabaztag	X	–	This study focused on the long-term acceptability of a social robot at home. After each of the ten-day interaction periods, three in total, the participants' experiences were assessed by means of semi-structured interviews. The questions were aimed at assessing all aspects of acceptability: usefulness, interaction, evolution of the relationship with the robot, discussions with other people about the robot, mode of use and well-being exercises Trial period: more than 30 days—3 phases of at least 10 days each	The results showed that incorporation into the domestic context depends on the user's perception of the robot. Prolonged use of Nabaztag increases appreciation of its usefulness and capabilities, as well as its ease of use. Enjoyment of social interactions seems to be the key factor in acceptability, and users often refer to this sphere when giving an evaluation. Usefulness is also a determining factor. In general, a positive evaluation of one of these aspects positively influences the others, and vice versa
Korchut et al. [21]	n = 264, 187 F/77 M 3 groups: • medical staff (n = 100) • potential users (n = 83) MCI = 67 AD = 16 • caregivers (n = 81) Age of the potential users: min 55, max 90	–	–	–	(1) Focus group with medical staff (2) From data emerged, a survey questionnaire was created for medical staff, potential users, and caregivers. Main aspects investigated: functional requirements; human–robot interaction, the design of the robotic assistant and aspects of social acceptance (3) Based on the answers, a prioritization of the requirements and needs regarding robotic assistants was made Trial period: 4 months	(1) A robot is useful during the routines of daily life, a caregiver can be replace by it (2) The functional requirements considered with a "high priority" level are those associated with user safety (3) All functions relate to patient safety should be activated autonomously (4) The user can interact with the robot, a "high priority" level has been assigned to voice-operated system (5) The robot should have an anthropomorphic appearance and a face with positive emotional expressions

(continued)

Table 1 (continued)

Authors and year	Participants in experimental group	Technology	Commercial	Prototype	Intervention	Results
Beuscher et al. [22]	n = 19 older adults; 11 F/8 M; Age: min 66, max 94, average 81.9 years MCI = 13 CIH = 6	Nao	X		The elderly interacted alone or in a pair with the robot for 30–60 min, participating in some cognitive and physical activities	Nao's results were generally accepted. Participants found it easy to understand (68%), appreciated its voice (74%) and its appearance (86%). They were able to hear and understand the robot's speech (79%). Furthermore, it kept them interested (95%) and having a pleasant. However, only 63% rated the interaction with the robot as comfortable
Ray et al. [23]	n = 47 older adults, Age: average 70.8 years 47 CIH	digital photo frame-based well-being monitoring system		X	This study involved all the stakeholders, including older adults, during an iterative process for the design and development of the device	Most of the participants showed that they were not anxious when using the tablet applications. They showed a positive attitude towards this technology. Continuous family involvement and motivation was found to have a positive impact on the elderly's willingness to use these applications
Cavallo et al. [24]	n = 45 older adults, 30 F/15 M Age: min 65, max 86, average 74.21 years MCI = 0 CIH = 45	Robot-Era (DORO, CORO, ORO)		X	The experiments were organized in two sessions, using three robots in three different environments: home, condominium and outdoors. Initially, a questionnaire was administered to the user to collect first impressions, then the usability and acceptability of each robotic service was evaluated. For this last evaluation phase, an ad hoc questionnaire was prepared, composed of 14 items evaluated on a 5-point Likert scale Trial period: 2 sessions, the second one 3 months later	In general, the aesthetics and functionality of the robots had a positive impact on the elderly. Furthermore, the results suggest that the positive perception of the aesthetics of the robot might play a role in increasing the acceptance of robotic services by the elderly. Finally, the system showed the potential to be developed as a socially acceptable robotic service to promote the ability of the elderly to remain in their homes

(continued)

Table 1 (continued)

Authors and year	Participants in experimental group	Technology	Commercial	Prototype	Intervention	Results
Boumans et al. [25]	$n = 42$ older adults, 19 F/23 M Age: average 77.1 years	Pepper	X		In the first session, one group of participants was interviewed by the robot and another group by the nurse. Then, after 2 weeks, the groups were switched. The interview consisted of the same 3 questions, in each session of the study Trial period: 15 min each session, washout period of 2 weeks between sessions	(1) Social robots can interview the older people independently and the data collected can be considered valid (2) No significant differences emerged either in the speed of conducting the interview or in the similarity of the data collected
Chen et al. [26]	$n = 103$ older adults with dementia, 82 F/21 M Experimental group $n = 52$, control group $n = 51$ Age: min. 67, max 108, average 87.2 years	Kabochan		X	4 phases: in the first and third phases, the experimental group received routine care, while in the first two weeks of the second phase (phases B), they were instructed in the functions and characteristics of Kabochan. During the remaining six weeks of the second phase (B) and the eight weeks of the fourth phase (B), Kabochan was introduced to the subjects individually and everyone was free to interact with him. The control group received standard care throughout the trial period (1) The STAM used to verify acceptance of the robot (2) Direct observation to measure subject involvement Trial period: 32 weeks	(1) Positive change in perceived ease of use: involvement with the robot actually has the potential to improve the perceived ease of use of the technology (2) No significant change in attitudes towards technology, perceived usefulness, facilitation conditions, technology anxiety and self-efficacy after exposure to Kabochan compared to the control group

(continued)

Table 1 (continued)

Authors and year	Participants in experimental group	Technology	Commercial	Prototype	Intervention	Results
Søraa et al. [27]	$n = 8$ older adults MCI = 8	eWare system: Tessa robot and SensaraCare	X		Each person was interviewed 1–6 times during the experimental period in which they used the eWare system in their own home	Two uses of the eWare system were observed: end-users who mostly related to the Tessa robot and informal caregivers who mostly related to the SensaraCare sensors. For older adult end-users, Tessa took on a certain personality. The set of caregivers benefited from the reorganization of social relations through technology. All dimensions of domestication overlap and influence each other. Although they are presented separately, they were analysed—and should be seen—as interconnected and complementary. Technological domestication is not an individual process, but relies on a wide variety of actors. Therefore, it would be meaningful to add a fourth level to the theory of domestication of technology—that of "social domestication."

M male; F female; CIH cognitively intact healthy; MCI mild or moderate cognitive impairment; AD Alzheimer's Disease; TAM Technology Acceptance Model; STAM Senior Technology Acceptance Model

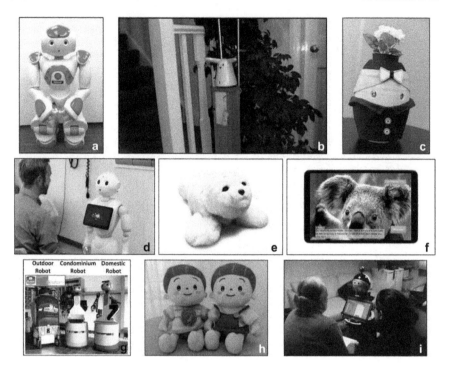

Fig. 1 Technologies involved in the studies analysed

invited to the laboratory once a week for four weeks. They interacted with the robot for about 1 h via voice or touch screen and performed 10 tasks to simulate its use in everyday life. To assess their acceptance, a questionnaire based on the Unified Theory of Acceptance and Use of Technology (UTAUT) model was developed, and time, the number of errors, and help required to perform the tasks were recorded. At the first session, participants expressed a low to moderate acceptance of Kompai. Low scores were given on four dimensions: intention to use, perceived usefulness, attitudes towards the robot, and images of an assistive robot. In contrast, ease of use, social influence, perceived enjoyment, and anxiety received relatively high scores. When comparing the first and fourth sessions, no significant differences emerged in the assessment of robot acceptance between the MCI and CIH groups.

Specifically, for acceptance, three themes emerged to capture users' attitudes and willingness to accept an assistive robot. For the interaction experience, all samples stated that Kompai had interesting features, while 7 out of 11 found its appearance pleasant. However, the weakest aspect of the robot was the voice control, due to technical failures of the system. It did not work well, and using it was frustrating, so much so that 3 users preferred to interact via the touch screen. Three MCIs also experienced cognitive difficulties, which were reflected in their inability to learn how to use the robot. Then, all unanimously reported that they were still independent and had no intention of using an assistive robot right away. With regard to future use, 7 out of 11 users were not enthusiastic. Furthermore, some barriers to acceptance were identified. For all of them, the use of an assistive robot was associated with negative aspects or with ageing, imagining this phase with fear. In addition, many users ($n = 8$) said they belonged to a generation not used to, or even averse to, technology. Finally, three participants raised ethical and social issues in relation to the use of robots, because they would feel observed or their privacy violated.

An American study conducted in 2014 by McGlynn et al. [19] aimed to investigate the perceived acceptance and usefulness of the Paro robot (Fig. 1 panel E) by healthy older people. It also investigated whether framing the social robot in three different ways, i.e. as a pet, a robot, or a toy, could influence these perceptions. Participants were 30 healthy older adults, 15 women and 15 men, aged between 67 and 80 years. Paro is a baby seal and specifically developed for therapeutic purposes, so its function is only to arouse positive emotions such as happiness and relaxation. Paro is covered in soft fur and has tactile, light, sound, and posture sensors, as well as being able to move its neck, fins, and eyelids. A special script was used to present the robot in each of the three framing conditions. Pre- and post-interaction attitudes towards Paro were assessed by adapting the Perceived Ease of Use and Perceived Usefulness scales from the Technology Acceptance Model (TAM) so that they were relevant to the study. Participants were asked eight questions before the interaction with the robot and eight questions afterwards. Analyses were conducted on the entire sample and focused on perceptions of usefulness after Paro had been switched on and participants had interacted with it. The mean perceived usefulness score was not significantly different from the neutral score, suggesting that participants found Paro neither likely nor unlikely to be useful to them. The perceived ease of use scores, both pre- and post-interaction, were significantly high, suggesting that participants found it quite likely that Paro would be easy to use both before and after interacting with it. Ultimately, the main finding of this study is that healthy older adults perceived the possible uses and benefits of Paro. The results showed that there were minimal effects from the different framing of the robot. Quantitative scores of perceived usefulness showed that healthy adults found it neither likely nor unlikely that Paro would be useful in their daily lives. Another trend was that the robot's usefulness was perceived to be contingent on whether a person was in a certain mood (e.g. "feeling down") or living situation (e.g. "care home" or "alone").

In 2014, de Graaf et al. [20] decided to study the long-term acceptance of social robots by older adults. For the research, six participants aged 50–76 years, healthy and without pre-existing conditions placing restrictions on exercise, were recruited. Two participants were retired, three were employed and one was visually impaired. The social robot used was Nabaztag (Fig. 1 panel B), a 30 cm tall bunny rabbit equipped with flashing LEDs, a motion sensor and a webcam to record interactions. Nabaztag was installed in homes for three phases of use, each lasting ten days. Participants were told that the aim of the study was to improve their health. After each phase, their experiences were evaluated by means of semi-structured interviews transcribed verbatim. Concerning utilitarian factors, most participants clarified that a specific purpose of use is essential for the success of robots. At the beginning, the participants were oriented towards understanding the usefulness of the robot and its functions, but did not perceive it as useful. So, they were more interested in ease of use and perceived intelligence. However, in the last phase, most revealed that they found it useful for keeping healthy, somewhat intelligent, and that it was important to be able to adapt it to their personal needs. On the enjoyment side, not all participants experienced fun and those who did enjoyed it least made it to the third stage. Also, on the appearance of the robot, some thought it was cute, while for others, this did not matter compared to the functionality. After the third phase, almost everyone started to be more positive about its social skills. The topic of conversation also became more important, so that some wanted a wider range of topics because they all saw the potential for companionship. Regarding the context of use, all participants at the end of the third phase talked more about the opinions their family and friends had about the robot, but these did not influence their attitude towards the use of Nabaztag. About privacy issues, one user indicated that having it in the house influenced the sense of invasion of privacy, two were concerned about the privacy of visitors or uncomfortable even walking past the robot, while two others were not concerned at all. Nabaztag's reliability was also a crucial issue for most participants: when the robot provided incorrect information, participants felt mistrust and wondered if they were using it correctly. Concerning individual characteristics, half of the participants mentioned age as an influential factor for using a robotic device. In addition, most stated that they still had some general interest in technology, which made them more receptive to the robot in the beginning. To analyse long-term acceptance, the theory of domestication [28] was used. It describes the process of adopting a new technology into everyday life and consists of three phases: appropriation, incorporation, and conversion. In the first phase, participants tried to get to know the robot and its functions, becoming familiar with its behaviour. Then, the novelty of Nabaztag wore off and they became accustomed to having it in their homes and integrating it into their daily lives. Finally, only two participants said they liked the robot and wanted to use it in the future, while half said it did not meet their needs unless there were technical improvements. Only one participant said they would not want it in their home because they had higher expectations.

Korchut et al. [21] recruited a user group consisting of people aged 55 to 90 years with MCI or diagnosed with Alzheimer's disease (AD) and administered a survey to them. This included questions on four sections (functional requirements; human–robot interaction, design of robotic assistants, and social acceptance aspects). Based on the answers given to the questions, the authors extracted the main requirements and needs regarding robotic assistants. Then, a certain priority level was assigned to these requirements (high, medium, and low priority level). The results show that more than 80% of the interviewees believe that a robot can be useful to support the daily life of the elderly people, and also caregivers were willing to accept to be partially replaced by a robotic assistant. Moreover, to increase acceptability, most respondents said it was essential that the robot could call for help if something happened to the user. Regarding the functional requirements, those with a high priority are associated with the potential safety of the user, those with a medium priority are those referring to basic daily activities, such as preparing food, dressing, finding what is needed. A low priority level was assigned to requirements related to entertainment, relaxation, and shopping. It is important that most of the daily activities are carried out by the elderly person, who in this way can remain active, in order to train cognitive functions and delay the worsening of dementia as much as possible. In this case, the robot should encourage the user to perform certain activities and remain active. In order to increase the level of interaction between man and robot, the robot should be able to answer questions, participate in dialogue with the user, understand their emotional and psychological state: For these reasons, communication based on voice commands was chosen as a priority. Regarding the robot's appearance, most of the respondents would like a robotic assistant to have an anthropomorphic appearance and be shorter than the user. Interestingly, when potential users were asked if they could imagine using a robot in their daily life, young adults gave more positive answers than adults over 65, while when asked if they would accept a robot that would help them maintain their independence, acceptance was higher among the elderly. Finally, it was noted that there are some differences in the willingness to accept a robotic assistant: for some, maintaining independence is crucial, so they would be willing to accept a robot that can help them in this, while others feel that the burden of caring for them lies with family members or the state, thus they do not accept the introduction of a robot into their daily life. It can be said that investigating and categorizing the factors that lead to the acceptance of a new technology is of primary importance, as these change depending on the type of user considered, their perception of old age and cognitive impairment, the idea users have of the robot, how it works and what it can and cannot do.

Beuscher et al. [22] evaluated older adults' acceptance of the commercialized NAO robot (Fig. 1 panel A). For this purpose, the new Robot Acceptance Survey (RAS) was proposed. The RAS consisted of a modified version of the UTAUT questionnaire, so that each item was mapped to one of following three constructs: performance expectancy, effort expectancy, and attitude. In this study 19 individuals over 66 years of age were recruited, most of whom were found to be highly educated. Six of them were diagnosed with mild cognitive impairment or dementia. However, all participants were able to interact with the robot for dialoguing or doing chair exercises. Eleven participants engaged with NAO for 45–60 min individually, whereas the remaining eight participated in a dual interaction (two older adults and the robot) for 30 min. In both experimental procedures, the elderly completed some cognitive, social, and physical tasks such as observing the robot dancing, doing chair exercises and answering math questions. The RAS was conducted in pre- post-experimental phases, and there was no statistical difference in the results depending on time of the interview. Participants appreciated several robot's features such as the voice, comprehensive speech, and general appearance. Thus, NAO was well accepted, and they enjoyed interacting with it, even though they either did not like or were neutral towards NAO's human-like attributes at first. Moreover, most of the activities were highly rated by the participants, especially those involving exercises.

Ray et al. [23] created a well-being monitoring system based on digital photo frame (Fig. 1 panel F) using an iterative approach during the design and development stage. This choice was due to ensure the usability of the final product for the elderly, in order to avoid early abandonment. The device should allow elderly people and their caregivers to share pictures or information about their status in a two-way communication. The proposed methodology for the design and implementation stages included three phases. In the first phase, a prototype was shown to four formal caregivers who gave some suggestions to optimize the device, based on their experience in elderly care services. Once the suggestions were implemented, in the second phase, eight elderly people were asked to use the prototype for 3 weeks. At the end of this period, they were interviewed to define their perspective in terms of attitude, ease of use, ease of learning and perception of usefulness. In the last phase, 50 older people were recruited to evaluate their acceptance of the system while sharing photographs and videoconferencing. Acceptance was measured by seven parameters: anxiety, attitude, facilitating condition, intention to use the system, self-efficacy, social influence, and usefulness. The results showed that most of the end-users had a positive attitude towards this technology and found it quite easy to use. Moreover, the possibility to get in contact with their relatives and their enthusiasm seemed to influence and motivate them positively in using the system. So, involving all users in every stage of design and development of a technological product could have a considerable positive impact on its acceptance and use.

Another study, conducted in Italy by Cavallo et al. [24], involved 45 elderly people aged 65–86, who had a normal mental assessment and the necessary autonomy to perform daily activities. The Robot-Era (GA 288899) system implemented six robotic services in three different environments: home, condominium, and outdoor. The robots were DORO, CORO, and ORO, respectively (Fig. 1 panel G). As evaluation tools, both for the acceptability of the robots and for the usability of the services, specific questionnaires based on a 5-point Likert scale were developed. At the end of each service tested, the System Usability Scale (SUS) was administered to the volunteers. Looking at the results, older adults expressed a more positive opinion on CORO and ORO, which generally do not operate in the home environment. Users with more technological experience also gave better ratings to these two robots, because they are aware that they can connect the outside world with their own home. In addition, ORO received a higher rating from men, because this outdoor robot was seen as more masculine in appearance. Almost all volunteers were positively impressed by the robots' facial features, saying that the presence of a head encourages interaction. They also said that the colours and size were appropriate for their purposes. All volunteers reported that they would use a robot if they lost their independence to perform daily activities. In addition, many would prefer to be assisted by a robot to avoid burdening relatives, or having to perform tedious household tasks, and that they would feel safer in the home with their presence. During the trial, the Robot-Era system did not evoke anxious or negative emotional reactions. Many admitted that they were initially worried about appearing inadequate if they were unable to complete the tests, but then felt relaxed and comfortable thanks to the explanations provided by the researchers. Moreover, the system was not too privacy-intrusive according to the users, as they were free to choose whether to use the proposed services. Participants suggested increasing the robots' vocabulary so that they could speak naturally without having to remember keywords. In addition, older adults suggested that robots should give more feedback on their status, such as a description of what they are doing, and tell the user if a command was understood. Finally, acceptance decreases with increasing age: Older individuals think that new technologies are too complicated, whereas younger older people are more likely to use them. However, if the technology meets their own needs, the effect of age on acceptance becomes less important.

Boumans et al. [25] conducted a study starting from the evidence that collecting PROM data, essential information on the person's health status, is a heavy and demanding task for healthcare professionals (HCP). For this reason, the idea was to support these operators by using the commercialized Pepper robot (Fig. 1 panel D), testing whether or not the time taken by the robot to conduct the interviews to obtain these data differs from that taken by HCP and whether or not the target user could accept this technology. To test these hypotheses, 42 participants aged over 70 years, who were leading independent lives without cognitive disabilities, were recruited. The experiment consisted of two sessions, and participants were divided into two groups: in the first session, one group answered three questionnaires administered by the nurse (NP), and the other group answered the same three questionnaires administered by the robot (RP); in the second session, the two groups were reversed. The primary outcome measure was the time required to complete the questionnaires in RP and NP interactions. The secondary outcome measures were the similarity of the data collected and the percentage of NP interactions completed alone, without HCP intervention. Participants were asked to score the acceptability of the robot using Almere questionnaires, which assessed: attitude towards the robot, facilitating conditions, anxiety, perceived sociability, social influence, perceived ease of use, social presence, perceived enjoyment, trust, and perceived usefulness. The results showed that the average interview duration of the NP group was not significantly shorter than that of the RP group, while the completion rate was 92.8% in the RP group and 100% in the NP group. Regarding acceptability, participants reported generally positive feelings towards the robot, also finding it easy to use. The results therefore suggest that social robots could actually interview seniors in an autonomous and acceptable way and collect reliable and valid PROM data, constituting a valuable aid for HCP. Furthermore, these results may be generalizable to elderly patients or patients visiting general practice, while this generalization is not valid for hospitalized patients with more severe functional and cognitive limitations.

Social robots have been shown to be effective in reducing loneliness and agitation in older people with dementia. However, the acceptance of this technology among this population is not particularly high. In this regard, Chen et al. [26] wondered whether direct exposure to a social robot could lead to positive changes in attitudes and acceptance of technology. For this purpose, 103 residents of long-term care facilities between 67 and 108 years, diagnosed with dementia, were recruited. The robot chosen for this study was Kabochan (Fig. 1 panel H), a robot resembling a 3-year-old child. The participants were divided into two groups, the experimental and the control group. The whole study lasted 32 weeks, divided into four phases: In the first and third phases, the experimental group received routine care, while in the first two weeks of the second phase, they were instructed in the functions and characteristics of Kabochan. During the remaining 6 weeks of the second phase and 8 weeks of the fourth phase, Kabochan was introduced to the subjects individually and everyone was free to interact with him without the involvement of staff or researchers. Participants assigned to the control group received standard care. To investigate the acceptance of the robot, the Senior Technology Acceptance Model (STAM) was used, which included a questionnaire with which six main domains were measured: attitudes towards technology, perceived usefulness, perceived ease of use, technology self-efficacy, technology anxiety, and facilitating conditions. Subject's involvement was measured by direct observation. The results showed a positive change in perceived ease of use. This indicates that involvement with the robot does indeed have the potential to improve the perceived ease of use of the technology, probably also depending on the type of robot used: Kabochan is a robot capable of stimulating an emotionally meaningful relationship with the person, as it does not require great cognitive skills and technological expertise. On the other hand, no significant changes in attitudes towards technology, perceived usefulness, facilitating conditions, technological anxiety, and self-efficacy were observed after exposure to Kabochan compared to the control group. The change in attitude towards technology probably occurs cognitive, and emotional dissonance can be produced with respect to previous attitudes and beliefs. In this case, as the study was conducted, this change did not occur.

Domestication theory states that users adopt technology through three separate dimensions: practical, symbolic, and cognitive domestication. Søraa et al. [27] observed and analysed the domestication of a social robot in private homes, i.e. how technology is acquired and integrated into the domestic sphere. In addition, this study considers a fourth dimension: social domestication. Eight elderly Norwegians (aged 66–89 years) with mild to moderate cognitive impairment were interviewed during their involvement in the eWare project (AAL-2016-s071). From a technological point of view, the eWare ecosystem consists of three interoperable devices: Tessa, a flowerpot-like non-mobile robot (Fig. 1 panel C), SensaraCare, a lifestyle monitoring technology, and eWare cloud computing system which elaborates data from the above sources. Formal and informal caregivers have access to the system through a tablet provided with the eWare mobile application. They can set goals for their elderly relatives and receive feedback. The Tessa robot acts as an advisor and reminder system for these goals and congratulates the elderly person when they accomplish an activity. The system is able to learn the user's behavioural patterns about bedtime, meals, and other daily activities, so that it can also notice unusual patterns and notify the caregiver, if necessary. Once the experimentation in a real-world setting was completed, users were interviewed with qualitative and quantitative questionnaires to obtain the following information: sociodemographic information, measurement of functional status, measurement of quality of life, attitude towards technology, and acceptance of the system (based on UTAUT scale). On the user experience side, the system was perceived as non-intrusive by the users. The main criticism on the functional aspect was audio: due to hearing impairment of some users or poor audio settings of Tessa, voice communication was sometimes poor. Regarding symbolic domestication, i.e. how the robot is perceived by the user, the robot was gradually considered as part of the house by the participants. In some cases, they even called it sweet nicknames, demonstrating a kind of relationship between them and Tessa. On the informal caregivers' side, SensaraCare and the eWare system were found useful, but it was noticed that only a technical error significantly decreased their trust. As regards cognitive dimension, this study had to consider that participants were affected by cognitive impairment and that the aim of the project was to mitigate the decline. This impairment had a clearly impact on learning to use: some users unplugged the robot, turning off the whole eWare system. Finally, it was noticed that the system had an impact on the social life of some users and caregivers. Indeed, a social interaction was established between older adults and caregivers through the system. This interaction has a mitigating effect on the user's loneliness and a positive effect on the quality of life of informal caregivers. On this basis, the concept of social dimension was introduced. When this interaction is established, the relational together-work becomes more important than the use of technology itself. Even though each user may approach and perceive the robot differently (practical, symbolic, and cognitive dimensions), the social dimension is crucial for successful technological domestication.

4 Discussion

Nowadays, there are several robots that have been developed to not only provide companionship to older adults, [29] but also to cooperate with them during health and lifestyle activities, such as facilitating reminiscence through cognitive stimulation [30], remembering tasks to do, monitoring vital signs and whether they fall down, while at the same time entertaining them [29–31].

Mataric et al. provided a detailed taxonomy for defining Social Assistive Robotics (SAR) and future challenges to provide care for the elderly [32]. From their definition, two main features of SARs can be evinced: the ability to assist the users through cooperation in daily activities and social interaction.

Despite the undeniable usefulness of SARs, developers are often forced to prioritise the improvement of specific technical features due to the unavailability of resources and the different degrees of flexibility and acceptability imposed by unstructured settings, as the private homes [33].

The above studies sought to explore the usability and acceptability of the latest technological solutions in the field of IoT and social assistive robotics for older people, taking into consideration the availability of results from both design stages and clinical trials, ensuring a patient-centred approach to older people.

In six studies, a fairly large number of older adults were interviewed [19, 21, 23–27], whereas in four [18, 20, 22, 27] the number of older adults who participated was small. Three studies [21, 26, 27] focused on older adults with moderate or mild cognitive impairment or dementia, while five studies [19, 20, 23–25] interviewed only healthy people. Two studies [18, 22] interviewed both categories.

As it is possible to notice, the ten studies differ from each other in several aspects. That means that there is no common and established procedure for designing social robots. However, it is possible to classify the reported studies in order to determine which are the key indicators to pursue the acceptability of the technology among elderly users.

Firstly, it can be noted that the human-like appearance of the robot seems to be a feature that influences acceptance [22, 24]. Although older adults sometimes do not consider entertainment or dialogue as primary functions [21], once they engage a robot, they suggest improvements in this field, due to the importance they give to companionship function [20–23]. In addition, errors during human–robot interaction (HRI) can frustrate and discourage users, significantly lowering acceptance and usability [18]. Thus, high-level voice interaction should be considered as a key element for a positive engagement between the older adult and technology.

Another factor that strongly supports acceptability, preventing early abandonment, is social domestication. Indeed, older adults find the robot more useful when relatives or caregivers are enthusiastic towards technology [21, 23, 27]. For this reason, it can be hypothesized that they are more incline to accept technology when there is an improvement in the quality of life of caregivers. Moreover, when a relationship between elderly and caregivers is established through the device, motivation increases, and in turn the efficiency of the whole system [27].

The most surprising result of our research is the low involvement of end-users in the design stage of a SAR.

Among the studies analysed, six were based on the use of commercialized technology [18, 19, 22, 25, 26], whereas three studies [23, 24, 27] tried to propose innovative prototypes. In one case [21] acceptability was determined only by means of questionnaires, without any simulation or experimentation.

During the aforementioned six studies, researchers analysed the acceptability of commercialized robots, trying to establish their suitability for certain care activities towards elderly people. In most cases, a commercialized robot does not consider a specific target population or a specific activity by design. Although some commercialized robots have commonly accepted features and can be programmed and adapted to any situation, this lack of focus may represent a barrier in achieving acceptability. In our review, only one study [23] reported that older adults and caregivers were interviewed from design stages, in order to personalize the device for the specific purpose, in contrast to recommendations from guidelines such as the Ambient Assisted Living Joint Programme, which consider mandatory the involvement of different end-users in all the design and development phases. This approach should be taken into account to maximize acceptability from a patient-centred perspective.

On the contrary, prototypes designed for a specific purpose show very good results in terms of acceptability and usability, as highlighted by the results of this paper. Indeed, in all three studies, the perspective of all the end-users was gathered from design stages to the final testing [34–38].

On the care side, designing new psychosocial interventions to support behavioural and psychological symptoms of dementia, promoting advance care planning, improving nutrition and quality of life, supporting the maintenance of physical and social functions, designing lifestyle interventions, and supporting frailty [39] are just some of the problems to be solved through SARs and IoT, that require a long-term interaction between technology and end-users.

5 Conclusions

This chapter has brought to light several outcomes and a number of interesting implications, which are important for the acceptance of social robots in different settings by older adults.

In particular, utilitarian factors, which are usefulness, ease of use, adaptability and intelligence, should be considered as key characteristics to ensure long-term interaction with technologies and continued use, in addition to coherence and simplicity of information provided to end-users.

Understanding how to integrate IoT and smart solutions in the care pathway and daily life of the end-users is still a challenge, especially for healthcare managers but also industries. Since the greatest benefit of SARs is that the elderly people are given the opportunity of remaining at home, it is fundamental to understand how to model the relationship between user and robot, to foster interaction in the closest "familiar" context.

Overall, IoT systems offer a potential solution to reduce costs, minimize the burden on caregivers and broaden the range of customers who can benefit from them [40, 41].

It is desirable that the number of studies grows in the future, in terms of number of participants and duration of the trial, but, more important, by involving a wider group of older people and caregivers by design. This will allow them to express their needs and ideas on aspects such as the role of the psychosocial characteristics of IoT and SARs, such as social presence and the level of usability. Finally, future studies in the field can benefit from the introduction of a new framework to properly understand the role of technology acceptance.

References

1. UN Department of Economic and Social Affairs: World Population Prospects: The 2019 Revision. UN Department of Economic and Social Affairs, New York (2019)
2. World Health Organization: The World Health Report 2002: Reducing Risks, Promoting Healthy Life. World Health Organization, Geneva (2002)
3. Murman, D.L.: The impact of age on cognition. Semin Hear. **36**(3), 111–121 (2015)
4. Ince, Y.M.: Economic and social consequences of population aging the dilemmas and opportunities in the twenty-first century. Appl. Res. Qual. Life **10**(4), 735–752 (2015)
5. Chen, X., Mao, G., Leng, S.X.: Frailty syndrome: an overview. Clin. Interv. Aging **9**, 433–441 (2014)
6. Abdi, J., Al-Hindawi, A., Ng, T., Vizcaychipi, M.P.: Scoping review on the use of socially assistive robot technology in elderly care. BMJ Open **8**(2), e018815 (2018)

7. National Academies of Sciences, Engineering, and Medicine: Social Isolation and Loneliness in Older Adults: Opportunities for the Health Care System. The National Academies Press, Washington, DC (2020)
8. Oh, C.S., Bailenson, J.N., Welch, G.F.: A Systematic review of social presence: definition, antecedents, and implications. Front Robot AI. **5**(114), 1–35 (2018)
9. Chita-Tegmark, M., Scheutz, M.: Assistive robots for the social management of health: a framework for robot design and human-robot interaction research. Int. J. Soc. Robot. **13**, 197–217 (2020)
10. Tickle-Degnen L., Scheutz M., Arkin R.C.: Collaborative robots in rehabilitation for social self-management of health, vol. 6 (2014)
11. Okamura, A.M., Mataric, M.J., Christensen, H.I.: Medical and health-care robotics. IEEE Robot Autom. Mag. **17**(3), 26–37 (2010)
12. Rabbitt, S.M., Kazdin, A.E., Scassellati, B.: Integrating socially assistive robotics into mental healthcare interventions: applications and recommendations for expanded use. Clin. Psychol. Rev. **35**, 35–46 (2015)
13. Moyle, W., Jones, C.J., Murfield, J.E., Thalib, L., Beattie, E.R.A., Shum, D.K.H., et al.: Use of a robotic seal as a therapeutic tool to improve dementia symptoms: a cluster-randomized controlled trial. J. Am. Med. Dir. Assoc. **18**, 766–773 (2017)
14. Seelye, A.M., Wild, K.V., Larimer, N., Maxwell, S., Kearns, P., Kaye, J.A.: Reactions to a remote-controlled video-communication robot in seniors' homes: a pilot study of feasibility and acceptance. Telemed. J. E Health **18**, 755–759 (2012)
15. Soler, M.V., Agüera-Ortiz, L., Rodríguez, J.O., Rebolledo, C.M., Muñoz, A.P., Pérez, I.R., Chillón, L.C.: Social robots in advanced dementia. Front. Aging Neurosci. **7**, 133 (2015)
16. Pu, L., Moyle, W., Jones, C., Todorovic, M.: The effectiveness of social robots for older adults: a systematic review and meta-analysis of randomized controlled studies. Gerontologist **59**(1), e37–e51 (2019)
17. Góngora, A.S., Hamrioui, S., de la Torre Díez, I., Motta, C.E., López-Coronado, M., Franco, M.: Social robots for people with aging and dementia: a systematic review of literature. Telemed. J. E Health **25**(7), 533–540 (2019)
18. Wu, Y.H., Wrobel, J., Cornuet, M., Kerhervé, H., Damnée, S., Rigaud, A.S.: Acceptance of an assistive robot in older adults: a mixed-method study of human-robot interaction over a 1-month period in the living lab setting. Clin. Interv. Aging **9**, 801–811 (2014)
19. McGlynn S.A., Kemple S.C., Mitzner T.L., King C.H., Rogers W.A.: Understanding older adults' perceptions of usefulness for the paro robot. Proc. Hum. Factors Ergon. Soc. Annu. Meet. **58**(1), 1914–1918 (2014)
20. Maartje M.A. de Graaf, Allouch S.B., Klamer T.: Sharing a life with harvey: exploring the acceptance of and relationship-building with a social robot. Comput. Human Behav. **43**, 1–14 (2015)
21. Korchut, A., Szklener, S., Abdelnour, C., Tantinya, N., Hernández-Farigola, J., Ribes, J.C., Skrobas, U., Grabowska-Aleksandrowicz, K., Szczęśniak-Stańczyk, D., Rejdak, K.: Challenges for service robots-requirements of elderly adults with cognitive impairments. Front. Neurol. **8**, 228 (2017)
22. Beuscher, L.M., Fan, J., Sarkar, N., Dietrich, M.S., Newhouse, P.A., Miller, K.F., Mion, L.C.: Socially assistive robots: measuring older adults' perceptions. J. Gerontol. Nurs. **43**(12), 35–43 (2017)
23. Ray, P., Li, J., Ariani, A., Kapadia, V.: Tablet-based well-being check for the elderly: development and evaluation of usability and acceptability. JMIR Hum. Factors **4**(2), 12 (2017)
24. Cavallo, F., Esposito, R., Limosani, R., Manzi, A., Bevilacqua, R., Felici, E., Di Nuovo, A., Cangelosi, A., Lattanzio, F., Dario, P.: Robotic services acceptance in smart environments with older adults: user satisfaction and acceptability study. J. Med. Internet Res. **20**(9), e264 (2018)
25. Boumans, R., van Meulen, F., Hindriks, K., Neerincx, M., Rikkert, M.G.M.: Robot for health data acquisition among older adults: a pilot randomised controlled cross-over trial. BMJ Qual. Saf. **28**(10), 793–799 (2019)

26. Chen, K., Lou, V.W., Tan, K.C., Wai, M.Y., Chan, L.L.: Changes in technology acceptance among older people with dementia: the role of social robot engagement. Int. J. Med. Inform. **141**, 104241 (2020)
27. Søraa, R.A., Nyvoll, P., Tøndel, G., Fosch-Villaronga, E., Serrano, J.A.: The social dimension of domesticating technology: Interactions between older adults, caregivers, and robots in the home. Technol. Forecast Soc. Change **167**, 120678 (2021)
28. Silverstone, R., Haddon, L.: Design and the domestication of ICTs: technical change and everyday life. In: Silverstone, R., Mansell, R. (eds.) Communication by Design. The Politics of Information and Communication Technologies, pp. 44–74. Oxford press, Oxford, UK (1996)
29. Robinson, H., MacDonald, B., Broadbent, E.: The role of healthcare robots for older adults at home: a review. Int. J. Soc. Rob. **6**, 575–591 (2014)
30. Robinson, H., MacDonald, B.A., Kerse, N., Broadbent, E.: Suitability of healthcare robots for a dementia unit and suggested improvements. J. Am. Med. Dir. Assoc. **14**, 34–40 (2013)
31. Broekens, J., Heerink, M., Rosendal, H.: Assistive social robots in elderly care: a review. Gerontechnology **8**, 94–103 (2009)
32. Feil-Seifer, D., Mataric M.J.: Defining socially assistive robotics. In: International Conference on Rehabilitation Robotics. Proceedings of the IEEE 9th International Conference on Rehabilitation Robotics. pp. 465–468 (2005)
33. Meng, Q., Lee, M.H.: Design issues for assistive robotics for the older adults. Adv. Eng. Inform. **20**, 171–186 (2006)
34. Casaccia S., Revel G.M., Scalise L., Bevilacqua R., Rossi L., Paauwe R.A., Karkowsky I., Ercol, I., Artur Serrano J., Suijkerbuijk S., Lukkien D., Nap H.H.: Social Robot and Sensor Network in Support of Activity of Daily Living for People with Dementia: Communications in Computer and Information Science. pp. 128–135 (2019)
35. Bevilacqua R., Felici E., Marcellini F., Glende S., Klemcke S., Conrad I., Esposito R., Cavallo F., Dario P.: Robot-era project: Preliminary results on the system usability Lecture Notes in Computer Science (including subseries Lecture Notes in Artificial Intelligence and Lecture Notes in Bioinformatics)., vol 9188, pp. 553–561 (2015)
36. Casaccia S., Bevilacqua R., Scalise L., Revel G.M., Astell A.J., Spinsante S., Rossi L.: Assistive sensor-based technology driven self-management for building resilience among people with early stage cognitive impairment. In: 2019 IEEE International Symposium on Measurements & Networking (M&N). pp. 1–5 (2019)
37. Cavallo, F., Esposito, R., Limosani, R., Manzi, A., Bevilacqua, R., Felici, E., Di Nuovo, A., Cangelosi, A., Lattanzio, F., Dario, P.: Robotic services acceptance in smart environments with older adults: user satisfaction and acceptability study. J. Med. Internet Res. **20**(9), e264 (2018)
38. Nap, H.H., Suijkerbuijk, S., Lukkien, D., Casaccia, S., Bevilacqua, R., Revel, G.M., Rossi, L., Scalise, L.: A social robot to support integrated person centered care. Int. J. Integr. Care. **18**, 120 (2018)
39. Livingston, G., Sommerlad, A., Costafreda, S., Huntley, J., Ames, D., Ballard, C., Banerjee, S., Burns, A., Cohen-Mansfield, J., Fox, N., Gitlin, L., Howard, R., Kales, H., Larson, E., Ritchie, K., Rockwood, K., Sampson, E., Mukadam, N.: Dementia prevention intervention and care. Lancet **390**, 2673–2734 (2017)
40. Bevilacqua, R., Casaccia, S., Cortellessa, G., Astell, A., Lattanzio, F., Corsonello, A., D'Ascoli, P., Paolini, S., Di Rosa, M., Rossi, L., Maranesi, E.: Coaching through technology: a systematic review into efficacy and effectiveness for the ageing population. Int. J. Environ. Res. Public Health **17**, 5930 (2020)
41. Lattanzio, F., Abbatecola, A.M., Bevilacqua, R., Chiatti, C., Corsonello, A., Rossi, L., Bustacchini, S., Bernabei, R.: Advanced technology care innovation for older people in Italy: necessity and opportunity to promote health and wellbeing. J. Am. Med. Dir. Assoc. **15**(7), 457–466 (2014)

Exoskeletons in Elderly Healthcare

Matteo Sposito, Tommaso Poliero, Christian Di Natali, Marianna Semprini, Giacinto Barresi, Matteo Laffranchi, Darwin Gordon Caldwell, Lorenzo De Michieli, and Jesús Ortiz

Abstract The older population is projected to quadruple between the years 2000 and 2050. Many of the elderly experience mobility impairments of varying degrees. These are caused by a physiological muscular decay or associated health conditions, such as stroke, which shows an increasing rate of incidence with the age of the subject. The introduction of exoskeletons in elderly healthcare scenarios, derived from the rehabilitation one, is becoming a promising approach. The opportunities and advantages of these systems in healthcare are of great interest. Most widely used systems are stationary, improving the outcomes of traditional approaches of rehabilitation. Fewer fully wearable systems are being used due to their cost, complexity, weight and performance. However, big steps have been done in the last years to improve them. The potential use of wearable untethered systems or exosuits in home environments opens new possibilities, especially in daily healthcare, promoting mobility and an active life. To promote exoskeleton's use, usability and acceptability are central factors in elderly healthcare scenario. This includes not only technical characteristics of the device (such as weight or level of assistance), but also aesthetics and compatibility with everyday activities. Considerable developments have been achieved in the area of user experience, mostly thanks to the use of industrial design and Human-Centered Design—HCD principles. These approaches put great emphasis in keeping the users in the design loop, ensuring that technical developments are focused on their real needs. Additionally, an effective use of the exoskeletons in unstructured environments requires to process information on the context and the activity being performed, enabling assistance in Activities of Daily Living—ADL. This can be done relying on the growing trend of wearable sensors and Internet of Things—IoT, exploiting the paradigm of ubiquitous computing, cloud storage, and intuitive human-machine interaction.

M. Sposito (✉) · T. Poliero · C. Di Natali · D. G. Caldwell · J. Ortiz
Advanced Robotics, Istituto Italiano di Tecnologia, via San Quirico 19D, 16163 Genova, Italy
e-mail: matteo.sposito@iit.it

M. Semprini · G. Barresi · M. Laffranchi · L. De Michieli
Rehab Technologies Lab, Istituto Italiano di Tecnologia, via Morego 30, 16163 Genova, Italy

1 Introduction

There is a steady increase of ageing population in all the countries worldwide: from 1980s to 2017 the population over-60 doubled to 962 million [1] and it is expected to see it almost doubled again by 2030, outnumbering children under the age of 10. The trend is growing much steeper in the developed countries, but 8 out of 10 of the oldest people will live in the developing countries. To face the challenges posed by a growing number of elderly, in the fields of public health, assistance and quality of life, the United Nations (UN) sets shared policies regarding housing, healthcare, employment and social protection [1]. In this frame, mobility is of paramount importance to guarantee a high quality of life, social inclusion and independence of the ageing population. Mobility is a key component of health across the lifespan and is necessary for older adults to maintain autonomy [2]. Proper solution to the mobility problem should take into consideration the needs of their users and the context of use. Indeed, more than 64% of all walking aid are used by over-65 [3]. Walking sticks, wheelchairs or walking frames offer reasonable assistance while walking, however most of elderly require assistance from a person even with walking aids. Indeed, unstable walking, muscle weakness and cognitive issues block elderly to maintain their independence [4].

Lately, wearable assisting technologies have risen as a promising solution to address the mobility problem. For instance, the assisting devices can guide the user and help them navigate unstructured spaces [5] or physically help the elderly in their movements [3]. Several devices have been assessed: they proved to have ability to reduce walking fatigue [6] or restore the partial loss of muscle control while not restricting freedom of movement in subjects with mild impairment [7]. Especially wearable robots, or exoskeletons, offer a versatile digital and connected platform to offer physical assistance to their *primary* users as mobility aids.

Exoskeletons have the potential to offer valuable services also to *secondary* and *tertiary* users that can benefit from data and alerts sent from the device. In fact, wearable connected devices offer a unique opportunity to enhance the monitoring and intervention abilities of medical staff and relatives, in case of life-threatening situations [8]. Indeed, smart wearable devices that deliver physical assistance must adapt to different activity scenarios (e.g. walking, sitting, climbing stairs or other ADL), thus requiring wearable and smart sensors that must be connected with the device. This data can be analyzed and sent to nurses, medical doctors and public health agencies for monitoring purposes. For such reason, the field of *Tele-Health* is exploring the emerging possibility to use wearable devices sensory capabilities. Exoskeletons offer a platform to collect and share data for continuous monitoring and analysis, in order to offer tailored drug treatment and other therapies, alongside with an existing ecosystem of other solutions spanning from remote video consultations to cloud based data sharing techniques [9], where the exoskeletons can act as user interface and a peripheral hub connected to edge-computing services.

In spite of the effectiveness of the solutions, what really determines their success is the final users' acceptance rate of the device. Acceptance is defined by several dimensions (e.g. ease of use, social stigma or expectations) that are affected by education, age and social status. To maximize acceptance rate, and so the adoption of devices intended to promote elderly well-being, it is central to design assisting solutions following approaches that involve the users and are capable to meet their particular needs [10, 11]. User-centered Design—UCD approaches, as part of the HCD paradigm, have been widely used in applications where the users and their needs are central to every design phase.

From the above considerations, it should emerge that when designing an exoskeleton meant for usage in elderly healthcare, skills from several domains are needed. As an example, mechatronics knowledge is useful for the design of the devices, medical and biomechanics understandings are helpful for its evaluation, and ergonomics for comprehending how the final users will interact with it. For such reason, the aim of this chapter is to present to a multidisciplinary target two use cases describing, from the developers' point of view, the steps taken to build and test two exoskeletons in elderly healthcare for severe and mild mobility impairments. The focus of the use cases will be on the technological improvements, the implementations and future directions, describing how to implement IoT assistive devices that try to meet the expectations of the final users.

This chapter is divided as follows. Section 2 introduces a brief description of the types of exoskeletons, their working principles and their benefits to healthy subjects and frail elderly. Then, the Section provides a background on the *Participatory Design* methodology and the *User-Centered Design* approach, that are implemented in the design phases of wearable robots. In Sect. 3.1 and Sect. 3.2 the two use cases are presented. The first describes the XoSoft exosuit, meant for assisting mild-impaired elderly. The second use case, instead, presents the TWIN exoskeleton, a device intended for providing support to severely impaired patients. To conclude, Sect. 4 reports the authors' point of view on future challenges to adoption, development and research on wearable robots, namely how to assess their acceptance and how to exploit the amount of data that such devices can produce.

2 Technical Background

This section gives an overview of the current state of the art exoskeletons, that are market available or are being developed in research institutions. Due to the variety of tasks that exoskeletons can assist, there are many specialized devices that are tailored for specific assistance. Thus, it is central for designers to approach the users as an active part of their process, to continuously confront with hands-on workshops and refine requirements. To this end, in 2.2 there is a description of the UCD approach and its activities and phases.

2.1 Exoskeletons and Exosuits

An exoskeleton is a wearable robot that assists with the execution of physical activities by delivering forces/torques at the human joints that are encompassed by the device itself, [12, 13]. There are two different drivers for this technology. On one side, the empowerment of healthy-bodied humans, typical of military or occupational scenarios [14–19]. On the other side, the restoration of mobility capacities in physically impaired persons, typical of rehabilitation and elderly care scenarios [20–23]. As an example, Fig. 1 displays examples of exoskeletons being used in operational scenarios. One important and very specific feature of exoskeletons is the intrinsic interaction between the human and the robot. Human–Robot Interaction - HRI is twofold: firstly, cognitive, because the human controls the robot that is providing the feedback to the human; secondly, a physical or biomechanical interaction leading to the application of controlled forces bidirectionally between the robot and the human [24]. The fact that a human is an integral part of the design is one of the most exciting aspects in the design of biomimetic and biomechatronic wearable robots. It does, however, impose several restrictions, challenges and demands on the design of this type of device since it involves the cooperation of two dynamic systems, i.e. human motor control and robot control, in a closed loop system. Additionally, both systems must be able to adapt to each other in order to stably achieve their common goal. Therefore, Human-Activity Recognition - HAR is required to understand what kind of action the user is performing [25–30].

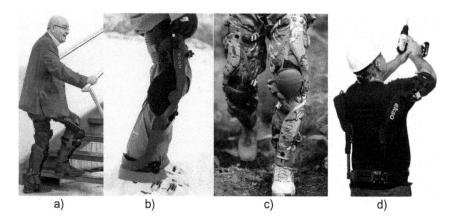

Fig. 1 Example of application fields for the exoskeleton technology. **a** Keeogo by B-Temia (B-TEMIA Inc., 4780 Rue Saint-F´elix 105, Saint-Augustinde-Desmaures, Canada), a powered knee exoskeleton for assisting people with mobility impairments. **b** Elevate by Roam Robotics (Roam Robotics, 650 Alabama Street, San Francisco, CA, 94110, USA), a powered exoskeleton for offloading knees and quads during skiing activities. **c** PowerWalk by Bionic Power (Bionic Power, 2661 Lillooet Street, Vancouver, BC, V5M 4P7, Canada), a passive knee exoskeleton for military applications. **d** Evo by Ekso Bionics (Ekso Bionics, 1414 Harbour Way S 1201, Richmond, CA 94804, USA), a passive arm and shoulder exoskeleton for supporting workers in industrial scenarios. All images are taken from Exoskeleton Report (https://exoskeletonreport.com)

Exoskeletons can be categorized in several ways. According to the presence or not of rigid elements, exoskeletons may be referred to as *rigid* or *soft*. Soft exoskeletons also known as *exosuits*, are lightweight and easily integrated in every-day clothing. They take advantage of compliant and soft elements such as webbing or elastic bands to provide forces to the wearer. On the contrary, in rigid exoskeletons, the presence of structural frames and links can be exploited not only to support part of the exoskeleton weight, but also to transmit forces and torques. Despite the footprint and the weight of rigid exoskeletons being higher than soft ones, they can provide higher forces. A further classification can be done according to the joint the exoskeleton assists, i.e., shoulder, neck, wrist, back, hip, knee, ankle, or any combination of the previous. Finally, according to their actuation principle, exoskeletons can be described as *passive, active* or *quasi-passive*. In particular, to deliver assistance, *passive* exoskeletons rely solely on mechanical elements—like springs or elastic bands [31]. This implies that, in specific phases of the movement, the device stores the energy coming from the user to, then, release it in successive phases. It follows that a passive actuation is not suited for paraplegic or severely impaired users since they have no residual strength to "charge" the mechanical elements. For these users, an *active* exoskeleton represents the optimal fit. Indeed, exploiting controllable elements—like electrical motors or pneumatic actuators—this class of devices can directly deliver assistance to the wearers, without first requiring them to store energy into the exoskeleton [32]. As a matter of fact, the energy is drawn from external sources like batteries or air reservoirs. The last category, *quasi-passive* exoskeletons, takes advantage of controllable elements not to directly provide assistance to the user but, rather, control the engagement of the connected passive elements [33]. In Sect. 3.1, we will present an example of quasi-passive exoskeleton XoSoft, and in Sect. 3.2 we will present an example of active exoskeleton TWIN.

2.2 User-Centered Design (UCD)

Wearable assisting devices must be designed with criteria imposed by Human Factors to adapt different subjects anthropometric measurements. This will be, arguably, the best method for a rehabilitation device used in clinics; where trained professionals can operate and fit the device properly.

But what about everyday assisting devices? How the designer can learn the new constraints that are set by unstructured home environment or usability from a naive user?

To take into account multiple user-set constraints, *Participatory Design* is the right approach to use. This design methodology can profitably collect constraints that are set by the users' capabilities, living or working context and activities. The paradigm of *Participatory design* is based on the concept of *co-design*. Final users become co-designers and are involved in the process: from setting and refining requirements in early-stage development to simulations with mockups in the mid-stages of design [34]. Involvement of the users is of paramount importance to collect and prioritize the device's characteristics that will impact most usability and acceptance, from the users' point of view. Final users are active figures in requirements synthesis and refinement rather than actors/personas in a determined scenario [35].

HCD and *UCD* are specialized design methodologies born from the participatory approaches. The term *UCD* was introduced during the 80s [36] and, particularly, focus on users' needs and device usability, while HCD implements a broader concept of design that aims to adapt devices to humans' capabilities, physical factors and skills.

UCD approach consists in an iterative design loop, as depicted in Fig. 2. During *Early-stage* phases 1, 2 and *End-stage* phases 5, 6 all users are always required, while in *Mid-stage* phases 3, 4 they may not be involved [37]. Indeed, in phase 1 designers define the problem to solve by analyzing the context of application (e.g. indoor or outdoor), users' needs (e.g. maximum weight for wearability) and other specifications (e.g. set by technical limitations). Users are, then, grouped in *Primary, Secondary* and *Tertiary* users. Primary users are the one who will use the device,

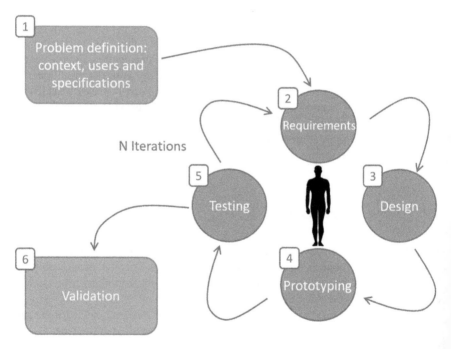

Fig. 2 Example of a UCD approach pipeline. Phases 1 and 6 are performed only once in the cycle of design, while phases from 2 to 5 are performed iteratively, until all requirement are set and implemented to match the device functionalities. *Early stage* phases consists definition of the users, context and technical specification of the device to build (phase 1) and the iterative phase of requirement refinement and handling. *Mid-stage* consists in design and prototyping phases where designers may involve users to test critical functions of the device as early as possible to test if the solution matches users' requirements. *End-stage* consists in testing and the final device validation. In the iterative testing phase, designers may work with a selected group of users

Secondary users are the one who will be involved in the use through an intermediary (e.g. nurses caring for elderly) and Tertiary users are the one that can be affected by the use of the device (e.g. health insurance companies) [37].

Primary and Secondary users may be involved through workshops and *handson* in the Design and Prototyping phases to further refine requirements and the critical parts of the device (e.g. user interfaces or data-communication protocol), especially in the first UCD iterations. On the other hand, all users will be involved in Testing and Validation phases through interviews (e.g. questions on usability or comfort), trials in the targeted scenario and sensors' data collection (e.g. movements reconstruction, metabolic consumption or muscular activation).

3 Use Cases

This section will present two use cases that represent the exoskeleton approach, TWIN, with rigid frame and actuators and the exosuit approach, XoSoft, with compliant structure and actuation units. The description will provide with a detailed explanation of their working principles and the design processes, with an emphasis on Participatory approaches. At the end of each paragraph, there are brief description of validation trials and application in life-like scenarios (e.g. nursing homes).

3.1 XoSoft for Mild-Impaired Elderly

The XoSoft exosuit targeted the development of a new generation of lower-limb modular soft exoskeletons for assistance of people with mobility impairment. These restrictions to movements can be due a partial loss of sensory or motor function [38] as a consequence of ageing or pathology. One of the main challenges of the project was to develop a complete soft system that provides assistance to the user accordingly with specific physical needs. During the development of the exoskeleton, focus was not only on the sensing and actuation technology, but also on understanding the user requirements and needs. Therefore, the UCD approach (see Sect. 2.2) provided important guidelines for an effective development of the exoskeleton prototypes. More in details, the identified requirements were:

- The system needs to be worn under the users' primary clothing. • The garment materials need to be easy to care for and dry cleanable. Thus fabric elements with electronic components or sensors that cannot be separated from the fabric must be designed accordingly with such need.
- Donning and doffing shall be achieved easily (preferably in less than 5 min and without external help). Male and female users must be able to go to the toilet on their own without external assistance, as wearer dignity and independence is of paramount importance.

- The garment shall facilitate the storage or carrying of the power source (battery or spring) for the XoSoft System. Power supply shall be interchangeable through simple user friendly procedures.

3.1.1 The XoSoft Exosuit Gamma Prototype

The Gamma prototype (see Fig. 3) is the most advanced iteration of the UCD approach and comprises of a garment where the technological components are integrated: the modular actuation units, electronic controls and soft sensors. The device meets the essential requirements and is classified as a *class 1 medical device* compliant with IEC 60601. The Gamma prototype involved a truly modular approach, allowing actuation of different joints, unilaterally or bilaterally, depending on the users' needs. To provide assistance, the XoSoft exosuit takes advantage of a Quasi-Passive Actuation—QPA, chosen according to a preliminary energy efficiency analysis, reported in [38]. More in details, whenever the pneumatic clutches (see Fig. 3a) in series with the passive element (see Fig. 3b) are engaged, the system stores energy. This energy is released in successive phases of the gait. Indeed, the pneumatic clutches are controlled according to the gait phases. Consequently, the core of the control system is a state machine that keeps track of the gait of the user. The gait

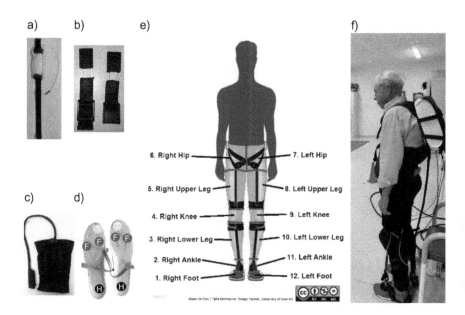

Fig. 3 XoSoft Gamma prototype and its components. **a** Pneumatic clutches. **b** Elastic bands. **c** Capacitive soft knee sensors. **d** Sensorized insoles. **e** Schematic representation of the Gamma prototype. **f** Elderly subject wearing the XoSoft Gamma during testing at the Geriatrics Centre Erlangen, Germany (GCE)

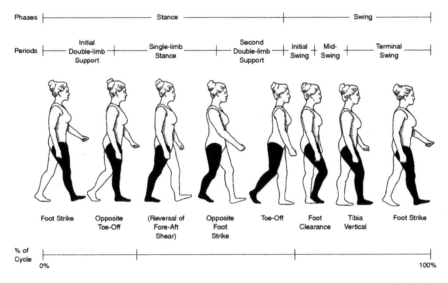

Fig. 4 Figure (adapted from [42]) representing human gait cycle. 0% corresponds to the heel strike and 100% represents the successive heel strike, for the same leg

cycle (time between two consecutive heel strikes, of the same lower limb, see Fig. 4) consists in two main phases:

1. Stance phase, that is the time between the heel strike of the foot and the toe off (from 0 to about 60%);
2. Swing phase, time between the toe off and its consecutive heel strike (from about 60 to 100%).

The transition between these phases is marked by the heel-strike and by the toe-off respectively. To gather this information, the device relies on sensorized insoles (see Fig. 3d) with pressure sensors in strategic places: (i) a rear sensor placed approximately under the heel, (ii) middle sensors placed between the heel and the toes, and (iii) a front sensor placed at the tip of the toes [39]. Additionally, soft capacitive strain sensors [40] ((see Fig. 3c)), embedded in commercial knee braces and worn in contact with the skin, under the exosuit. These sensors are used to further refine the segmentation of the gait cycle, considering up to six events, namely Heel Strike—HS, Flat Foot—FlF, Front Foot FrF, Toe Off—TO, Positive Speed Inflection—PSI and Negative Speed Inflection—NSI [41]. The control strategy for the XoSoft exosuit can be selected based on the required assistance for specific lower limbs joints and task. During an initial phase there is the energy storage to elongate the elastic band. In this case the user has to fight against the resistance force generated by the actuator. Once the joint starts rotating in the opposite direction, the system releases the accumulated mechanical energy. In this phase, the system provides assistance to the user until the leg segment returns to the initial position. Therefore, it is possible to store and deliver different amounts of energy by modulating the timing of clutch engagement.

3.1.2 XoSoft Experimental Validation

The XoSoft exosuit was tested to assess functionality, validity and reliability [39, 43–46]. Concerning the device, it emerged that:

- There is no need for a high-power actuation system. Indeed, it is worth noting that while the healthy human gait is highly optimized with only a small margin for improvement, for patients with a small/medium degree of disability, a quasi-passive actuation system has the potential for significant improvement.
- The energy efficiency of the system (and consequently the autonomy) can be substantially improved.
- Alternative actuation mechanisms, that are more suitable for a soft system, need to be explored.

A variety of primary users were targeted to test wearing the Gamma. The platform has been subject to laboratory testing on specific scenarios: Walking on level surface; Sit-to-stand/stand-to-sit; Balance (e.g. standing and reaching; postural sway; Walking on an incline plane; Obstacles; Individual steps (step up & down); Donning/Doffing). In laboratory six primary users, with different levels of impairment (1 stroke, 3 with incomplete spinal cord injury, 2 frail elderly), were tested [47]. For all participants, a baseline gait analysis without XoSoft was performed in order to gain insight into their specific gait pattern. Participants had a garment custom fitted to their anthropometrics. The baseline gait analysis and the garment fitting were done between 1 and 4 months before data collection with the XoSoft prototypes. However, both frail elderly participants were not able to do the data collection with the exosuit due to serious health issues unrelated to the data collection.

The clinical validation [48, 49] was performed with nine participants: two participants with stroke and two participants with incomplete Spinal Cord Injury iSCI were measured with the Gamma prototype at RRD (Netherlands), and five frail elderly participants were measured with the Gamma prototype at GCE (Germany). Different actuation protocols were used, depending on the individual user needs. Results show that the actuation resulted in improved kinematics of the actuated joint, and in some cases also affected the other joints of the assisted limb. The amount of improvement varied between the participants. Improvement of foot clearance was found in one of the participants with iSCI, which was also the participant with the most striking improvements in gait kinematics. All participants commented that the system was supporting their leg, such that it took less effort to walk compared to walking without a soft exoskeleton. With respect to usability of the Gamma prototype, all participants reported that the Gamma prototype was too large and too bulky to be used in daily life. However, these comments include the size and weight of the backpack and the use of an external compressor (with accompanying noise and umbilical cord). In addition, participants reported that in the future, the "one-size-fits-all" garment needs to be improved to a customized garment. This includes the size of the garment, but also relates to the individual needs for a specific patient. Participants commented that they would only like to have features included in the garment that are beneficial for them. For example, straps and attachment points on the unaffected lower limb, or around joints that are not actuated, need to be removed from the garment in future designs. This will increase the usability of the garment with respect to donning and doffing and comfort of wearing the garment.

Based on our experiences with the Gamma prototype in stroke, iSCI and frail elderly, we would like to make some recommendations for future developments of soft exoskeletons. Besides the above mentioned aspects on usability mentioned by the participants who used to device, the actuation mechanisms are important to consider in future developments. So far, the Gamma prototype did not succeed in actuating knee flexion during swing. As sufficient knee flexion is an important mechanism to accomplish foot clearance in swing, actuating knee flexion during swing is expected to contribute to improved gait in participants who have problems with their foot clearance, for example as a result of a stiff-knee gait. Instead of actuating knee flexion during swing, it was possible to actuate hip flexion with the current Gamma prototype. Positive effects of hip actuation were found, resulting in increased hip flexion during swing, and a more upright position of the trunk. Actuation of the hip could only be included in a small number of participants. In daily clinical practice, no devices are available to support hip function in participants facing problems concerning this joint. This is in contrast to for example the ankle, where many different types of ankle–foot orthoses are available to support ankle movement during gait.

3.2 TWIN for Severely-Impaired Elderly

TWIN is a lower limb exoskeleton powered at knee and hip, originally designed for Spinal Cord Injured—SCI patients [50]. TWIN is the result of a joint effort coming from the tight cooperation between engineers, industrial designers, physical therapists, physiatrists and SCI patients, which jointly collaborated to develop the device, employing a user-centered approach.

3.2.1 The TWIN Lower Limb Exoskeleton

The developmental process of TWIN initially involved investigation of user needs with SCI subjects and a tight cooperation with physiatrists and physical therapists from two major rehabilitation clinics in Italy throughout the whole development. At first, SCI subjects were requested to express typical needs in their daily life and opinions regarding personal use of an exoskeleton. In a second stage, this information was employed for drafting the general layout of the exoskeleton and the requirements of the device to guide its development.

Overall, what emerged from the analysis of user needs were specific suggestions for an effective application of robotics to people with spinal cord injury. Their feedback could be summarized in two main key needs, i.e. the device should be used autonomously and should be practical to facilitate its employment during its daily usage. The developmental phase followed these specific requirements.

The distinctive feature of the TWIN system (Fig. 5) is indeed its full modularity: the four motors (hips and knee) can be easily donned on and off by means of eight lateral quick release connectors placed on both ends of each actuation module. These connectors realize a dual function: they can both bear the structural mechanical load and serve as electrical interface between the different parts of the exoskeleton. Implementation of this quick release system posed many challenges. It is in fact essential to guarantee the support of the complex, multi-axial, force-torque load imposed on the structure, while at the same time ensuring patient safety, high structural stiffness, power supply and continuity of data streaming. Furthermore, although the "in-line" coupling layout seemed preferable because it bears both axial load and bending moments well, this choice was discarded to prioritize the usability of the device and ease of donning through side mounting. The lateral rapid safety system has indeed been designed to require the patient to make a minimum effort during use, while ensuring high mechanical and electrical safety, following the IEC 60601 safety standard for electro-medical devices [51].

The TWIN system allows the user to set the gait parameters through a mobile device-based GUI, whereas the steps are driven by means of an Inertial Measurement Unit—IMU based trigger. The actuation units employed to power all four joints, are based on flat Maxon motors coupled with 100:1 CSD Harmonic Drive gearboxes. This solution guarantees limited lateral encumbrance and can support patients weighing up to 110 kg.

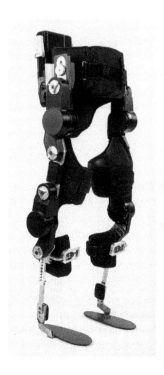

Fig. 5 The TWIN lower limb exoskeleton

The structural parts of the exoskeleton (pelvis, femur, tibia) come with different sizes to adapt the device to the anatomy of the patient. Furthermore, a battery pack located at the back of the device, guarantees up to four hours of continuous operation, whereas a motherboard located next to it is employed as central control unit to send/receive commands and measurements to/from each of the motors. This unit takes care of the high level control that is executed by a TI TM4C123GH6PM TIVA microcontroller.

As for device control, we chose a position control-based scheme to provide full support to the SCI patients during use. As in [50], we used predefined gait trajectories, generated in Cartesian space, by using a basis function interpolation method which was designed so as to maximize stable walk. This indeed was one of the main gait pattern features requested by SCI subjects. The steps are triggered by reaching a set of two torso inclination thresholds. Torso inclination angles are measured by the IMU sensor located in backpack of the device. The step is triggered by the user by means of elaborating the signals coming from the IMU. The pitch and roll angles are defined as the tilt of the waist unit with respect to the frontal and Sagittal planes, respectively. When these angles both pass the frontal and lateral threshold values, the step trigger is activated. These two parameters can be set according to patient needs.

The evaluation of the device's mechatronics as well as the usability of TWIN have been initially carried out by testing the device on healthy subjects (see Fig. 6). A group of ten healthy volunteers participated to the experiment. They had no neurological or muscular diseases. The goal of this phase was to obtain feedback on comfort, usability and safety of the device and its control throughout the development process to allow design adjustments and improvements in a timely manner.

The experimental evaluation was carried out in empty areas, under the supervision of qualified personnel to ensure the safety of the subjects. Both subjects and supervisors were instructed on how to use the exoskeleton. The subjects were asked to perform straight walk from a starting point to a final point located ten meters away, at their preferred speed. Usability and safety were evaluated qualitatively by obtaining feedback from the subjects and the physical therapists. Overall, the device was assessed positively by the two user groups, both from the comfort/ergonomics perspective and feasibility of the walking pattern.

The TWIN exoskeleton is now used in a clinical trial aimed at assessing its usability by patients with incomplete SCI. Usability is evaluated in terms of safety,

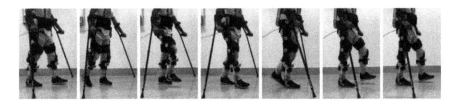

Fig. 6 Testing of the TWIN exoskeleton. Image adapted from [50]

ease of use and intended use. The level of satisfaction of the device by both patients and therapists will also be assessed. More recently, the TWIN exoskeleton has also been adapted to rehabilitation of stroke subjects and a clinical trial is currently being performed, specifically aimed at investigating its usability and user acceptance for neurological rehabilitation.

3.2.2 Potential Use of TWIN for Applications on the Elderly

Preliminary results on the tested population of healthy subjects and of patients from ongoing clinical trials have indicated the potential of the TWIN exoskeleton for rehabilitation of subjects with motor impairments due to traumatic or neurological nature. One obvious exploitation of this technology would thus be its application in the context of motor impairment not due to a pathological condition, but to the physiological motor decline, typical of ageing. Indeed, it is likely that in future years the elderly population will constitute the majority of exoskeletons users, not only because neurological diseases with motor consequence typically affect older adults, but also because ageing is characterized by a progressive deterioration of motor functions, walking being one of them [52].

Given its high modularity and usability, TWIN could serve as a portable device for at home use. Numerous studies has pointed out the importance of aerobic exercise, such as walking, for maintenance of cognitive abilities in superagers [53]. However, older adults are often limited in the execution of physical exercise because of fear of falling. A supporting device such as TWIN might thus promote the execution of walking training also for those subjects whose motor limitations made motor exercise impossible without the assistance of physiotherapists. Moreover, just as a physiotherapist would do, TWIN control can be regulated such as to adjust the gait parameters (i.e. step length, speed and so on) according to the subject's need.

However, in order to effectively adapt current robotic devices to use on the elderly population, we once again stress the importance of understanding user needs and of designing exoskeletal solutions tailored to this specific application.

4 Future Challenges and Trends

In the previous section, we have shown the results obtained with two exoskeletons that can be used also for elderly assistance. In the following, we would like to focus on two trends/open challenges for the future: make sure the exoskeletons are actually used and promote their widespread adoption; and take advantage of the great amount of data that can be collected not only from the exoskeleton but also the final user. The first challenge is addressed in Sect. 4.1 concerning technology acceptance; the second in Sect. 4.2 focusing on tele-health applications and data monitoring.

4.1 Technology Acceptance

A preliminary step to introduce exoskeletons for older people in real contexts is definitely the user's acceptance of such systems. In [54] is reported why adoption and use of wearable robots by older adults is not yet properly understood and analyzed by Technology Acceptance Models—TAMs. TAMs represent the factors that must be considered before to design any assistive technology [55–58], even in case of older people [59, 60], whose attitude toward learning to use and actually employ a novel aid also depends on their decline in sensory, motor, and cognitive skills alongside the challenged constituted by a novel aid.

For instance, the adoption of a system and the intention to use it can be influenced by its perceived usefulness and ease of use from the point of view of the user, whose anxiety, expectations on the device performance, beliefs on its reliability, and experience of social pressure can affect the curiosity and enjoyment in trying the proposed solution. Furthermore, these factors directly influence the key aspect of self-efficacy—the subjective judgment of one's capability to face a certain situation—which is critically relevant in many cases of robot acceptance [61].

Considering this premise, the authors of [54] state the need of older UCD methodologies to create novel wearable geron technologies. Adapting TAMs like Almere [59] or STAM [60] to exoskeletons for elderly could be a strategy for improving the user-centered design techniques, interpreting qualitative and quantitative data on the specific needs and reactions of older people.

Accordingly, [62] proposed the Exoscore as an iterative design and evaluation method to evaluate the exoskeleton acceptance in order to optimize it for elder people (they tested this approach to assess a prototype of a soft lower limb exoskeleton—XoSoft). This method is based on 3 phases—Perception Evaluation, Experience Evaluation, Perceived Impact Evaluation—characterized by a progressive user-centered assessment of the device through visual exposure, usability testing, questionnaires. Importantly, the authors introduced novel constructs, discussed in [63] too. Experiential Perception describes how the user perceives the interaction with the device, including aspects like the embarrassment and the excitement for wearing the exoskeleton alongside physical comfort issues related to weight or noise. Self-Liberty is constituted by the user's belief of being able to independently manage the device. Quality of Life Enhancement is based on the value attributed to the system according to its impact in daily activities. The authors also suggested that robotic assisting devices must adapt to the individual changes in health and life condition during the aging process. Overall, an acceptable exoskeleton must also be usable, trusted, and comfortable to promote the user's motivation to perform trial-and-error learning processes, achieving improved control skills, self-efficacy, and autonomy of use. In order to achieve this outcome, the product designers must also identify the unmet needs of older adults in order to avoid frustration, embarrassment and the abandonment of the devices.

The designers and developers must also care for de-stigmatizing the devices themselves, which risk to mark the user's condition with signs of deteriorating health and autonomy [64]. In order to solve this issue, [65] suggested to hide or integrate the exoskeleton with regular clothing, considering also the potential of personalization in improving the technology acceptance. Making a system truly user-specific constitutes a response to the variability demonstrated by older adults in judging their current need of adopting a wearable robotic system in daily activities. Overall, an appropriate training alongside an intuitive design could overcome the general difficulties of the users. On the other hand, the doubts of specific users can be solved through customization options, demonstrating to consider the individual needs in real contexts. In order to anticipate the heterogeneous needs of the users and increase the technology acceptance, the authors suggest to actively involve the older adults in the decision to adopt an exoskeleton, supporting such a decision-making process through the advice of experts.

Finally, the technology acceptance issues may also be related to the physicians and the therapists, which are involved in co-design processes to estimate the opportunity of using exoskeletons in assistance and rehabilitation. Mortenson et al. [66] observed how using a lower limb exoskeleton may reduce the physical demand on therapists during repetitive, effortful exercises. The authors highlighted anyway how clinicians must manage the patient's expectations about the outcome of the exoskeleton usage. Furthermore, the therapists must face issues related to the cost of the device, the system calibration time, and the intensive training required to employ the technology with the patients.

4.2 Tele-Health and IoT

Tele-health allows to connect remotely the different subjects involved in the rehabilitation process. This includes not only the patients (primary users), but also clinicians (secondary users) and others (tertiary users). In particular, the tele-health systems allow different kind of interactions. In [67], the main interactions are divided in three groups: (i) clinician to clinician, (ii) clinician to patient and (iii) patient to mobile health technology. Each of them have a different purpose and requirements.

A typical rehabilitation scenario where tele-health can provide an important benefit is when the patient is not able to travel to the clinical setup, due to distance limitations or other external factors. Furthermore, the COVID-19 situation has made this scenario even more plausible [68–70], and a tele-rehabilitation system where the person can exercise remotely without the need to coming in person to the clinic offers important advantages from the infection prevention point of view. Nevertheless, not all the rehabilitation procedures can be done remotely, or they would require an excessively complex system.

A second application of tele-health is the continuous monitoring. The data collection from the rehabilitation exercises help the clinicians to evaluate the progress of the patient. While more classical tele-health approaches make use of simpler technologies such as phone, email or video-chat, latest IoT technologies allow continuous monitoring and feedback of the rehabilitation process [71–73]. As an example in the

XoSoft project, we developed the XoSoft Connected Monitor system—XCM [74] that remotely monitors all data generated by the sensors and control hardware, and also records full 3D kinematic data of the lower body and trunk. The first type of data is envisioned for unsupervised use in the final product, and the latter type of data for clinical device calibration and fitting, patient training and patient assessment. The XCM also doubles as a tool for testing of the Gamma version of the XoSoft exosuit in simulated home environment ADL tasks. The XCM has been shown to provide complete, relevant, robust and flexible monitoring and control functionality and interfacing and has been shown to provide accurate, reliable, reproducible data handling and analysis with a high level of automation [74].

Despite the multiple benefits of the tele-health technologies in rehabilitation, there are several obstacles that prevent from a wider implementation. The cost of these technologies is still a barrier, but with the spread of the IoT technologies more and more devices are easier to integrate into a tele-health system. However, physical rehabilitation still often requires specific expensive devices. Reimbursements from National health systems or health insurance companies can only cover part of the expenses.

The second barrier is related with what was described in the previous section, namely the technology acceptance in elderly groups. In this particular case the acceptance is linked with the use of handheld devices for monitoring or using the tele-rehabilitation setup. While new generations are comfortable with the use of handheld devices, older patients might need more time to adapt and they could even reject these solutions. Important efforts have been put in the development of intuitive and easy to use user interfaces to improve the introduction of these technologies [75, 76].

5 Discussion

In this chapter we presented two different exoskeletons, aimed to relieve subjects affected by different levels mobility impairments: XoSoft and TWIN.

XoSoft is a soft exoskeleton that targets subjects with low to mild mobility impairments. It offers modularity to assist only unhealthy joints of the lower limbs, improving pathological gait. The user can feel the assistance from the device that is delivered only when the user needs it, allowing the subject to move unconstrained. To do so, the device is a soft garment with harnesses and its control structure relies on the identification of the users' gait pattern.

Conversely, TWIN is a rigid exoskeleton that aims to assist users that cannot autonomously move anymore. Severe impairments to the lower limbs, such as SCI and other pathological muscle illness, require strong assistance, elaborated control strategies and a rigid structure to support users and let move freely.

These devices are primarily intended to physically assist elderly with pathological or natural muscle tone reduction (sarcopenia) to give them back the possibility to perform activities of daily living autonomously. Indeed, with the increase of ageing population is of utmost importance to develop and deploy devices to allow wellness and active life of this population. Indeed, it is argued that an active lifestyle helps in preventing additional severe diseases and decay, promoting a healthy-ageing [1, 2].

Secondarily, exoskeletons comprise digital and communication devices that can monitor users' biometric parameters. Indeed, exoskeleton must collect data regarding gait phases and balance of the users for their correct functionality. However, computing and connection capabilities allow exoskeleton to act as a hub to collect data from different biometric sensors that can monitor other health parameters (e.g. blood glucose level). There are endless possibilities to monitor health parameters through various sensors connected with the exoskeleton through local body area networks (e.g. Bluetooth Low Energy—BLE), among the most important there are:

- central hub streaming a continuous data flow will allow researchers and clinician to monitor effects of prolonged use of wearable assistive devices, possibly bridging the gap to show efficacy of wearable assistive devices;
- continuous monitoring allowing caregivers and emergency to rapidly intervene in case of sudden illness;
- allow for detection of illness from the appearance of early signs that can be correlated to severe or impairing pathologies.

Despite the promising primary and secondary benefits, exoskeletons still need to face potential challenges to fill the gap to the market. To this end, we believe that a multidisciplinary UCD approach, extended to all direct and indirect users of the device, is the best way to promote impactful development of the current prototypes. Indeed, an effective communication to all stakeholders could become a strong driver for promoting application and further progress in the physical assistive devices field.

6 Conclusions

Exoskeleton and exosuits are moving from tethered rehabilitation devices to walking aids, emerging as a valid solution to maintain independence and mobility for an ageing society. Wearable robots act twofold: physically assisting the user and collecting biometric data. Therefore, wearables robots offer the possibility to develop connected digital services, promoting continuous monitoring and tailored medical treatments. Potential applications target elderly, caretakers and public or private institutions. To reach a widespread adoption of wearable assistive devices, researchers are addressing two main challenges. Firstly, enhancing the acceptability, predicted through TAMs for elderly. Secondly, providing to all the stakeholders involved in elderly healthcare an intuitive and integrated platform to access biometric data collected from the wearable robots.

References

1. D. o. E. United Nations and S. Affairs: World population ageing 2017 highlights. Last accessed on 11 Mar 2021 (2017)
2. Richardson, C.A., Glynn, N.W., Ferrucci, L.G., Mackey, D.C.: Walking energetics, fatigability, and fatigue in older adults: the study of energy and aging pilot. J. Gerontol Series A: Biomed. Sci. Med. Sci. **70**(4), 487–494 (2015)
3. Graf, B.: An adaptive guidance system for robotic walking aids. J. Comput. Inf. Technol. **17**(1), 109–120 (2009)
4. Charron, P.M., Kirby, R.L., MacLeod, D.: Epidemiology of walker-related injuries and deaths in the United States (1995)
5. Priplata, A.A., Niemi, J.B., Harry, J.D., Lipsitz, L.A., Collins, J.J.: Vibrating insoles and balance control in elderly people. lancet **362**(9390), 1123–1124 (2003)
6. Martini, E., Crea, S., Parri, A., Bastiani, L., Faraguna, U., McKinney, Z., Molino-Lova, R., Pratali, L., Vitiello, N.: Gait training using a robotic hip exoskeleton improves metabolic gait efficiency in the elderly. Sci. Rep. **9**, 1–12 (2019)
7. Séguin, E., Doumit, M.: Review and assessment of walking assist exoskeleton knee joints. In: 2020 IEEE International Conference on Systems, Man, and Cybernetics (SMC), IEEE, pp. 1230–1235 (2020)
8. Kekade, S., Hseieh, C.-H., Islam, M.M., Atique, S., Khalfan, A.M., Li, Y.-C., Abdul, S.S.: The usefulness and actual use of wearable devices among the elderly population. Comput. Methods Programs Biomed. **153**, 137–159 (2018)
9. Tuckson, R.V., Edmunds, M., Hodgkins, M.L.: Telehealth. N. Engl. J. Med. **377**, 1585–1592 (2017)
10. Sanders, E.B.-N.: From user-centered to participatory design approaches. In: Design and the social sciences, pp. 18–25, CRC Press (2002)
11. Power, V., de Eyto, A., Hartigan, B., Ortiz, J., O'Sullivan, L.W.: Application of a user-centered design approach to the development of xosoft—a lower body soft exoskeleton. In: International Symposium on Wearable Robotics, Springer, pp. 44–48 (2018)
12. J. L. Pons, Wearable robots: biomechatronic exoskeletons. Wiley (2008)
13. Toxiri, S., Näf, M.B., Lazzaroni, M., Fernández, J., Sposito, M., Poliero, T., Monica, L., Anastasi, S., Caldwell, D.G., Ortiz, J.: Back-support exoskeletons for occupational use: an overview of technological advances and trends. IISE Trans. Occup. Ergonomics Human Factors **7**(3–4), 237–249 (2019)
14. Bogue, R.: Exoskeletons and robotic prosthetics: a review of recent developments. Ind. Robot: Int. J. (2009)
15. Nussbaum, M.A., Lowe, B.D. de Looze, M., Harris-Adamson, C., Smets, M.: An introduction to the special issue on occupational exoskeletons (2019)
16. Proud, J.K., Lai, D.T., Mudie, K.L., Carstairs, G.L., Billing, D.C., Garofolini, A., Begg, R.K.: Exoskeleton application to military manual handling tasks. Human Factors 0018720820957467 (2020)
17. Kermavnar, T., de Vries, A.W., de Looze, M.P., O'Sullivan, L.W.: Effects of industrial back-support exoskeletons on body loading and user experience: an updated systematic review. Ergonomics 1–48 (2020)
18. Gull, M.A., Bai, S., Bak, T.: A review on design of upper limb exoskeletons. Robotics **9**(1), 16 (2020)
19. Toxiri, S., Anastasi, S.: Occupational exoskeletons: a new challenge for human factors, ergonomics and safety disciplines in the workplace of the future. In: Proceedings of the 21st Congress of the International Ergonomics Association (IEA 2021): Volume IV: Healthcare and Healthy Work, vol. 222, p. 118, Springer (2021)
20. Dollar, A.M., Herr, H.: Lower extremity exoskeletons and active orthoses: challenges and state-of-the-art. IEEE Trans. Rob. **24**(1), 144–158 (2008)
21. Kapsalyamov, A., Jamwal, P.K., Hussain, S., Ghayesh, M.H.: State of the art lower limb robotic exoskeletons for elderly assistance. IEEE Access **7**, 95075–95086 (2019)

22. Shi, D., Zhang, W., Zhang, W., Ding, X.: A review on lower limb rehabilitation exoskeleton robots. Chin. J. Mech. Eng. **32**(1), 1–11 (2019)
23. Thalman, C., Artemiadis, P: A review of soft wearable robots that provide active assistance: trends, common actuation methods, fabrication, and applications. Wearable Technol. **1** (2020)
24. Rocon, E., Pons, J.L.: Exoskeletons in rehabilitation robotics: Tremor suppression, vol. 69. Springer (2011)
25. Lim, D.-H., Kim, W.-S., Kim, H.-J., Han, C.-S.: Development of real-time gait phase detection system for a lower extremity exoskeleton robot. Int. J. Precis. Eng. Manuf. **18**(5), 681–687 (2017)
26. Khan, A.M., Yun, D.-W., Zuhaib, K.M., Iqbal, J., Yan, R.-J., Khan, F., Han, C.: Estimation of desired motion intention and compliance control for upper limb assist exoskeleton. Int. J. Control Autom. Syst. **15**(2), 802–814 (2017)
27. Recher, F., Banos, O., Nikamp, C.D., Schaake, L., Baten, C.T., Buurkc, J.H.: Optimizing activity recognition in stroke survivors for wearable exoskeletons. In: 2018 7th IEEE International Conference on Biomedical Robotics and Biomechatronics (Biorob), pp. 173–178, IEEE (2018)
28. Poliero, T., Mancini, L., Caldwell, D.G., Ortiz, J.: Enhancing back-support exoskeleton versatility based on human activity recognition. In: 2019 Wearable Robotics Association Conference (WearRAcon), pp. 86–91, IEEE (2019)
29. Jamˇsek, M., Petriˇc, T., Babiˇc, J.: Gaussian mixture models for control of quasi-passive spinal exoskeletons. Sensors **20**(9), 2705 (2020)
30. Porta, M., Kim, S., Pau, M., Nussbaum, M.A.: Classifying diverse manual material handling tasks using a single wearable sensor. Appl. Ergonomics **93**, 103386 (2021)
31. Huysamen, K., Bosch, T., de Looze, M., Stadler, K.S., Graf, E., O'Sullivan, L.W.: Evaluation of a passive exoskeleton for static upper limb activities. Appl. Ergon. **70**, 148–155 (2018)
32. Toxiri, S., Koopman, A.S., Lazzaroni, M., Ortiz, J., Power, V., de Looze, M.P., O'Sullivan, L., Caldwell, D.G.: Rationale, implementation and evaluation of assistive strategies for an active back-support exoskeleton. Front. Robot. AI **5**, 53 (2018)
33. Diller, S., Majidi, C., Collins, S.H.: A lightweight, low-power electroadhesive clutch and spring for exoskeleton actuation. In: 2016 IEEE International Conference on Robotics and Automation (ICRA), pp. 682–689, IEEE (2016)
34. Binder, T., De Michelis, G., Ehn, P., Jacucci, G., Linde, P., Wagner, I.: Participation in design things. In: Design Things, The MIT Press (2011)
35. Bannon, L.J.: From human factors to human actors: the role of psychology and human-computer interaction studies in system design. In: Readings in Human–Computer Interaction, pp. 205–214 (1995)
36. Anderson, N.S., Norman, D.A., Draper, S.W.: User centered system design: new perspectives on human-computer interaction. Am. J. Psychol. (1988)
37. Abras, C., Maloney-Krichmar, D., et al.: User-centered design. Bainbridge (2004)
38. Ortiz, J., Di Natali, C., Caldwell, D.G.: Xosoft-iterative design of a modular soft lower limb exoskeleton. In: International Symposium on Wearable Robotics, pp. 351–355, Springer (2018)
39. Poliero, T., Di Natali, C., Sposito, M., Ortiz, J., Graf, E., Pauli, C., Bottenberg, E., De Eyto, A., Caldwell, D.G.: Soft wearable device for lower limb assistance: assessment of an optimized energy efficient actuation prototype. In: 2018 IEEE International Conference on Soft Robotics (RoboSoft), pp. 559–564, IEEE (2018)
40. Totaro, M., Poliero, T., Mondini, A., Lucarotti, C., Cairoli, G., Ortiz, J., Beccai, L.: Soft smart garments for lower limb joint position analysis. Sensors **17**(10), 2314 (2017)
41. De Rossi, S.M., Crea, S., Donati, M., Reberˇsek, P., Novak, D., Vitiello, N., Lenzi, T., Podobnik, J., Munih, M., Carrozza, M.C.: Gait segmentation using bipedal foot pressure patterns. In: 2012 4th IEEE RAS & EMBS International Conference on Biomedical Robotics and Biomechatronics (BioRob), pp. 361–366, IEEE (2012)
42. Hrones, J.A., Nelson, G.L.: Analysis of the four-bar linkage: its application to the synthesis of mechanisms. Published jointly by the Technology Press of the Massachusetts Institute of Technology, Wiley, New York (1951)

43. Kermavnar, T., Power, V., de Eyto, A., O'Sullivan, L.W.: Computerized cuff pressure algometry as guidance for circumferential tissue compression for wearable soft robotic applications: a systematic review. Soft Rob. **5**(1), 1–16 (2018)
44. Sadeghi, A., Mondini, A., Mazzolai, B.: Preliminary experimental study on variable stiffness structures based on textile jamming for wearable robotics. In: International Symposium on Wearable Robotics, pp. 49–52, Springer (2018)
45. Sposito, M., Poliero, T., Di Natali, C., Ortiz, J., Pauli, C., Graf, E., De Eyto, A., Bottenberg, E., Caldwell, D.: Evaluation of xosoft beta-1 lower limb exoskeleton on a post stroke patient. In: Sixth National Congress of Bioengineering (Milan) (2018)
46. Di Natali, C., Poliero, T., Sposito, M., Graf, E., Bauer, C., Pauli, C., Bottenberg, E., De Eyto, A., O'Sullivan, L., Hidalgo, A.F., et al.: Design and evaluation of a soft assistive lower limb exoskeleton. Robotica **37**(12), 2014–2034 (2019)
47. Graf, E., Bauer, C., Schüˈlein, S., de Eyto, A., Power, V., Bottenberg, E., Weyermann, B., O'Sullivan, L., Wirz, M.: Assessing usability of a prototype soft exoskeleton by involving people with gait impairments. In: World Confederation for Physical Therapy Congress (WCPT), Geneva, 1013 May 2019, ZHAW Zuˈrcher Hochschule fuˈr Angewandte Wissenschaften (2019)
48. Schuelein, S, Gassmann, K.-G.: "xosoft" a soft-exoskeleton for people with moderate gait insecurities. In: *ZEITSCHRIFT FUR GERONTOLOGIE UND GERIATRIE*, vol. 50, pp. S138–S138, Springer Heidelberg TIERGARTENSTRASSE 17, D-69121 Heidelberg, Germany (2017)
49. Shore, L., Power, V., Hartigan, B., Schüˈlein, S., Graf, E., de Eyto, A., O'Sullivan, L.: Exoscore: a design tool to evaluate factors associated with technology acceptance of soft lower limb exosuits by older adults. Human Factors **62**(3), 391–410 (2020)
50. Vassallo, C., De Giuseppe, S., Piezzo, C., Maludrottu, S., Cerruti, G.M. L. D'Angelo, E. Gruppioni, C. Marchese, S. Castellano, E. Guanziroli, F. Molteni, M. Laffranchi, De Michieli, L.: Gait patterns generation based on basis functions interpolation for the twin lower-limb exoskeleton*. In: 2020 IEEE International Conference on Robotics and Automation (ICRA), pp. 1778–1784 (2020)
51. Eic 60601 medical electrical equipment (2021)
52. Verrusio, W., Renzi, A., Ripani, M., Cacciafesta, M.: An exoskeleton in the rehabilitation of institutionalized elderly patients at high risk of falls: a pilot study. J. Am. Med. Dir. Assoc. **19**(9), 807–809 (2018)
53. Kim, B.R., Kwon, H., Chun, M.Y., Park, K.D., Lim, S.M., Jeong, J.H., Kim, G.H.: White matter integrity is associated with the amount of physical activity in older adults with super-aging. Frontiers in Aging Neuroscience **12**, 294 (2020)
54. Shore, L., Power, V., de Eyto, A., O'Sullivan, L.W.: Technology acceptance and user-centred design of assistive exoskeletons for older adults: a commentary. Robotics **7**(1) (2018)
55. Azjen, I.: Understanding attitudes and predicting social behavior. Englewood Cliffs (1980)
56. Ajzen, I.: From intentions to actions: a theory of planned behavior. In: Action control, pp. 11–39, Springer (1985)
57. Davis, F.D.: A technology acceptance model for empirically testing new end-user information systems: Theory and results. PhD thesis, Massachusetts Institute of Technology (1985)
58. Venkatesh, V., Morris, M.G., Davis, G.B., Davis, F.D.: User acceptance of information technology: toward a unified view. MIS Quarterly 425–478 (2003)
59. Heerink, M., Kröse, B., Evers, V., Wielinga, B.: Assessing acceptance of assistive social agent technology by older adults: the almere model. Int. J. Soc. Robot. **2**(4), 361–375 (2010)
60. Chen, K., Chan, A.H.S.: Gerontechnology acceptance by elderly hong kong chinese: a senior technology acceptance model (stam). Ergonomics **57**(5), 635–652 (2014)
61. Latikka, R., Turja, T., Oksanen, A.: Self-efficacy and acceptance of robots. Comput. Hum. Behav. **93**, 157–163 (2019)
62. Shore, L., Power, V., Hartigan, B., Schüˈlein, S., Graf, E., de Eyto, A., O'Sullivan, L.: Exoscore: a design tool to evaluate factors associated with technology acceptance of soft lower limb exosuits by older adults. Human Factors (2019)

63. Shore, L., de Eyto, A., O'Sullivan, L.: Technology acceptance and perceptions of robotic assistive devices by older adults–implications for exoskeleton design. Disabil. Rehabil.: Assistive Technol. 1–9 (2020)
64. Hill, D., Holloway, C.S., Ramirez, D.Z.M., Smitham, P., Pappas, Y.: What are user perspectives of exoskeleton technology? A literature review (2017)
65. Jung, M.M., Ludden, G.D.: What do older adults and clinicians think about traditional mobility aids and exoskeleton technology? ACM Trans. Human-Robot Interact (THRI) **8**(2), 1–17 (2019)
66. Mortenson, W.B., Pysklywec, A., Chau, L., Prescott, M., Townson, A.: Therapists' experience of training and implementing an exoskeleton in a rehabilitation centre. Disabil. Rehabil. 1–7 (2020)
67. Reed, T., Tuckson, V., Edmunds, M., Hodgkins, M.L.: (No Title). Tech. Rep. (2017)
68. Chang, M.C., Boudier-Rev´eret, M.: Usefulness of telerehabilitation for stroke patients during the covid-19 pandemic. Am. J. Phys. Med. Rehabil. (2020)
69. Prvu Bettger, J., Resnik, L.J.: Telerehabilitation in the age of covid19: an opportunity for learning health system research. Phys. Ther. **100**(11), 1913–1916 (2020)
70. Leochico, C.F.D.: Adoption of telerehabilitation in a developing country before and during the covid-19 pandemic. Annals Phys. Rehabil. Med. (2020)
71. De Marchi, F., Contaldi, E., Magistrelli, L., Cantello, R., Comi, C., Mazzini, L.: Telehealth in neurodegenerative diseases: opportunities and challenges for patients and physicians. Brain Sci. **11**(2), 237 (2021)
72. Dabiri, F., Massey, T., Noshadi, H., Hagopian, H., Lin, C., Tan, R., Schmidt, J., Sarrafzadeh, M.: A telehealth architecture for networked embedded systems: a case study in in vivo health monitoring. IEEE Trans. Inf Technol. Biomed. **13**(3), 351–359 (2009)
73. Atashzar, S.F., Carriere, J., Tavakoli, M.: Review: how can intelligent robots and smart mechatronic modules facilitate remote assessment, assistance, and rehabilitation for isolated adults with Neuro-Musculoskeletal conditions? (Apr 2021)
74. Baten, C.T., de Vries, W., Schaake, L., Witteveen, J., Scherly, D., Stadler, K., Sanchez, A.H., Rocon, E., Bos, D.P.O., Linssen, J.: XoSoft connected monitor (XCM) unsupervised monitoring and feedback in soft exoskeletons of 3D kinematics, kinetics, behavioral context and control system status. In: Biosystems and Biorobotics, vol. 22, pp. 391–395, Springer International Publishing (Oct 2019)
75. Dodd, C., Athauda, R., Adam, M.: Designing user interfaces for the elderly: a systematic literature review (2017)
76. Rot, A., Kutera, R., Gryncewicz, W.: Design and assessment of user interface optimized for elderly people. a case study of actgo-gate platform. In: ICT4AgeingWell, 157–163 (2017)

Video Games for Positive Aging: Playfully Engaging Older Adults

Sasha Blue Godfrey and Giacinto Barresi

Abstract One of the biggest challenges in the near future will be finding strategies to promote positive aging, that is, aging with a high quality of life with respect to both mental and physical health. Video games appear to be one of the most appealing interactive technologies for empowering older adults and assisting them to overcome health issues. As underlined by recent studies, computer games can improve seniors' quality of life in several areas, including training of cognitive abilities, relaxation, socializing, and motivating healthy behaviors such as physical activity. Their capability to engage people is especially useful in clinical settings, enhancing patient adherence to therapy exercises, perhaps even more so when they can employ recent advances in Extended Reality, Internet of Things, and Tele-Health. Furthermore, emerging domains, like Digital Health, offer revolutionary ways to make games more effective, ubiquitous, adaptive, and personalized, empowering the user-centered (and senior-centered) design of these systems. Within this context, this chapter discusses the role of video games to foster positive aging, analyzing how they can enhance mental and physical health in the elderly population.

Keywords Video games · Older adults · Serious games · Gamification · Internet of Things · Digital Health

1 Introduction

The promise of technological applications for the elderly in general, and computer and serious games in particular, has long been recognized [1]. We now live in an era where the ubiquity of and familiarity with technology makes that promise more achievable than ever. In this chapter, we will explore the use of various kinds of

---

S. B. Godfrey (✉)
Research and Development, SimTec MD Inc., Lethbridge, Canada
e-mail: sasha@simtecmd.ca

G. Barresi
Rehab Technologies Lab, Istituto Italiano di Tecnologia, Genoa, Italy

video games to improve the health, well-being, and lives of senior citizens, an ever-increasing segment of the global population.

One of the main advantages, in the opinion of the authors, of using video games to address a specific need is the engagement with the user. In rehabilitation, whether physical or cognitive, exercises can become monotonous or boring over time, even for individuals that understand the benefits of therapy and are motivated to improve. High repetition is often key to reaping the positive benefits of rehabilitation. Through the use of video games, this repetition can become less tedious and more fun.

Similarly, video games (and, in certain cases, the stories they tell) can be a powerful tool to draw people in helping them identify with the scenario presented, making it an effective avenue for promoting healthy habits and meaningful lifestyle changes [2]. Finally, video games can be used to tackle mental health challenges. Sometimes, it can be difficult to face mental health issues head-on in conventional therapy, but, similar to healthy habit promotion, stories and games can help the player engage with and work through these difficult subjects. Overall, the health of seniors will be the main target of the systems we describe, but game-based solutions can be exploited in many other fields to engage older adults with direct and indirect effects on their well-being. The choice to focus on health-related applications derives from the need to prioritize managing and potentially countering the effects of aging and age-related challenges. These applications may in turn enable other aspects of older people's daily life. In this chapter, we will explore these applications and others, considering how they can be empowered by technologies for Extended Reality, Internet of Things, and Tele-Health. Furthermore, we will explore senior-centered design and how it can improve these applications. We will touch on the wide variety of game modalities, their connection to the individual's interests, and how the user must be considered as a whole regardless of the specific focus, health or otherwise, of the application. Embracing and exploring this variety can help discover novel strategies for engaging seniors. Finally, we will discuss how these systems intertwine with exemplary innovations in Digital Health to promote positive aging through ubiquitous personalization features.

2 Engagement and Game Systems

Video games are interactive systems characterized by a remarkable ability to involve players, intrinsically motivating them both to persist in their use and to fully engage their mental and physical skills to improve their performance and achieve a goal. A proper game design is rich in elements (e.g., rules, challenges, feedback, rewards, difficulty levels, and objectives) that generate this kind of personal involvement [3]. Neuroscientific studies on video game interactivity have shown how such engagement is a rewarding (and therefore motivating) experience that goes beyond the multisensory stimulation of the game [4].

2.1 Engagement, Game Features, and Well-Being

Literature offers interpretative models of video game engagement processes, considering [5] and in line with the self-determination theory [6] (SDT, Fig. 1), and how it depends on the satisfaction of specific player needs: (i) competence, as the feeling of being an expert in an activity; (ii) autonomy, as the feeling of being who determines what happens; (ii) relatedness, as the feeling of being involved in interactions and bonds with other individuals.

The SDT offers a versatile key for understanding how certain tasks and situations are intrinsically motivating, thus engaging. Considering an example outside the context of video games, Lee et al. [7] presented the results of a successful 13 month SDT-based plan promoting physical exercise adherence and resulting in improvements in physical fitness and quality of life in older adults. When SDT is adopted to engage players of video games, its effects are enhanced by the interactivity of this class of media. Games generate a motivational pull [8] based on the enjoyment that depends on the type of feedback adopted, the rules characterizing the game, and the social features enriching it—matching, respectively, the three dimensions of SDT: competence, autonomy, and relatedness.

Overall, game literature suggests multiple ways of engaging the user through scientifically informed choices of game design [9]. An example is offered by Guardini et al. [10], who show how it is possible to increase the perceived competence and enjoyment of the player by simply increasing the visualized amount of XP (experience points, the points that determine the growth of the character) accumulated during the game sessions.

Considering this, it is advantageous to introduce game features in systems traditionally unrelated to leisure contexts [11] for improving users' motivation, their engagement in executing tasks, and, consequently, the expected benefits of such solutions. Especially effective is the approach of gamification [12]: applying video game elements to a system not designed to entertain the user (for instance for professional

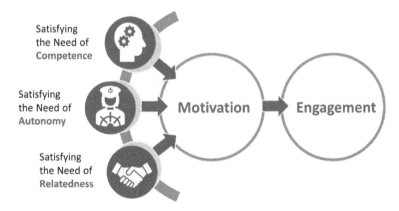

Fig. 1 From the factors of motivation in self-determination theory to engagement

training) in order to make its use more engaging. Another perspective is that of serious games [13]: actual games designed for purposes not only related to entertainment (such as stimulating and promoting physical exercise, in the case of exergames).

However, this classification tends to be excessively rigid if we look at the integration of game features in applied contexts. Indeed, game-based systems (a term we use often in this chapter) can be considered as gamified solutions or serious games depending on the way they are presented to the user.

Considering their health-related applications, systems based on video game-inspired paradigms (real games or their elements) are often used to motivate students to learn [14] or patients in the execution of both diagnostic tests [15] and therapeutic-rehabilitative exercises [16, 17] that are often repetitive or frustrating. Video game solutions can also be used to distract patients from pain [18] due to pathologies or clinical interventions. They are also used to treat anxiety disorders and phobias [19] and, in particular, post-traumatic stress disorder (PTSD), as in the case of veterans [20].

Interactive digital entertainment paradigms can also be offered to people whose motor and cognitive activities must be stimulated or whose habits must be changed in order to promote their well-being. This is the case of video games that entertain the elderly [21] by presenting a set of activities able to physically and mentally challenge them in order to counter the effects of aging, or by driving lifestyle changes for people with chronic conditions, such as diabetes [22], or by facilitating relaxation through biofeedback [23].

It is important to highlight how game-based solutions offer high versatility to engage older adults in activities aiming at improving their quality of life [24]. Elements such as feedback and rewards in video game tasks enable various clinical and health-supporting protocols that enhance and assist the adherence of those who must perform the required procedures. As noted above, this is especially the case of older adults, who need specific stimulation for countering the effects of aging on their life and skills or changing their habits to prevent the worsening of chronic diseases, in particular clinical exercises for monitoring and treating pathological conditions. Thus, the versatility of game-based systems is particularly valuable for exploring and creating novel strategies to approach elderly needs.

However, such strategies depend on the technologies we consider for implementing game elements, which must be appropriate for the individual needs, especially in health-related contexts [25]. The technological systems enabling game-based solutions constitute both constraints and opportunities for the designers and developers. The next sub-section will introduce technological platforms that will be recurring themes in this chapter.

2.2 *Engagement and Game Technology Innovation*

Video games and, in general, game-based solutions can exploit engaging features and specific design choices [26] with a potential that increases with the growing development of affordable and accessible technologies (from headsets to projectors) for virtual reality (VR, when the perceived setting is fully computer-generated, even within a screen in the case of non-immersive settings) [27]. In addition to VR, games may be played in mixed reality (MR, when within the perceived setting real and virtual items coexist) solutions like the ones for augmented reality (AR, when computer-generated items are experienced within a real environment) [28].

The definitions of these settings are continuously updated according to the innovations in interaction technologies. For instance, Palmas et al. [29] considers VR, AR (depicted just in terms of informational overlay), and MR (represented as a fully interactive augmented setting where the computer-generated objects behave like physical ones) to be different examples of Extended Reality (XR), a concept that can be expanded according to the emergence of novel interaction paradigms in various fields, including health [30].

Overall, virtual and augmented environments constitute ideal game settings for generating engagement derived from different degrees of immersion (related to sensory fidelity) and presence (the feeling of being within a mediated environment and the belief that virtual events are actually occurring), both of which are strictly connected to psychological concepts like the flow state [31–33]. Since immersion and presence positively affect engagement, adopting virtual and augmented environments for designing games is quite advantageous for maximizing the player's motivation [34]. Such advantages are clear, especially considering how low-cost leisure products supporting XR are (e.g., smartphones) or are becoming (e.g., headsets for computers and consoles) quite common on the market and ever more affordable.

The potential of XR can be magnified in conjunction with other systems. In particular, Internet of Things (IoT) solutions [38] constitute a key enabler to connect different kinds of technologies—e.g., mobile devices [35], wearable systems [36], and sensor networks [37]—to allow automated adaptation of the game features to the individual and for making these features follow the user in different settings. These technologies can thus generate the conditions for sensor-based virtual coaching [39] and pervasive computing [40], both of which can have integrated game features. Thus, they have a central role in making novel interaction patterns emerge within the domain of games for older adults, taking advantage of IoT functions to gain a degree of autonomy lost with the age-related decline of sensory, motor, and cognitive abilities.

The interplay between IoT and serious games is currently being explored [41] to achieve personalized interventions (empowering user-specific benefits of games for health) based on data collected, for instance, at home through environmental and wearable sensor networks and analyzed by machine learning systems.

This kind of process enables the adjustment of user interfaces and feedback to individual behaviors and physiological reactions. IoT sensors can feed AI systems that guide game mechanics to adapt games to the person's lifestyle through continuous monitoring or to improve the effectiveness of a game-based treatment of the consequences of events like a stroke [42] through a computational intelligence guiding the game mechanics. AI solutions can also use user data to adjust the activity of artificial agents working as coaches that stimulate mental and physical activity of elder people within gamified platforms for assessment and training [43].

Tung [44] proposed this kind of solution within a human–robot interaction framework where a home robot worked as an exercise companion that can accomplish its functions in any room, anytime. The robotic system is connected to an IoT sensor network including a smart watch that collects physiological data as the output of the exercise routine alongside motion data collected through a computer vision system. The robot suggests exercise videos, follows the execution, and gives accomplishment points (a gamification solution, represented through flower diagrams) according to the data collected through the IoT systems.

Interestingly, the convergence between robotic systems and game systems can also be observed outside the domain of IoT, with serious games enhancing the execution of rehabilitative exercises guided by mechatronic solutions [45]. In addition, robotic systems can trigger and facilitate game dynamics that also lead to social interactions between older adults, for example in virtual environments [46].

Furthermore, IoT can also be connected to virtual and augmented environments, as demonstrated by the work in [47], which used it with MR to generate a novel assistive technology paradigm for the elderly. The authors presented these systems for assisting older people with sensory impairments, using analysis of the environment, the search and recognition of objects, navigation and wayfinding to make the user relatively independent in activities of daily living.

These IoT solutions are not explicitly designed for gaming, but they offer a high-potential framework to tailor game-based features in its MR component, offering a design space for supporting an engaging guide to stimulate an active life. This can happen everywhere, since IoT systems [48] can support monitoring of the elderly in natural settings through virtually any object near the individual in everyday life, with great potential benefits for telemedicine and serious game-based telerehabilitation [49].

Figure 2 shows the recent COCARE project as an example of a senior-centered Tele-Health initiative adopting game-based solutions. COCARE is conducted by

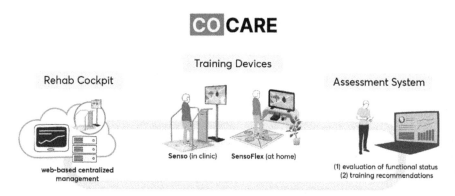

Fig. 2 COCARE: an example of a Tele-Health platform for elderly, including game-based training solutions. Illustration courtesy of COCARE project. https://cocare.rehab

Dividat AG (Switzerland, coordinator), IRCCS Fondazione Don Carlo Gnocchi (Italy), ETH Zürich (Switzerland), and Materia Agecare (Cyprus) within the framework of the Ambient Assisted Living (AAL) European Program. This project proposes a user-friendly technological ecosystem for geriatric continuum-of-care and telerehabilitation. In COCARE, game-based training systems are used to engage patients, and they can also mediate the diagnostic and monitoring activity of remote clinicians.

Considering the potential of multiple technological approaches for engaging seniors, the next sections will highlight exemplary applications of game-based solutions for the well-being of older adults. Our goal is to demonstrate the potential of such solutions across different aspects of daily life and across the spectrum of clinical applications. We then will discuss perspectives on game design for older adults, considering the opportunities offered by disruptive technologies poised to interact with and influence this research field.

3 Video Games for Older Adults' Well-Being

The term "well-being" can encompass all aspects of life: physical, emotional, and mental. A person's experience may clearly affect their well-being on all these levels, which literally can become "playing fields" to improve the quality of an older person's life through video games and game-based systems (including gamification solutions) [50]. The next sub-sections will introduce a non-exhaustive list of application fields for game-based systems.

3.1 Promoting Healthy Habits

Maintaining or improving fitness in the healthy elderly population can help prevent some of the physical deterioration associated with aging, and the effects of physical activity extend beyond fitness to mental and brain health [51, 52]. Fitness and physical activity are increasingly becoming gamified. A wide variety of mobile apps and console games targeting nutrition and physical activity are commercially available, and the industry continues to grow. Larsen et al. examined the availability and effectiveness of exergames in the healthy elderly [53]. While methodological differences between studies make an extensive meta-analysis of results challenging, six of the seven randomized, controlled studies they reviewed suggested that exergames can produce positive physical outcomes in the elderly. It is worth noting that five of these studies utilized commercial gaming solutions in their interventions. The wide availability of this technology could help research facilities that are not well-versed in game and/or software development examine similar strategies with larger sample sizes and dose-matched control groups to further this knowledge base.

Medication use is a potential future area of serious game development for the elderly population. Abraham et al. [54] reviewed 12 games for medication adherence, education, and safety in studies published between 2003 and 2019. Most of these games were targeted at children and/or young adults, and as a nascent field, results are still limited and variable. However, it is a promising avenue to explore. Elderly individuals may find themselves having to manage a complicated medication schedule, and they may be uncertain what, if any, over the counter medications they can take as needed. Serious games could complement technology already in use to assist medication adherence and provide an engaging and flexible learning environment in which to understand medication safety and interactions. This approach can be extended to treatments that work to change habits like smoking or diet, as in the case of diabetes [55]. Establishing and maintaining healthy habits is an area particularly ripe for IoT and pervasive and ubiquitous systems. In [56], researchers explored the potential of using a virtual pet (animal or tree) whose state reflected the relative health of the meals submitted via photograph to encourage healthy eating. While this solution was aimed at children, the ease of use of the system (submitting a photograph of a meal rather than typing in foods or selecting from a list) as well as the non-intimidating and easy to interpret output makes this kind of system easily modifiable for an older population. Similarly, Takahashi et al. in [57] explored a mobile walking game to encourage seniors to leave the house and engage with the community; a game that can fit in nearly each of the clinical applications covered in this section. Overall, digital solutions like games can be a powerful tool for educating patients to adopt and maintain healthy behaviors [58] like physical exercise.

3.2 *Physical Activity Stimulation and Motor Rehabilitation*

Physical activity, as discussed in previous paragraphs, is a very active area of game (or more specifically, exergame) development and commercialization. Roughly two thirds of studies published on (serious) games for rehabilitation used commercial technology, while the remaining third used games designed for the express purpose of rehabilitation. Bonnechère [59] examined the breakdown of studies using games for physical rehabilitation across over 200 studies and nearly 8000 subjects and found the breakdown of study topics coherent with the incidence of the pathologies and topics of study. Twenty-nine percent of the subjects included participated in studies on games for aging. Twenty-two percent of subjects participated in studies on topics that typically disproportionately affect the elderly (19% for rehabilitation post-stroke and 3% targeting Parkinson's disease). An additional 16% of subjects participated in studies on balance, which included subjects of all ages and various conditions, including elderly subjects. The remainder of the studies focused on obesity and cerebral palsy, by and large targeting a younger population. The sheer size of this field precludes it from being covered extensively in this chapter; we will highlight key examples and applications here, and the reader is invited to explore references [53, 59–61].

A particularly rich area of application of game-based physical rehabilitation is with individuals post-stroke. Games for rehabilitation post-stroke have been tested to target a variety of stroke sequelae, including upper and lower limb function as well as balance and general motor function [59]. In [62], Doumas et al. presented a meta-analysis of the effects of using games for upper limb stroke rehabilitation. Across 42 trials and 1760 subjects, interventions using serious games resulted in better outcomes than conventional therapy in upper limb function and activity; these results, while significant, had low effect size. Looking ahead to the development of future games for stroke rehabilitation, Doumas et al. observed a moderate effect size when considering only a subgroup of the above studies that included at least 8 (out of 11) identified neurorehabilitation principles. These principles include type and quantity of practice and feedback, among others; the interested reader is directed to [63] for further information.

Both healthy aging and certain pathologies prevalent in the elderly can increase the risk of falling. A review by Choi et al. [64] examined 25 articles on exergames for fall prevention in the elderly. The vast majority of these used commercially available technology, primarily the Nintendo Wii (14) and Microsoft XBox Kinect (5), often with commercial games focused on balance or sports. Results of using exergames largely (24 out of 25 studies) showed improvements in at least one outcome measure, suggesting that these activities are likely effective. From the available data, it is not yet clear whether this intervention is more effective than conventional exercise. The video game industry is growing rapidly, with increasingly advanced technology and an enormous market share. Taking advantage of these advances, for example by using commercial games and technology, could facilitate widespread adoption and home use.

It is also worth noting that many of the newest game-based solutions take advantage of novel technology. Two prime examples are XR technology, introduced in Sect. 2 above, and haptic technology. Haptic technology gives the perception of touch and thus can be a powerful method to provide feedback and increase immersion; while beyond the scope of this work, the reader is invited to examine the effects of haptic feedback in rehabilitation using VR in [58]. IoT technology is also increasingly being used for physical rehabilitation [65]. Wearable devices and cloud technology are increasingly being employed to enable patients to meet their rehabilitation goals. Early results suggest that IoT is well accepted in this context, but much research is still needed to understand the cultural, economic, and other nuanced aspects of incorporating this new technology. Exergames tend also to be an effective component in telerehabilitation [66], which can also support cognitive training.

3.3 Cognitive Stimulation and Rehabilitation

Changes in cognitive function are known to occur with aging and begin relatively early in adult life, with many markers, such as selective attention, working memory, processing speed, reasoning, and spatial cognition, showing a decline [67]. However, these changes, posited in part to be compensated for by lifestyle changes and increases in function in other areas, such as experience and knowledge [68], are rarely noticed until they become more significant later in life. In healthy seniors, video games could promote cognitive stimulation through brain training [69] and edutainment activities [70]. However, the literature still shows a debate on the impact of game-based cognitive stimulation.

Two recent Cochrane reviews examined the effect of computerized cognitive training on maintaining cognitive function in cognitively healthy, elderly individuals [71] and on preventing dementia in individuals with mild cognitive impairment [72]. Both reviews compared against active and inactive control interventions and looked at global cognitive functioning as well as several subdomains, such as episodic memory, processing speed, executive function, working memory, and verbal fluency. Computerized cognitive training was found to have a small, positive effect on cognitive function overall in both groups. However, the quality of the evidence was generally deemed low or very low, suggesting that further study is essential to understanding and validating these effects.

It must be considered that computerized cognitive training solutions are a heterogenous family that includes a variety of design concepts and implementation solutions, and these aspects could be critically important for engaging the players during the procedures. This observation could be the premise to a larger study to correlate the user engagement of a cognitive training game and its impact on the targeted cognitive processes. It is possible that not all games are engaging enough to trigger the expected effect, and a user-centered game design [73] is the key to tailoring appropriate solutions to a diverse sector of the population like people with different cognitive impairments, especially when they are intertwined with the aging processes. This could explain how certain cognitive training games (e.g., brain training apps that enhance the cognitive performance and processing speed in older adults) [74] could be significantly more effective than others.

The importance of engagement is even more evident if we think about cognitive rehabilitation games. Park et al. [75] highlight how the existing computer-assisted cognitive rehabilitation systems are mostly constituted by repetitive exercises lacking actual fun for the players. Thus, they designed and developed a serious game called "Rejuvenesce Village," tested by 100 elderly people over 5 months. The results of this study showed an improvement in cognitive performance and life satisfaction with a decrease of depression symptoms. The study presented in this paper demonstrates the potential benefits of user-centered design of the game platform, focusing on the older person engagement to achieve the expected results.

Such systems can also be advantageously implemented in XR settings with advanced personalization features for proficiently matching the individual needs in cognitive and motor training and rehabilitation of older adults, addressing the diversity within this population [76]. This field is still open to be explored according to the emergence of convergent technologies: in [77] a brain training solution including games was based on wearable systems, AR, and IoT, for example, and it was designed according to neuroplasticity principles.

The possibility to scale such results through telerehabilitation solutions [78] for enabling older people to perform exercises at home is an invaluable opportunity that can be extended to general mental healthcare.

3.4 Mental and Social Well-Being

Interest is growing in using games to treat and manage mental health issues. Lau et al. [79] in 2017 conducted a meta-analysis of 9 studies targeting various aspects of mental health at various stages of life and found that this kind of intervention may be effective at reducing symptoms. This review examined results from games targeting alcohol use disorder, attention deficit hyperactivity disorder, autism spectrum disorder, cognitive functioning, depression, and post-traumatic stress disorder. This list shows the wide variety of potential applications of this technique. Furthermore, individuals from certain backgrounds or cultures may be more resistant to seeking help for psychological difficulties and disorders. Serious games may allow these individuals to tackle an otherwise-unapproachable issue in a way that feels safe and private. Additionally, certain disorders may be difficult to manage effectively with conventional methods and may benefit from this innovative approach.

Considering the case of older adults, Hall et al. [80] discuss the health benefits of digital games for elder people. The authors highlight in their systematic review how the most frequently reported significant effects of video game interventions for seniors were on their mental health (e.g., depression). Furthermore, Montana et al. [81] reviewed the advantages of emotion regulation techniques (including biofeedback and neurofeedback) in virtual environments to improve the well-being of adults and older adults through game-based settings designed to assist the individual in coping with stress and anxiety [82]. Moreover, Bojan et al. [83] demonstrated the positive effect of games on the emotions of people with dementia: in severe conditions, this strategy can be successful to facilitate the patients' acceptance for more traditional cognitive stimulation procedures.

The psychological well-being of older people must be considered in psychosocial and relational terms too, especially considering issues like loneliness [85]. As discussed also in Sect. 4 on game design, social interaction is a key factor to stimulate the gaming activity of elderly people. Social interactions can be achieved with multiple effects on seniors' health, especially when they are promoted by exergaming [86]. Furthermore, video games can foster intergenerational dynamics that engage older adults and their young relatives (Fig. 3). Video games can also be specifically designed for engaging older and younger people in personalized roles and activities within the same setting according to the each player's age (e.g., Age Invaders) [87]. In [88], the authors proposed this approach as a way to generate positive changes in intergroup anxiety and attitudes as well as intergenerational perceptions. Nguyen et al. [89] include three social interaction games targeting the elderly population in their 2017 review, two of which target intergenerational interactions. The third of these games [90] targets self-esteem in individuals with Alzheimer's or dementia

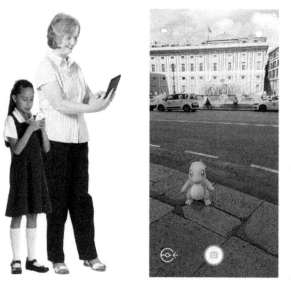
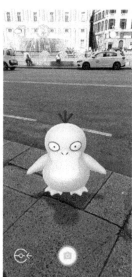

Fig. 3 An intergenerational scenario based on the Niantic Pokémon Go mobile game, which demonstrated multiple positive effects on elderly well-being [84]

with the dual goal of improving the individual's self-image and thereby improving social interaction between the individual and their caregiver. Additionally, Zhang and Kaufman [91] and Osmanovic and Pecchioni [92] discuss that social interaction can be a positive effect, and sometimes the goal, of playing. This concept reinforces the notion in [93] that social interaction can act as a motivating factor in games for other purposes, such as rehabilitation. From these examples, we see how social interaction in play can be powerful force, whether as the aim itself, a desired downstream effect, or a motivating factor, and is an aspect worth exploring and incorporating in future games for the elderly.

Considering emerging and disruptive technologies, there are many potential applications. In Sect. 3.1, we saw how pervasive gaming can be used to help seniors develop healthy exercise habits and increase socialization to avoid isolation [57]. IoT systems can also enable a detection of obsessive–compulsive disorder (OCD) symptoms and activate games designed to mitigate them in elderly [95]. Finally, the addition of distractive features in virtual reality games can be useful to ease treatments for elder people, as in the case of anxiety caused by chemotherapy [96].

3.5 Clinical Diagnosis, Monitoring, and Assessment

Most video games offer scores and progress measures that can be used to evaluate the conditions of the player. This is especially useful for monitoring the effects of senescence on the individual skills, health, and well-being. For instance, [97] presented an exemplary multiplatform serious game for rehabilitation of people with musculoskeletal issues following surgeries or fractures or the effects of aging. The goal of the authors was to present an engaging way to make the users perform physical exercises, while their physiological parameters (e.g., heart rate and temperature) were monitored in real time by remote caregivers. Such an approach is quite effective for the cognitive assessment of older adults [98], overcoming issues like the under-diagnosis of cognitive impairments, especially in ecologically-valid settings where activities of daily living (like cooking) can be accomplished through effortful multitasking processes [99].

Another exemplary case is offered by [100], who proposed to use video games played by healthy older adults to detect early signs of dementia within a framework of preventive medicine. They performed a neuroimaging study to successfully validate their approach, correlating MRI observations of atrophy with lower scores in a memory game and in the PAL test. This demonstrated how impactful memory games can be for the early screening of pathological cognitive decline, highlighting their advantages in terms of accessibility and cost-effectiveness.

Overall, all opportunities offered to collect data via games for the elderly can be useful for monitoring and diagnostic functions: actions performed by the players can be correlated to other indices, including the ones detected through IoT sensor networks (this would enable the emergence of novel, hybrid biomarkers). Such systems are described in Sect. 4.2, based on the idea that senior-centered game design (a focus of Sect. 4.1) can include personalization features that require heterogenous data for understanding the individual's needs.

4 Perspectives on Senior-Centered Game Design

Designing game-based solutions for seniors requires the consideration of age-specific factors to predict the adoption of this kind of system. Ijsselsteijn et al. [101] discussed this topic after presenting the premise that older people play digital games less than younger cohorts. The authors state that this is not directly connected to a lack of availability of new technology or lack of interest on the part of older adults; however, this technology must be useful for their own purposes without costs like substituting social contacts in person with technology-mediated ones.

Furthermore, the authors consider the critical impact of age-related changes that, in both normal senescence and pathological conditions, can lead to mild-to-severe impairments in sensory (e.g., difficulties in visual acuity and accommodation, and in auditory acuity and sensitivity), motor (e.g., slower response times, disruption of coordination and balance), and cognitive (e.g., deficits in attention, executive function, and working memory) skills that are necessary to appropriately use and enjoy a game or a system implementing game-based features. All these aspects (further described in works like [102]) must guide the design of user interfaces, input and output systems, and games for elderly in order to improve their usability and accessibility.

Overall, it is important to consider how to implement the guidelines derived from these observations within a structural model of a video game or of a game-based feature that will be designed for older adults. Gerling et al. [103] described the formal elements of video games according to previous models [104, 105], depicting the user interface (interaction model and feedback model) as the mediator between the player and the core game mechanics (procedures, rules, objectives, conflict) that produce the outcome visualized through the user interface itself. Following this model, the authors must start from the older adults' needs (e.g., socialization through cooperative games) and limitations (e.g., the decline in attention span, short-term memory, and sensorimotor skills), which must lead the design of the game mechanics, possibly making them individually adjustable for including older players. The user interface should be designed according to the changes in motor skills caused by aging: for example, institutionalized older people may have difficulty in handling certain input devices (e.g., pressing buttons). Graphically (e.g., visual item sizes, contrast), the user interface elements and the feedback design should be adjusted to the perceptual difficulties of the users. Overall, the complexity of the commands required by the game should be reduced according to the cognitive impairments of the older players, which should also guide the design of the game mechanics. Avoiding a high cognitive load is compulsory, and quick reactions cannot be expected in older players. Learning can be facilitated by adopting daily life-based metaphors, while objectives and feedback should be explicit and clear, especially to inform the player about the game outcome (e.g., the success score thresholds should be adjustable according to the user's limitations).

IJsselsteijn et al. [101] also highlight the different experience of older adults with Information and Communication Technologies (ICTs) when compared to younger individuals. Many retired without the need of using computers for their activities, and they approach technological devices thoughtfully more than by trial-and-error. These issues can directly affect the self-efficacy of seniors in playing or starting to play a game. Such an issue requires appropriate positive feedback to encourage the older players to master a game. This allows for overcoming their anxiety through a game design that offers adequate time, a set of feasible learning goals, and a focus on mastery more than judgment to make them build their abilities and strategies. Finally, the authors of [101] consider how retirement can be experienced as an opportunity for further exploration in life, and game design must be tailored to user needs. Age-related changes in mind, body, and roles should be analyzed with the heterogenous skills, knowledge, preferences, interests, and background of seniors. This effort requires appropriate models and frameworks to interpret the data collected through qualitative and quantitative research methods, especially for promoting game technology acceptance by recognizing the individual motives for playing—like seeking a challenge [106], self-growth and learning [107], and socialization [108].

Gaming in general is gaining a wider audience, sparking the question of how to design a game for a non-gamer. Many games have similar control systems that feel familiar to habitual players; as new users flock to games, it is becoming increasingly important to aid the control- and play-learning process. Tactics used successfully in commercial games can be ported, with some modifications, to game design for older players in order to ease their transition. Two simple examples [109]: including a map of keys to each UI element always on screen (such as in Fortnite) or frequently showing command reminders or hints, especially within the context of the controller layout (such as in Breath of the Wild). The above notion is compounded when considering game design for older individuals who have limited to no experience with gaming. Exploring playability and player experience in older adults is a nascent field [110] but is essential to crafting games for this population. Indeed, considering all of the aspects mentioned above, a wholistic approach to game design must be taken, accounting for player motivations and goals as well as physical and cognitive abilities.

Such an approach needs a deep understanding of personal needs in real contexts in order to tailor game solutions that can engage seniors and provide them functions. Next paragraphs will propose potential strategies for senior engagement before introducing the IoT-based opportunities offered by Digital Health in terms of personalization.

4.1 Engagement Requirements and Strategies

In order to better understand older player motivations as prerequisites to game acceptance, Wang and Sun [111] proposed an Extended Technology Acceptance Model (ETAM) to predict the effects of a set of factors on the gameplay intentions of older adults. Comparing this to general Technology Acceptance Models (TAMs) tailored to the needs and beliefs of the elderly [112], it is possible to identify the novelties of the ETAM (Fig. 4). It introduces factors like game narrative (a meaningful game experience is useful to alleviate boredom and stimulate curiosity), social interactions (the possibility to establish contacts with other people through the game is probably the most important predictor of gaming), and physical conditions (people who are used to exercise tend to try games more than others).

Furthermore, age, gender, and previous experience can have a moderating effect on game intention factors. For instance, the perceived usefulness of gaming can be modulated by past exposure to interactive technologies. This factor will become more and more important as the cohorts of digital natives age, who are generally used to express themselves through interactive systems, facilitating the future introduction of games for positive aging. Interestingly, the growing practice with and exposure of elderly people to virtual contexts lead to specific research studies involving them as

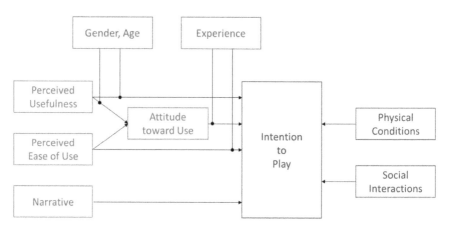

Fig. 4 Extended Technology Acceptance Model (ETAM)—based on [111]

in [113], where the authors examined their moral foundations in decision making, and their subsequent enjoyment, within an interactive setting. Models like the ETAM in [111] can support the design process of games (making them more user-friendly and adaptive) for older adults in order to promote their self-esteem, entertainment, physical activity, and social interaction (in particular benefitting those who live alone) with a positive impact on well-being. As mentioned above, social interaction is a key factor to stimulate the gaming activity of elderly people. An ideal example of this factor are games designed to foster intergenerational dynamics that engage older adults and their young relatives with personalized roles and activities within the same setting [87, 88].

Alongside social contact, another design principle exploitable to make games engaging for the elderly is familiarity, which strictly depends on the experience of each individual. Zhang et al. [114] proposed to counter the age-related perceived digital divide and promote the use of exergames by inserting design features connected to familiarity: the relationship between a person and a memory of salient past feelings and experiences. These memories are typically recollected without attentive effort, automatically. In particular, the authors analyzed five sub-constructs of familiarity: previous experience with a certain stimulus, positive emotions elicited by such a stimulus, the frequency of its occurrence, the depth and complexity of the memory it generated, the stimulus memory retention rate (especially how much it decreases between two occurrences of the same stimulus). Coherently, the authors, presented five guidelines of familiarity design of stimuli, which should: (1) correspond with real world, (2) trigger positive emotion, (3) be meaningful, (4) have been presented repeatedly, and (5) recently in individual experience.

Alongside the individual knowledge defining familiarity, the basic skills of each person should be considered before forcing any training to use a system. Accordingly, game solutions can be enriched by features like natural control modalities based on gestures [115] or tangible user interfaces [116], which offer intuitive solutions that help older adults interact with the device and improve usability if they are appropriately designed [117], especially in video games [118]. Overall, these technologies create high engagement when they involve the body [119] through motor tasks [120] or multisensory (and especially haptic) feedback [121]. Thus, an intuitive design based on body motion and physical stimulations can provide highly engaging solutions in game design for elderly.

Furthermore, all design solutions should be specified according to individual preferences. The type of games that are preferred by older people must also be considered following the principles of participatory design [122]: according to literature, older adults prefer casual games and the features of this preference were investigated by [123] through the Gaming Experience Questionnaire (CEGEQ) [124] (based on the self-evaluation of how much older people enjoyed the game, understood its gameplay rules, learned to control the game, and made it their own). The preference for casual games can be explained by a high compatibility with the decreased cognitive skills of most seniors. Indeed, casual games are usually characterized by high learnability, memorability, intuitive control, and simple mechanics. In particular, casual puzzle games generate higher enjoyment than casual simulation games; both categories overtook casual action games (which require quicker reactions) in this aspect. Furthermore, casual puzzle games were easier to control than casual simulation and action games. Casual puzzle games and casual strategy games were also perceived with higher ownership than casual action games.

These conclusions refer to a sample belonging to a particular cohort, characterized by a certain set of experiences. The widespread diffusion of interaction technologies among young people will require a continuous update of such studies because the preferences for games will mature earlier and earlier in generations initially exposed to these media during childhood. Furthermore, cohort studies must consider cross-cultural differences alongside the individual preferences: the acceptance of video games, especially in health-related contexts, can be affected by cultural factors. For instance, Pyae et al. [125] observed differences in the overall positive experiences of senior citizens of Finland and Japan who played a skiing video game. Finnish subjects showed relatively negative opinions and attitudes about digital games before the study. Conversely, Japanese subjects appreciated video games before participating in this study. After the experimental sessions, both groups showed an improved interest in digital games: in particular, Japanese subjects recommended them as impactful options for physical exercise. However, Finnish subjects recommended games as an alternative training just when traditional physical activities are not available.

This area deserves further investigation for understanding how the self-representation of the elder person's conditions can affect the adoption of an apparently leisurely activity as a treatment. Similar to the example presented above is the possibility that different sub-populations may respond to and engage with a game in a different way. For example, several studies on games have been conducted specifically in elderly military veterans; one aimed to treat PTSD, as mentioned in Sect. 2.1 above, another aimed to increase physical activity [126], while a third aimed to improve balance [127]. It is worth investigating if the same intervention would produce the same results in a broader population (or different sub-population) or if the principles of user-centered game design could be applied to a specific group to guide different themes or features in these games to improve their appeal.

Overall, the heterogeneous traits of older adults must guide user-centered game design, especially accounting for the changes caused by senescence processes. It must be observed how most perspectives presented in this section are related to the requirements of healthy older adults with limited impairments. However, the severity of certain chronic or acute pathologies generates further requirements that must be strictly investigated before designing a game for clinical testing and therapy (or to gamify existing procedures). Thus, the heterogenous medical conditions of older adults require specific approaches (as described in the sub-sections on clinical treatments and assessments), while extending general guidelines like using somatosensory games [128] to engage older adults with disabilities too must be calibrated to the individual needs and difficulties. Moreover, since senescence facilitates the emergence of a wide range of health issues, some of which may be severe, further research must be accomplished to find innovative solutions.

Finally, customization and, possibly, personalization strategies could be quite effective to improve game usability and game user experience through a (respectively) voluntary and automated adjustment to the user needs. In particular, personalization can be based on data collected and analyzed through IoT solutions, (as introduced in Sect. 2.2) [41]. Accordingly, the next sub-section will describe promising technological opportunities with high potential for innovating games for older adults through personalization features based on concepts of pervasive data collection and interaction.

4.2 Toward Ubiquitous Personalization

The technological trends discussed in this chapter offer promising opportunities for empowering the capability of game systems (and gamified systems) to improve quality of life for older adults and for positive aging. In particular, this sub-section will present technologies that are not necessarily adopted for game-related uses or tailored to elderly needs. However, they present unique features that can be exploited for innovating game technologies for older adults.

It must be highlighted that these innovation trends take advantage of the drive provided by the advances in entertainment systems, which are progressively introducing low-cost XR solutions. These systems require careful design improvements for adapting them to older adults, for instance regarding the comfort of head-mounted displays or the risk of cybersickness for the user [129], which can lead some to prefer non-immersive solutions [130]. Virtual and augmented environments offer a high capacity to adapt to the user's activity and conditions while managing the interaction of the individual with different layers of reality. They probably constitute one of the most promising domains of enabling technologies for positive aging, with fertile opportunities for re-defining the XR domain itself with new perspectives [131].

However, particular events, like the COVID-19 emergency, can push the development of these interactive solutions too: for example, in terms of telemedicine for enabling healthcare services without any hazardous contact in person, countering the extreme conditions in which elder people found themselves. Older adults were the main victims of this emergency because of their difficulty to fight the disease. Furthermore, conditions of social isolation and loneliness worsened during the lockdown periods [132], affecting the well-being of older adults especially in terms of mental health. Gabbiadini et al. [133] discussed the helpful contribution of digital communication technologies—including online games—during a lockdown in Italy to enhance the perception of social support and, consequently, mitigate the effects of isolation on mental wellness, which is confirmed by [134] with specific reference to older adults. These gerontechnologies helped to nurture a sense of connection between older people and relatives, friends, and caregivers. Furthermore, during the COVID-19 emergency, video games also stimulated the engagement of older people in meaningful and healthy activities, like physical exercise [135].

Within the context of COVID-19, special attention was paid to IoT solutions because of their capability to monitor the conditions of the elderly and to enhance their autonomy. This type of solution offers great opportunities to make games truly centered around older people.

This scenario creates an opportunity for extending the pervasive impact of a game system (for instance a virtual coach proposing tests or exercises in different rooms) within a ubiquitous computing framework (possibly also connecting remote caregivers and relatives). Literally, the game would follow (and engage) the older person around the home and can adapt itself to the individual and environmental conditions according to the data collected and interpreted in real time (Fig. 5). Such a scenario requires further investigation, especially in terms of user-centered design, to become an acceptable and engaging solution for the elderly.

It is worth highlighting that location-based pervasive game frameworks have already been investigated for mobile solutions and their impact on elder people's health and social activities [136]. The potential of this area is enormous, in particular if we consider how game-based solutions can be implemented within human–robot interaction frameworks too [137, 138].

Through appropriate technological platforms [139], this approach could harness the power of big data analytics (already used in other domains of game user research) [140]. In this way, it would be possible to collect data in meaningful contexts and tasks for detecting or predicting health issues through the involvement of multiple elder players, especially considering the connection with the approach of Digital Health.

The convergence of heterogenous technological solutions is progressively exploited by novel approaches that address health and healthcare challenges, such as Digital Health [141, 142]. These are systems that, for instance, can engage users to improve their lifestyle and health, managing health-related data, and supporting biomedical research and clinical activities. This approach is followed by Digital Therapeutics (DTx) [143]: evidence-based, software-driven treatments designed to

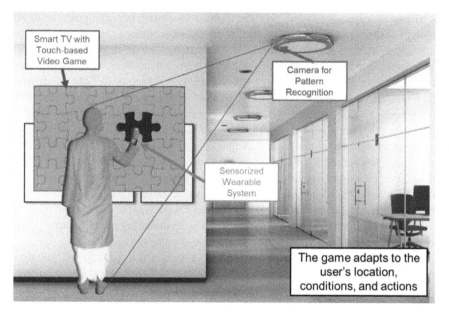

Fig. 5 Example IoT-enhanced game session

prevent and manage medical disorders or diseases, such as the recent case with official approval of health institutions [144] for video game therapy.

Recchia et al. [145] discuss how Digital Health solutions can optimize the efficiency, quality, and safety of care activities, improving their costs and access. Within Digital Health, DTx solutions are designed to have a "digital active ingredient" (the procedure, test or exercise, that generates the clinical outcome) and a "digital excipient," constituted by technological features like reminders or rewards that can be typically implemented through game-based solutions or through full-fledged games to engage the patients. Overall, the DTx systems can be implemented in most digital platforms, from smartphone apps to virtual environments. This approach can radically change the management of issues that typically hit older adults, due for instance to neurodegenerative conditions [146] like Alzheimer's disease or chronic metabolic diseases [147] like diabetes, providing medical doctors with a preliminary option to improve the clinical adherence of their patients through game-based engagement.

The trend of DTx can show its pervasive power especially through games based on mobile and wearable systems: their portability enables any patient to perform their treatments with low-cost devices that can be updated through an app connected to the caregivers who are monitoring the individual conditions [148]. As suggested previously, exploiting the approach of digital therapeutics to collect and analyze big data during the daily life of the patient can help to discover "digital biomarkers" that can be used, always within the Digital Health domain, in diagnostic and prognostic processes and to evaluate the outcome of more traditional medical treatments. For instance, [149] adopted this approach to identify the condition of mild cognitive

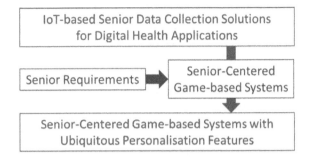

Fig. 6 IoT and Digital Health solutions improve senior-centered game-based systems with ubiquitous personalization features

impairment (MCI). MCI is typically constituted by a perceived cognitive decline that deeply affects the quality of elderly people's life and can steadily progress to dementia if clinicians do not detect it in time. The authors proposed to integrate the classical neuropsychological tests with VR (to create an ecologically controlled simulation) and AI solutions to analyze the collected data (patients' kinematics) while the user performed instrumental activities of daily living (IADL). The digital biomarkers are based on the collected data, enabling the generation of predictive models that identify MCI-specific patterns of motor and cognitive deficits to anticipate the most appropriate clinical interventions. These topics are discussed in another chapter of this book—"Neuro-Gerontechnologies: Applications and Opportunities."

Overall, the opportunities offered by IoT sensors for collecting individual data and of Digital Health for interpreting such information in clinically relevant terms enable a better understanding of the senior user's requirements and empower ubiquitous personalization features (Fig. 6). These solutions can be used for improving the general well-being of older adults (optimizing the game experience or making it persuasive to improve their habits) or for facilitating the execution of certain rehabilitation procedures for elderly patients. A ubiquitous game experience that can adapt to each individual is a decidedly powerful solution for caring and monitoring a person via engaging and unobtrusive solutions.

5 Discussion

This chapter presented the potential of video game systems to promote positive aging. As observed in literature, results are promising, but many hurdles remain, and further investigation is warranted to establish the potential of game-based solutions in improving the quality of seniors' lives. We considered the engagement achieved through game-based systems, their power to improve the quality of life of the elderly, and the possibility to further promote engagement through virtual and augmented settings. However, engagement as a function of gaming should not be taken for granted. Indeed, user-centered game design perspectives were presented, providing insight and solutions for improving the game acceptance of older people alongside their experience and engagement. Design approaches should focus on adapting game strategies to specific needs of older people, especially in the case of pathological conditions. Furthermore, such designs should always consider the recommendations of experts to implement appropriate procedures based on valid principles and evidence [150], contributing to a senior-centered selection of game elements.

Along with the design of the games and gamified solutions themselves, new methods are also required for evaluating the impact and the outcome of such game-based systems in healthcare contexts. Evaluating the results of these novel technologies, for example by conducting a meta-analysis, may not always be straightforward, as some of the reviews in this chapter mention, in large part due to the variety of outcome measures used. As innovations like IoT, XR, and DTx become more and more well-known and common, implementing these solutions in a home or similar environment will become increasingly more feasible. From the available literature on the power of games and game-based systems in general and applied specifically to the elderly as explored in this chapter, we believe there is cause for optimism. It is also prudent for the field to exercise caution in deploying these novel technologies before they are thoroughly vetted. Many elements need to be considered in evaluating these novel solutions, and they must be compared to each other as well as to traditional methods in both effectiveness and efficiency to be applied safely and ensure maximum benefit for the seniors who use them.

6 Conclusion

In this chapter, we considered the engagement achieved through game-based systems, its power to improve the quality of life of the elderly, and the possibility to further promote engagement through virtual and augmented settings as well as user-centered design. A (non-exhaustive) set of application domains of this approach for older people along with several specific applications were highlighted to give a sense of the range and creativity of this growing field. We also presented two promising areas of technological development to empower video games for seniors: connecting systems through IoT systems supported by AI for making games pervasive and adaptive; creating Digital Health solutions like DTx for treating health issues through game-based features that can lead to the discovery of novel digital biomarkers of diseases progression and therapy effectiveness. This relatively new field must continue to evolve to adapt to the increased familiarity of the next generations of elderly individuals and to incorporate the latest advances in technology. Combining technology, user-centered design, and games has the power to dramatically improve the lives of older people and help them age positively.

References

1. Whitcomb, G.R.: Computer games for the elderly. In: Proceedings of the Conference on

Computers and the Quality of Life, pp. 112–115 (1990)
2. DeSmet, A., Van Ryckeghem, D., Compernolle, S., Baranowski, T., Thompson, D., Crombez, G., Poels, K., Van Lippevelde, W., Bastiaensens, S., Van Cleemput, K.: A meta-analysis of serious digital games for healthy lifestyle promotion. Prev. Med. **69**, 95–107 (2014)
3. Lyons, E.J.: Cultivating engagement and enjoyment in exergames using feedback, challenge, and rewards. Games Health J. **4**(1), 12–18 (2015)
4. Cole, S.W., Yoo, D.J., Knutson, B.: Interactivity and reward-related neural activation during a serious videogame. PLoS one **7**(3), e33909 (2012)
5. Przybylski, A.K., Rigby, C.S., Ryan, R.M.: A motivational model of video game engagement. Rev. Gen. Psychol. **14**(2), 154–166 (2010)
6. Deci, E.L., Ryan, R.M.: Self-determination. In: The Corsini Encyclopedia of Psychology, pp. 1–2 (2010)
7. Lee, M., Kim, M.J., Suh, D., Kim, J., Jo, E., Yoon, B.: Feasibility of a self-determination theory-based exercise program in community-dwelling South Korean older adults: experiences from a 13-month trial. J. Aging Phys. Act. **24**(1), 8–21 (2016)
8. Rogers, R.: The motivational pull of video game feedback, rules, and social interaction: another self-determination theory approach. Comput. Hum. Behav. **73**, 446–450 (2017)
9. Hodent, C.: The Gamer's Brain: How Neuroscience and UX Can Impact Video Game Design. CRC Press (2017)
10. Guardini, P., De Simone, D., Actis-Grosso, R.: Faster is better: the speed of player character growth affects enjoyment and perceived competence. In: GHITALY@ CHItaly (2019)
11. Wenk, N., Gobron, S.: Reinforcing the difference between simulation, gamification, and serious game. In: Proceedings of the Gamification and Serious Game Symposium, pp. 1–3 (2017)
12. Stieglitz, S., Lattemann, C., Robra-Bissantz, S., Zarnekow, R., Brockmann, T.: Gamification. Springer (2017)
13. Göbel, S.: Serious games. Springer (2018)
14. Farrell, D., Moffat, D.: Applying the self determination theory of motivation in games based Learning. In: European Conference on Games Based Learning, p. 118. Academic Conferences International Limited (2014)
15. Tong, T., Chignell, M., Tierney, M.C., Lee, J.: A serious game for clinical assessment of cognitive status: validation study. JMIR Serious Games **4**(1), e7 (2016)
16. Dulau, E., Botha-Ravyse, C.R., Luimula, M.: Virtual reality for physical rehabilitation: a pilot study How will virtual reality change physical therapy? In: 2019 10th IEEE International Conference on Cognitive Infocommunications (CogInfoCom), pp. 277–282. IEEE (2019)
17. Mantovani, E., Zucchella, C., Bottiroli, S., Federico, A., Giugno, R., Sandrini, G., Chiamulera, C., Tamburin, S.: Telemedicine and virtual reality for cognitive rehabilitation: a roadmap for the COVID-19 pandemic. Frontiers Neurol. **11** (2020)
18. Fairclough, S.H., Stamp, K., Dobbins, C., Poole, H.M.: Computer games as distraction from PAIN: effects of hardware and difficulty on pain tolerance and subjective IMMERSION. Int. J. Human-Computer Stud. **139**, 102427 (2020)
19. Balan, O., Moise, G., Moldoveanu, A., Moldoveanu, F., Leordeanu, M.: Automatic adaptation of exposure intensity in VR acrophobia therapy, based on deep neural networks (2019)
20. Banks, J., Kowert, R., Colleen Gillespie, B., Latkin, C.: Connection, meaning, and distraction: a qualitative study of video game play and mental health recovery in veterans treated for mental and/or behavioral health problems (2018)
21. Xu, W., Liang, H.-N., Baghaei, N., Wu Berberich, B., Yue, Y.: Health benefits of digital videogames for the aging population: a systematic review. Games Health J. **9**(6), 389–404 (2020)
22. Joubert, M., Guillaume, A.: Videogames in diabetes. In: Handbook of Diabetes Technology, pp. 111–117. Springer (2019)
23. Agrawal, V., Naik, V., Duggirala, M., Athavale, S.: Calm a mobile based deep breathing game with biofeedback. In: Extended Abstracts of the 2020 Annual Symposium on Computer-Human Interaction in Play, pp. 153–157 (2020)

24. Wortley, D., An, J.-Y., Heshmati, A.: Tackling the challenge of the aging society: detecting and preventing cognitive and physical decline through games and consumer technologies. Healthcare Inform. Res. **23**(2), 87 (2017)
25. Ferreira-Brito, F., Fialho, M., Virgolino, A., Neves, I., Miranda, A.C., Sousa-Santos, N., Caneiras, C., Carrico, L., Verdelho, A., Santos, O.: Game-based interventions for neuropsychological assessment, training and rehabilitation: Which game-elements to use? A systematic review. J. Biomed. Inform. **98**, 103287 (2019)
26. Gamberini, L., Alcaniz, M., Barresi, G., Fabregat, M., Prontu, L., Seraglia, B.: Playing for a real bonus: videogames to empower elderly people. J. Cyberther. Rehabil. **1**(1), 37–48 (2008)
27. Robertson, G.G., Card, S.K., Mackinlay, J.D.: Three views of virtual reality: nonimmersive virtual reality. Computer **26**(2), 81 (1993)
28. Kamieth, F., Arca, A., Villalar, J.L., Arredondo, M.T., Dähne, P., Wichert, R., Jimenez-Mixco, V.: Exploring the Potential of Virtual Reality for the Elderly and People with Disabilities. INTECH Open Access Publisher (2010)
29. Palmas, F., Klinker, G.: Defining extended reality training: a long-term definition for all industries. In: 2020 IEEE 20th International Conference on Advanced Learning Technologies (ICALT), pp. 322–324. IEEE (2020)
30. Venkatesan, M., Mohan, H., Ryan, J.R., Schürch, C.M., Nolan, G.P., Frakes, D.H., Coskun, A.F.: Virtual and augmented reality for biomedical applications. Cell Rep. Med. **2**(7), 100348 (2021)
31. Sanchez-Vives, M.V., Slater, M.: From presence to consciousness through virtual reality. Nat. Rev. Neurosci. **6**(4), 332–339 (2005)
32. Pillai, J.S., Schmidt, C., Richir, S.: Achieving presence through evoked reality. Front. Psychol. **4**, 86 (2013)
33. Takatalo, J., Häkkinen, J., Kaistinen, J., Nyman, G.: Presence, involvement, and flow in digital games. In: Evaluating User Experience in Games, pp. 23–46. Springer (2010)
34. Boyle, E.A., Connolly, T.M., Hainey, T., Boyle, J.M.: Engagement in digital entertainment games: a systematic review. Comput. Hum. Behav. **28**(3), 771–780 (2012)
35. Sunwoo, J., Yuen, W., Lutteroth, C., Wünsche, B.: Mobile games for elderly healthcare. In: Proceedings of the 11th International Conference of the NZ Chapter of the ACM Special Interest Group on Human-Computer Interaction, pp. 73–76 (2010)
36. de Morais, W.O., Sant'Anna, A., Wickström, N.: A wearable accelerometer based platform to encourage physical activity for the elderly. Gerontechnol. Int. J. Fund. Aspects Technol. Serve Ageing Soc. **7**(02), 129–181 (2008)
37. Lawrence, E., Sax, C., Navarro, K.F., Qiao, M.: Interactive games to improve quality of life for the elderly: towards integration into a WSN monitoring system. In: 2010 Second International Conference on eHealth, Telemedicine, and Social Medicine. IEEE, pp. 106–112 (2010)
38. de Belen, R.A.J., Del Favero, D., Bednarz, T.: Combining mixed reality and Internet of Things: an interaction design research on developing assistive technologies for elderly people. In: International Conference on Human-Computer Interaction, pp. 291–304. Springer (2019)
39. Lete, N., Beristain, A., García-Alonso, A.: Survey on virtual coaching for older adults. Health Inform. J. **26**(4), 3231–3249 (2020)
40. Ebling, M.R.: Pervasive computing and the internet of things. IEEE Perv. Comput. **15**(1), 2–4 (2016)
41. Konstantinidis, E.I., Billis, A.S., Paraskevopoulos, I.T., Bamidis, P.D.: The interplay between IoT and serious games towards personalised healthcare. In: 2017 9th International Conference on Virtual Worlds and Games for Serious Applications (VS-Games), pp. 249–252. IEEE (2017)
42. Borghese, N.A., Pirovano, M., Lanzi, P.L., Wüest, S., de Bruin, E.D.: Computational intelligence and game design for effective at-home stroke rehabilitation. Games Health Res. Dev. Clin. Appl. **2**(2), 81–88 (2013)
43. Martinho, D., Carneiro, J., Corchado, J.M., Marreiros, G.: A systematic review of gamification techniques applied to elderly care. Artif. Intell. Rev. 1–39 (2020)

44. Tung, W.-F.: GEC-HR: gamification exercise companion for home robot with IoT. In: International Conference on Human-Computer Interaction, pp. 141–145. Springer (2019)
45. Roy, A., Mavuduri, P.: Future and impact of rehabilitation robotics on post-stroke care and recovery. In: Technology and Global Public Health, pp. 353–372. Springer (2020)
46. Lin, Y., Fan, J., Dietrich, M., Beuscher, L., Newhouse, P., Sarkar, N., Mion, L.: Can robots encourage social engagement among older adults? Innov. Aging 4(Suppl 1), 193–193 (2020)
47. de Belen, R.A.J., Bednarz, T., Favero, D.D.: Integrating mixed reality and Internet of Things as an assistive technology for elderly people living in a smart home. In: The 17th International Conference on Virtual-Reality Continuum and its Applications in Industry, pp. 1–2 (2019)
48. Buzzi, M.: Breaking interaction barriers: monitoring elderly in natural settings exploiting everyday objects. In: Human Computer Interaction and Emerging Technologies: Adjunct Proceedings from: 13
49. Amorim, P., Santos, B.S., Dias, P., Silva, S., Martins, H.: Serious games for stroke telerehabilitation of upper limb—a review for future research. Int. J. Telerehabil. **12**(2), 65–76 (2020)
50. Rienzo, A., Cubillos, C.: Research of gamification techniques and their application in digital games for older adults. In: 2019 IEEE CHILEAN Conference on Electrical, Electronics Engineering, Information and Communication Technologies (CHILECON), pp. 1–7. IEEE (2019)
51. Lautenschlager, N.T., Almeida, O.P., Flicker, L., Janca, A.: Can physical activity improve the mental health of older adults? Ann. Gen Hosp. Psychiatry **3**(1), 1–5 (2004)
52. Erickson, K.I., Hillman, C.H., Kramer, A.F.: Physical activity, brain, and cognition. Curr. Opin. Behav. Sci. **4**, 27–32 (2015)
53. Larsen, L.H., Schou, L., Lund, H.H., Langberg, H.: The physical effect of exergames in healthy elderly—a systematic review. Games Health Res. Dev. Clin. Appl. **2**(4), 205–212 (2013)
54. Abraham, O., LeMay, S., Bittner, S., Thakur, T., Stafford, H., Brown, R.: Investigating serious games that incorporate medication use for patients: systematic literature review. JMIR Serious Games **8**(2), e16096 (2020)
55. Wiemeyer, J., Kliem, A.: Serious games in prevention and rehabilitation—a new panacea for elderly people? Eur. Rev. Aging Phys. Activity **9**(1), 41–50 (2012)
56. Pollak, J., Gay, G., Byrne, S., Wagner, E., Retelny, D., Humphreys, L.: It's time to eat! Using mobile games to promote healthy eating. IEEE Perv. Comput. **9**(3), 21–27 (2010)
57. Takahashi, M., Kawasaki, H., Maeda, A., Nakamura, M.: Mobile walking game and group-walking program to enhance going out for older adults. In: Proceedings of the 2016 ACM International Joint Conference on Pervasive and Ubiquitous Computing: Adjunct, pp. 1372–1380 (2016)
58. Kuwabara, A., Su, S., Krauss, J.: Utilizing digital health technologies for patient education in lifestyle medicine. Am. J. Lifestyle Med. **14**(2), 137–142 (2020)
59. Bonnechère, B.: Serious Games in Physical Rehabilitation. Springer International Publishing, pp. 72–78 (2018)
60. Randriambelonoro, M., Perrin, C., Blocquet, A., Kozak, D., Fernandez, J.T., Marfaing, T., Bolomey, E., Benhissen, Z., Frangos, E., Geissbuhler, A.: Hospital-to-home transition for older patients: using serious games to improve the motivation for rehabilitation—a qualitative study. J. Population Ageing 1–19 (2020)
61. Bossavit, B.: Serious games in physical rehabilitation. J. Enabling Technol. (2019)
62. Doumas, I., Everard, G., Dehem, S., Lejeune, T.: Serious games for upper limb rehabilitation after stroke: a meta-analysis. J. Neuroeng. Rehabil. **18**(1), 1–16 (2021)
63. Maier, M., Ballester, B.R., Verschure, P.F.: Principles of neurorehabilitation after stroke based on motor learning and brain plasticity mechanisms. Front. Syst. Neurosci. **13**, 74 (2019)
64. Choi, S.D., Guo, L., Kang, D., Xiong, S.: Exergame technology and interactive interventions for elderly fall prevention: a systematic literature review. Appl. Ergon. **65**, 570–581 (2017)
65. Gradim, L.C.C., José, M.A., da Cruz, D.M.C., de Deus, L.R.: IoT services and applications in rehabilitation: an interdisciplinary and meta-analysis review. IEEE Trans. Neural Syst. Rehabil. Eng. **28**(9), 2043–2052 (2020)

66. Cikajlo, I., Hukić, A., Zajc, D.: Exergaming as part of the telerehabilitation can be adequate to the outpatient training: preliminary findings of a non-randomized pilot study in Parkinson's disease. Front. Neurol. **12**, 280 (2021)
67. Salthouse, T.A.: Neuroanatomical substrates of age-related cognitive decline. Psychol. Bull. **137**(5), 753 (2011)
68. Salthouse, T.A.: What and when of cognitive aging. Curr. Dir. Psychol. Sci. **13**(4), 140–144 (2004)
69. Ballesteros, S., Prieto, A., Mayas, J., Toril, P., Pita, C., Ponce de León, L., Reales, J.M., Waterworth, J.: Brain training with non-action video games enhances aspects of cognition in older adults: a randomized controlled trial. Frontiers Aging Neurosci. **6**, 277 (2014)
70. Kim, H., Roh, Y., Kim, J.-I.: An immersive motion interface with edutainment contents for elderly people. In: International Workshop on Motion in Games, pp. 154–165. Springer (2008)
71. Gates, N.J., Rutjes, A.W., Di Nisio, M., Karim, S., Chong, L.Y., March, E., Martínez, G., Vernooij, R.W.: Computerised cognitive training for 12 or more weeks for maintaining cognitive function in cognitively healthy people in late life. Cochrane Database Syst. Rev. (2) (2020)
72. Gates, N.J., Vernooij, R.W., Di Nisio, M., Karim, S., March, E., Martinez, G., Rutjes, A.W.: Computerised cognitive training for preventing dementia in people with mild cognitive impairment. Cochrane Database Syst. Rev. (3) (2019)
73. Viudes-Carbonell, S.J., Gallego-Durán, F.J., Llorens-Largo, F., Molina-Carmona, R.: Towards an iterative design for serious games. Sustainability **13**(6), 3290 (2021)
74. Bonnechère, B., Klass, M., Langley, C., Sahakian, B.J.: Brain training using cognitive apps can improve cognitive performance and processing speed in older adults. Sci. Rep. **11**(1), 1–11 (2021)
75. Park, S.-J., Chang, H.-D., Kim, K.: Effectiveness of the serious game 'Rejuvenesce Village' in cognitive rehabilitation for the elderly. Int. J. E-Health Med. Commun. (IJEHMC) **6**(1), 48–57 (2015)
76. Chen, W.: Towards personalized XR training and rehabilitation applications for older adults. In: 9th International Conference on Software Development and Technologies for Enhancing Accessibility and Fighting Info-exclusion, pp. 163–167 (2020)
77. Swan, M., Kido, T., Ruckenstein, M.: BRAINY—multi-modal brain training app for Google glass: cognitive enhancement, wearable computing, and the Internet-of-Things extend personal data analytics. In: Workshop on Personal Data Analytics in the Internet of Things 40th International Conference on Very Large Databases (2014)
78. Rodrigo, M.Á.A., Ángel, M., Rújula, P.F., Romero, O., Farreny, M.Á., del Carmen Buen, M., Llano, B., Ponce, E., Vidal, P.: Play for health: videogame platform for motor and cognitive telerehabilitation of patients (2011)
79. Lau, H.M., Smit, J.H., Fleming, T.M., Riper, H.: Serious games for mental health: are they accessible, feasible, and effective? A systematic review and meta-analysis. Front. Psych. **7**, 209 (2017)
80. Hall, A.K., Chavarria, E., Maneeratana, V., Chaney, B.H., Bernhardt, J.M.: Health benefits of digital videogames for older adults: a systematic review of the literature. Games Health Res. Dev. Clin. Appl. **1**(6), 402–410 (2012)
81. Montana, J.I., Matamala-Gomez, M., Maisto, M., Mavrodiev, P.A., Cavalera, C.M., Diana, B., Mantovani, F., Realdon, O.: The benefits of emotion regulation interventions in virtual reality for the improvement of wellbeing in adults and older adults: a systematic review. J. Clin. Med. **9**(2), 500 (2020)
82. Weerdmeester, J., van Rooij, M., Harris, O., Smit, N., Engels, R.C., Granic, I.: Exploring the role of self-efficacy in biofeedback video games. In: Extended Abstracts Publication of the Annual Symposium on Computer-Human Interaction in Play, pp. 453–461 (2017)
83. Bojan, K., Stavropoulos, T.G., Lazarou, I., Nikolopoulos, S., Kompatsiaris, I., Tsolaki, M., Mukaetova-Ladinska, E., Christogianni, A.: The effects of playing the COSMA cognitive games in dementia (2021)

84. Wang, A.I.: Systematic literature review on health effects of playing Pokémon Go. Entertain. Comput. **38**, 100411 (2021)
85. Hazer, O., Boylu, A.A.: The examination of the factors affecting the feeling of loneliness of the elderly. Procedia Soc. Behav. Sci. **9**, 2083–2089 (2010)
86. Li, J., Erdt, M., Chen, L., Cao, Y., Lee, S.-Q., Theng, Y.-L.: The social effects of exergames on older adults: systematic review and metric analysis. J. Med. Internet Res. **20**(6), e10486 (2018)
87. Khoo, E.T., Cheok, A.D., Nguyen, T.H.D., Pan, Z.: Age invaders: social and physical intergenerational mixed reality family entertainment. Virtual Reality **12**(1), 3–16 (2008)
88. Chua, P.-H., Jung, Y., Lwin, M.O., Theng, Y.-L.: Let's play together: effects of video-game play on intergenerational perceptions among youth and elderly participants. Comput. Hum. Behav. **29**(6), 2303–2311 (2013)
89. Nguyen, T.T.H., Ishmatova, D., Tapanainen, T., Liukkonen, T.N., Katajapuu, N., Makila, T., Luimula, M.: Impact of serious games on health and well-being of elderly: a systematic review. In: Proceedings of the 50th Hawaii International Conference on System Sciences (2017)
90. Benveniste, S., Jouvelot, P., Péquignot, R.: The MINWii Project: renarcissization of patients suffering from Alzheimer's disease through video game-based music therapy. In: International Conference on Entertainment Computing, pp. 79–90. Springer (2010)
91. Zhang, F., Kaufman, D.: Older adults' social interactions in massively multiplayer online role-playing games (MMORPGs). Games Culture **11**(1–2), 150–169 (2016)
92. Osmanovic, S., Pecchioni, L.: Beyond entertainment: motivations and outcomes of video game playing by older adults and their younger family members. Games Culture **11**(1–2), 130–149 (2016)
93. Barbosa, H., Castro, A.V., Carrapatoso, E.: Serious games and rehabilitation for elderly adults. GSJ **6**(1), 275 (2018)
94. Siddiqui, S., Khan, A.A., Nait-Abdesselam, F., Dey, I.: Anxiety and depression management for elderly using internet of things and symphonic melodies. In: ICC 2021-IEEE International Conference on Communications, pp. 1–6. IEEE (2021)
95. Spyrou, E., Mitrakos, D.: Cognitive game for OCD effects minimisation using IoT. In: 2019 15th International Conference on Distributed Computing in Sensor Systems (DCOSS), pp. 182–184. IEEE (2019)
96. Schneider, S.M., Ellis, M., Coombs, W.T., Shonkwiler, E.L., Folsom, L.C.: Virtual reality intervention for older women with breast cancer. Cyberpsychol. Behav. **6**(3), 301–307 (2003)
97. Shapoval, S., García Zapirain, B., Mendez Zorrilla, A., Mugueta-Aguinaga, I.: Biofeedback applied to interactive serious games to monitor frailty in an elderly population. Appl. Sci. **11**(8), 3502 (2021)
98. Tong, T., Chignell, M., Lam, P., Tierney, M.C., Lee, J.: Designing serious games for cognitive assessment of the elderly. In: Proceedings of the International Symposium on Human Factors and Ergonomics in Health Care, vol. 1, pp. 28–35. SAGE Publications Sage CA, Los Angeles, CA (2014)
99. Vallejo, V., Wyss, P., Chesham, A., Mitache, A.V., Müri, R.M., Mosimann, U.P., Nef, T.: Evaluation of a new serious game based multitasking assessment tool for cognition and activities of daily living: comparison with a real cooking task. Comput. Hum. Behav. **70**, 500–506 (2017)
100. Sirály, E., Szabó, Á., Szita, B., Kovács, V., Fodor, Z., Marosi, C., Salacz, P., Hidasi, Z., Maros, V., Hanák, P.: Monitoring the early signs of cognitive decline in elderly by computer games: an MRI study. Plos One **10**(2), e0117918 (2015)
101. Ijsselsteijn, W., Nap, H.H., de Kort, Y., Poels, K.: Digital game design for elderly users. In: Proceedings of the 2007 Conference on Future Play, pp. 17–22 (2007)
102. Gamberini, L., Raya, M.A., Barresi, G., Fabregat, M., Ibanez, F., Prontu, L.: Cognition, technology and games for the elderly: an introduction to ELDERGAMES Project. Psychnol. J. **4**(3), 285–308 (2006)
103. Gerling, K.M., Schulte, F.P., Smeddinck, J., Masuch, M.: Game design for older adults: effects of age-related changes on structural elements of digital games. In: International Conference on Entertainment Computing, pp. 235–242. Springer (2012)

104. Adams, E.: Fundamentals of Game Design, New Riders. Pearson Education Inc, Berkeley (2010)
105. Fullerton, T.: A playcentric approach to creating innovative games. In: Game Design Workshop (2008)
106. De Schutter, B.: Never too old to play: the appeal of digital games to an older audience. Games Cult. **6**(2), 155–170 (2011)
107. Delwiche, A.A., Henderson, J.J.: The players they are a-changin': the rise of older MMO gamers. J. Broadcast. Electron. Media **57**(2), 205–223 (2013)
108. Brown, J.A.: Let's play: understanding the role and meaning of digital games in the lives of older adults. In: Proceedings of the International Conference on the Foundations of Digital Games, pp. 273–275 (2012)
109. Schmidt, N.: How Do We Design Games for the Non-Gamer? (2020). https://medium.com/@s.natalie25/how-do-we-design-games-for-the-non-gamer-f1d306fc7ccc. Accessed 21 June 2021
110. Rienzo, A., Cubillos, C.: Playability and player experience in digital games for elderly: a systematic literature review. Sensors **20**(14), 3958 (2020)
111. Wang, Q., Sun, X.: Investigating gameplay intention of the elderly using an Extended Technology Acceptance Model (ETAM). Technol. Forecast. Soc. Chang. **107**, 59–68 (2016)
112. Chen, K., Chan, A.H.S.: Gerontechnology acceptance by elderly Hong Kong Chinese: a senior technology acceptance model (STAM). Ergonomics **57**(5), 635–652 (2014)
113. Dogruel, L., Joeckel, S., Bowman, N.D.: Elderly people and morality in virtual worlds: a cross-cultural analysis of elderly people's morality in interactive media. New Media Soc. **15**(2), 276–293 (2013)
114. Zhang, H., Wu, Q., Miao, C., Shen, Z., Leung, C.: Towards age-friendly exergame design: the role of familiarity. In: Proceedings of the Annual Symposium on Computer-Human Interaction in Play, pp. 45–57 (2019)
115. Oudah, M., Al-Naji, A., Chahl, J.: Hand gestures for elderly care using a microsoft Kinect. Nano. Biomed. Eng. **12**(3), 197–204 (2020)
116. Bong, W.K., Chen, W., Bergland, A.: Tangible user interface for social interactions for the elderly: a review of literature. Adv. Human-Computer Interact. (2018)
117. Cáliz, D., Alamán, X., Martínez, L., Cáliz, R., Terán, C., Peñafiel, V.: Examining the usability of touch screen gestures for elderly people. In: International Conference on Ubiquitous Computing and Ambient Intelligence, pp. 419–429. Springer (2016)
118. McCallum, S., Boletsis, C.: Augmented reality and gesture-based architecture in games for the elderly. Stud. Health Technol. Inform. **189**, 139–144 (2013)
119. Besombes, N., Maillot, P.: Body involvement in video gaming as a support for physical and cognitive learning. Games Cult. **15**(5), 565–584 (2020)
120. de Bruin, E.D., Schoene, D., Pichierri, G., Smith, S.T.: Use of virtual reality technique for the training of motor control in the elderly. Zeitschrift für Gerontologie und Geriatrie **43**(4), 229–234 (2010)
121. Nault, E., Baillie, L., Broz, F.: Auditory and haptic feedback in a socially assistive robot memory game. In: Companion of the 2020 ACM/IEEE International Conference on Human-Robot Interaction, pp. 369–371 (2020)
122. Vanden Abeele, V.A., Van Rompaey, V.: Introducing human-centered research to game design: designing game concepts for and with senior citizens. In: CHI'06 Extended Abstracts on Human Factors in Computing Systems, pp 1469–1474 (2006)
123. Chesham, A., Wyss, P., Müri, R.M., Mosimann, U.P., Nef, T.: What older people like to play: genre preferences and acceptance of casual games. JMIR Ser. Games **5**(2), e8 (2017)
124. IJsselsteijn, W.A., de Kort, Y.A., Poels, K.: The game experience questionnaire. Eindhoven: Technische Universiteit Eindhoven **46**(1) (2013)
125. Pyae, A., Joelsson, T., Saarenpää, T., Mika, L., Kattimeri, C., Pitkäkangas, P., Granholm, P., Smed, J.: Lessons learned from two usability studies of digital skiing game with elderly people in Finland and Japan. Int. J. Serious Games **4**(4) (2017)

126. Chiang, I.-T.: Old dogs can learn new tricks: exploring effective strategies to facilitate somatosensory video games for institutionalized older veterans. In: Transactions on Edutainment VIII, pp. 88–100. Springer (2012)
127. Padala, K.P., Padala, P.R., Lensing, S.Y., Dennis, R.A., Bopp, M.M., Parkes, C.M., Garrison, M.K., Dubbert, P.M., Roberson, P.K., Sullivan, D.H.: Efficacy of Wii-Fit on static and dynamic balance in community dwelling older veterans: a randomized controlled pilot trial. J. Aging Res. (2017)
128. Chen, S.-T., Huang, Y.-G.L., Chiang, I.-T.: Using somatosensory video games to promote quality of life for the elderly with disabilities. In: 2012 IEEE Fourth International Conference on Digital Game and Intelligent Toy Enhanced Learning, pp. 258–262. IEEE (2012)
129. Seifert, A., Schlomann, A.: The use of virtual and augmented reality by older adults: potentials and challenges. Frontiers Virtual Reality **2**, 51 (2021)
130. Bevilacqua, R., Maranesi, E., Riccardi, G.R., Di Donna, V., Pelliccioni, P., Luzi, R., Lattanzio, F., Pelliccioni, G.: Non-immersive virtual reality for rehabilitation of the older people: a systematic review into efficacy and effectiveness. J. Clin. Med. **8**(11), 1882 (2019)
131. Carroll, J., Hopper, L., Farrelly, A.M., Lombard-Vance, R., Bamidis, P.D., Konstantinidis, E.I.: A scoping review of augmented/virtual reality health and wellbeing interventions for older adults: redefining immersive virtual reality. Frontiers Virtual Reality **2**, 61 (2021)
132. Berg-Weger, M., Morley, J.E.: Loneliness and Social Isolation in Older Adults During the COVID-19 Pandemic: Implications for Gerontological Social Work. Springer (2020)
133. Gabbiadini, A., Baldissarri, C., Durante, F., Valtorta, R.R., De Rosa, M., Gallucci, M.: Together apart: the mitigating role of digital communication technologies on negative affect during the COVID-19 outbreak in Italy. Front. Psychol. **11**, 2763 (2020)
134. Chen, K.: Use of gerontechnology to assist older adults to cope with the COVID-19 Pandemic. J. Am. Med. Dir. Assoc. **21**(7), 983–984 (2020)
135. Hammami, A., Harrabi, B., Mohr, M., Krustrup, P.: Physical activity and coronavirus disease 2019 (COVID-19): specific recommendations for home-based physical training. Manag. Sport Leisure 1–6 (2020)
136. Santos, L.H., Okamoto, K., Hiragi, S., Yamamoto, G., Sugiyama, O., Aoyama, T., Kuroda, T.: Pervasive game design to evaluate social interaction effects on levels of physical activity among older adults. J. Rehabil. Assistive Technol. Eng. **6**, 2055668319844443 (2019)
137. Sawami, K., Kimura, M., Kitamura, T., Kawaguchi, M., Furusumi, M., Suishu, C., Morisaki, N., Hattori, S.: Robots visit homes for elderly people who have difficulty going out and practice brain training. EJMED **2**, 1–4 (2020)
138. Andriella, A., Torras, C., Alenya, G.: Cognitive system framework for brain-training exercise based on human-robot interaction. Cogn. Comput. **12**(4), 793–810 (2020)
139. Lazzaroni, L., Mazzara, A., Bellotti, F., De Gloria, A., Berta, R.: Employing an IoT framework as a generic serious games analytics engine. In: International Conference on Games and Learning Allianc, pp. 79–88. Springer (2020)
140. Egliston, B.: Big playerbase, big data: on data analytics methodologies and their applicability to studying multiplayer games and culture. First Monday **21**(7) (2016)
141. Mathews, S.C., McShea, M.J., Hanley, C.L., Ravitz, A., Labrique, A.B., Cohen, A.B.: Digital health: a path to validation. NPJ Dig. Med. **2**(1), 1–9 (2019)
142. Organization, W.H.: Classification of Digital Health Interventions v1. 0: A Shared Language to Describe the Uses of Digital Technology for Health. World Health Organization (2018)
143. Dang, A., Arora, D., Rane, P.: Role of digital therapeutics and the changing future of healthcare. J. Family Med. Primary Care **9**(5), 2207 (2020)
144. Traynor, K.: FDA Authorizes Marketing of Video Game-Based Therapy. Oxford University Press US (2020)
145. Recchia, G., Capuano, D.M., Mistri, N., Verna, R.: Digital therapeutics—what they are, what they will be. Acta Sci. Med. Sci. **4**, 1–9 (2020)
146. Abbadessa, G., Brigo, F., Clerico, M., De Mercanti, S., Trojsi, F., Tedeschi, G., Bonavita, S., Lavorgna, L.: Digital therapeutics in neurology. J. Neurol. 1–16 (2021)

147. Kaufman, N.: Digital therapeutics: leading the way to improved outcomes for people with diabetes. Diabetes Spectrum **32**(4), 301–303 (2019)
148. Kaldy, J.: Digital therapeutics: health care wired for the future. Senior Care Pharmacist **35**(8), 338–344 (2020)
149. Cavedoni, S., Chirico, A., Pedroli, E., Cipresso, P., Riva, G.: Digital Biomarkers for the early detection of mild cognitive impairment: artificial intelligence meets virtual reality. Frontiers Human Neurosci. **14** (2020)
150. Robert, P., König, A., Amieva, H., Andrieu, S., Bremond, F., Bullock, R., Ceccaldi, M., Dubois, B., Gauthier, S., Kenigsberg, P.-A.: Recommendations for the use of serious games in people with Alzheimer's disease, related disorders and frailty. Frontiers Aging Neurosci. **6**, 54 (2014)

Lightning Source UK Ltd.
Milton Keynes UK
UKHW020615020323
417913UK00002B/6